Medicare: Facts, Myths, Problems, Promise

Medicare: Facts, Myths, Problems, Promise

Edited by Bruce Campbell
and Greg Marchildon

James Lorimer & Company Ltd., Publishers
Toronto

James Lorimer & Company Ltd. acknowledges the support of the Ontario Arts
Council. We acknowledge the support of the Government of Canada through
the Book Publishing Industry Development Program (BPIDP) for our publishing activities. We acknowledge the support of the Canada Council for the
Arts for our publishing program. We acknowledge the support of the Government of Ontario through the Ontario Media Development Corporation's
Ontario Book Initiative.

Cover design: Kate Moore

Library and Archives Canada Cataloguing in Publication

    Medicare : facts, myths, problems, promise / edited by Bruce Campbell
& Greg Marchildon.

ISBN 10: 1-55277-000-1   ISBN 13: 978-1-55277-000-9

    1. Medical care--Canada. 2. Medical policy--Canada. 3. Public health-
-Canada.
I. Campbell, Bruce, 1948- II. Marchildon, Gregory P., 1956-

RA412.5.C3M418 2007   362.10971   C2007-906290-3

James Lorimer & Company Ltd.,
Publishers
317 Adelaide Street West, Suite #1002
Toronto, Ontario
M5V 1P9
www.lorimer.ca

Printed and bound in Canada.

CONTENTS

PREFACE

Medicare can be a confusing word. Historically, it meant public coverage for physician services in Canada. Because medicare followed on the heels of public hospital insurance — or hospitalization as it was popularly known — it quickly became identified with universal public coverage for both. Then with the expansion of public health services — particularly primary health care — in the 1970s, and the passage of the Canada Health Act in 1984, medicare came to mean all health services provided on a universal basis without user fees to all Canadians.

Medicare has also become shorthand for the terms and conditions under which Canadians receive a defined basket of health services. These are best summarized in the five principles — public administration, universality, accessibility, portability, and comprehensiveness — which underpin the Canada Health Act. At the same time, the word medicare is used to describe the thirteen tax-funded, single-payer systems administered by the provincial and territorial governments.

Occasionally, medicare in Canada is confused with the identically named social security program in the United States, but both the principles and the administrative systems which typify Canadian medicare differentiate it from the American program. Finally, medicare in Canada is not an insurance program where payments (premiums) are received in return for a range of benefits. It is a defined set of services administered and delivered provincially under a national framework and paid for through taxes paid to both provincial and federal governments.

The first phase of Canadian medicare was built on the pioneering efforts of the province of Saskatchewan, first in introducing universal hospitalization in 1947, then in implementing universal "medical care insurance" in 1962. For it to become national in scope, however, medicare depended heavily on the leadership role of the federal government. Ottawa not only shared costs but defined the critical principles and conditions under which the provincial systems would operate so that Canadians, irrespective of where they lived, would enjoy the principled consistency of a national framework.

When the Canada Health Act was passed in order to clarify and strengthen the national dimensions of medicare it was a rearguard action to protect what had been achieved in the 1950s and 1960s. The small but powerful anti-medicare coalition that had lost the struggle to prevent medicare began its campaign to discredit and undermine medicare soon after its implementation. Over time, this coalition succeeded in defining the terms of the debate as defending the status quo versus fixing medicare by introducing market mechanisms including "patient participation" through the introduction of user fees. We feel that the time is overdue for the broad pro-medicare coalition in this country to change the terms of this corrosive and misleading debate. It is time for those who believe in the principles of medicare and who understand the benefits of single-payer administration to take the offensive.

The individuals who have been brought together for this book are proponents of public medicare. At various times, they have vigorously defended the principles behind the Canadian model of medicare. But some have also been outspoken about some of the deficiencies in the administration and delivery of medicare, particularly since the onset of government cutbacks to health care in the early to mid-1990s. While they see the first phase of medicare as an important step in our self-definition as a country, they want to look beyond history and build the future. They want to expand medicare well beyond doctors and hospitals. They also want to re-orient public health care around primary health care, community care and what we now know about the social determinants of health. Based on their knowledge and experience, they describe the elements of what they think should constitute the second phase of medicare. They offer strategic advice on how to construct this second phase in terms of programs and politics. They also deflate the myths that have grown up around medicare. These myths have been created in part to undermine confidence in medicare's foundation: in particular, the single-payer mechanism, and the principles of public administration, universality and accessibility.

The origins of this book lie in a remarkable conference that took place in Regina on May 3–4, 2007. SOS Medicare 2: Looking Forward, Building on Tommy Douglas's Vision of Medicare was an event like no other. Beyond bringing together some of the leading thinkers and activists in Canada and the world, the conference and the interactive dialogue it generated created a sense of hope about the future that has been all too rare in recent years. After years of being on the defensive, the almost seven hundred participants returned home ready to take the offensive — ready to begin building the second phase of medicare.

The conference had its genesis in a grant by the Douglas-Coldwell Foundation to celebrate Tommy Douglas being voted "the greatest Canadian" in a CBC TV poll. The founding vision of Tommy Douglas — rightly seen by Canadians as the Father of Medicare — is an assertion of the fundamental value of equality. It has come to represent our crowning national achievement, an essential element of our identity as a just and caring society.

The Canadian Health Coalition and the Canadian Centre for Policy Alternatives were awarded the Douglas–Coldwell grant for their proposal to hold a conference that would honour Tommy's legacy by addressing his vision of medicare. The first phase of his vision was the removal of financial barriers between those giving the service and those receiving it. The second phase would restructure our health care delivery system and focus on prevention and the social determinants of health. This second phase remains largely undone. Thus, the challenge is how to complete Tommy's vision for medicare.

We decided to frame the conference as the sequel to the 1979 SOS Medicare One conference, which had brought together a broad coalition of medicare advocates to defend against forces that were attempting at that time to erode medicare, and to build on existing accomplishments. So too in 2007, the forces of for-profit, two-tier medicine are again gathering strength. Once again — as it was in the 1980s with user fees and in the 1960s with the doctors' strike — the right to health care as a fundamental right of citizenship is being challenged.

The Johnson-Shoyama Graduate School of Public Policy at the University of Regina joined the project shortly after as the third member of the organizing triumvirate. Later, the Faculty of Law at the University of Toronto agreed to be the conference co-host.

The conference brought together an unprecedented cast of luminaries: from Shirley Douglas, Monique Bégin, and Tom Kent, to Allan Blakeney, Roy Romanow, and Stephen Lewis. It included leading health policy experts, legal authorities and economists; union and other social justice activists; the whole spectrum of health care providers and support workers from nurses, home care and mental health workers, to medical technologists, rehab counsellors and physicians; government bureaucrats; provincial and federal politicians; and experts from the US, Europe, and Asia, all bound together by a passion for preserving and improving medicare.

We are indebted to many people and organizations for their role in the making of this book, which is an essential part of the legacy of the conference. The two are indivisible.

We would first and foremost like to thank Michael McBane,

coordinator of the Canadian Health Coalition and a formidable advocate for public health care. Mike was the initiator and a driving force behind the conference every step of the way. It was his vision that produced and then sustained the conference and this book.

We are also much indebted to Colleen Flood of the Faculty of Law at the University of Toronto — Canada's leading expert on the impact of the *Chaoulli* decision of the Supreme Court — who worked extensively with us in developing the intellectual content of the conference program and this book.

An undertaking of this magnitude would not have been possible without the more than forty organizations that stepped forward as sponsors: unions and other non-government organizations, provincial governments, and foundations. We thank you.

We would also like to extend our thanks to the following people: at the Douglas Coldwell Foundation, Pat Kerwin; at the Canadian Health Coalition, Brad Duplessis; at the CCPA National Office, Diane Touchette, Kerri Finn, Ed Finn, and Trish Hennessey; at the CCPA Saskatchewan office, Lynn Gidluck and the many volunteers in Regina; at the University of Regina, Devon Anderson and the student volunteers from the university; and at James Lorimer & Company, Catherine MacIntosh, Chris Keen, Mary Newberry, and of course, Jim Lorimer for recognizing the value of this project in educating Canadians about their most treasured social program.

And finally we would like to thank all the contributors to this book for their belief in the importance of this project, and for their discipline in getting back to us revised versions of their papers under very tight deadlines.

Roy Romanow, head of the 2002 Royal Commission on the Future of Health Care, told the conference that the struggle for reforms to medicare would be centrally determined by values.

There are two competing visions and guiding values
about health care. Each would take our nation down a
fundamentally different path. One view, high on rhetoric but low on evidence and masquerading as
something new, is based on the premise that health care
is a commodity — that medical needs ebb and flow
with markets, and they determine who gets care, when,
and how.

The other vision, rooted in our narrative as a nation,
backed by evidence and public opinion, strongly
believes that health care is a "public good." It believes
that democratically elected governments, as representatives of the public, not corporate bottom lines, should
define common needs, provide equitable services, and a
reasonable allocation of resources. Fairness, equity, compassion, and solidarity: these are the values that were
adopted and nurtured throughout Canada's history of
shared destiny.

These values gain their expression in our core belief
that everyone should have access to our health care system on the same terms and conditions, and that this
access is ultimately a right of Canadian citizenship.
These values are manifested through our view that
Medicare is a truly national program — a nation-defining and nation-building enterprise.

Tommy Douglas wrote after the 1979 SOS Medicare conference that its lasting value would be in the concerted organized
effort to apply pressure to provincial and federal governments.

Shirley Douglas warned our conference that unless those of us who believe in medicare raise our voices, and mobilize our friends and neighbours and communities in an all-out campaign to save medicare, we risk seeing it dismantled.

We hope that this book will be a useful resource for Canadians working together in the broadest possible coalition, to move Tommy Douglas's vision for medicare closer to reality.

Bruce Campbell (Ottawa) and
Greg Marchildon (Regina) August 2007

PART I

*Tommy Douglas'
Vision and the
Future of Medicare*

CHAPTER 1

SOS Medicare: A (Cautionary) Tale of Two Conferences

Shirley Douglas

My father would be thrilled to see what we did at the SOS Medicare 2 conference, but also probably dismayed that such an effort is still needed to preserve the legacy of public health care that he left us. But he would have understood why, too. He knew better than anyone the powerful forces arrayed against medicare, and he also knew that they would continue to weaken and subvert it even after it was installed as Canada's most treasured social program.

As I looked around the conference room, I saw many of the stalwarts who fought for so long to establish and improve our health care system — many of whom attended the national conference on health care in 1979, SOS Medicare 1. We all came for a reason: because we believe in something bigger than ourselves and because we are committed to work together, to muster our energy and resources to ensure that public health care is not destroyed in this country.

We face a formidable challenge to the preservation of medicare. Canada now has a prime minister who spent years heading the National Citizens' Coalition (NCC). The NCC was set up by insurance mogul Colin Brown in the early 1960s with the sole purpose of stopping Saskatchewan from establishing public health care. That initial anti-medicare campaign failed, but the NCC, under Stephen Harper, never stopped trying to undermine it. Now, as prime minister, he is in a position to do a lot more damage, even if it is mainly by refusing to enforce the Canada Health Act and thus allowing more privatization, lower standards, and less accessibility.

Medicare is a program that requires continuous and unstinting effort to protect it. Tommy Douglas knew that. Even after public health care was adopted all across the country, Tommy kept making speeches stressing the need always to be on guard against attacks both open and insidious — about the need to improve and extend health care with drug coverage and more clinics and other advances, instead of just fighting to maintain the basic system. And this at a time when most Canadians were satisfied with their health care and didn't think there was anything wrong with it.

My father was always aware of the enormous influence of the insurance companies, the pharmaceutical companies, entrepreneurial physicians, and the political, academic, and media ideologues who still did not want public health care. He kept telling us that if we failed to recognize and oppose these powerful enemies of medicare, we could lose it.

We must heed his warning. We know that medicare is being eroded and sabotaged today even more relentlessly than it was when my father was alive. We know that unless those of us who believe in medicare raise our voices, mobilize our friends and neighbours and communities in an all-out campaign to save medicare, we risk seeing it dismantled.

Remember his words: "I, for one, will not sit idly by and see that happen. I helped to establish the first medicare program in Canada and, even at my age, I'll trek this country from the Atlantic to the Pacific to stop medicare from being destroyed." I believe that all of us can and should do no less. We must go forth and find hundreds, thousands, and millions of our fellow Canadians to join us in this struggle. Whether they know it or not, all 33 million people in this country are counting on us.

There is a lot of money to be made in breaking medicare. I believe this is the reason Dr. Brian Day is promoting private, for-profit clinics. Dr. Day is currently the president of the Canadian Medical Association (CMA). We need to remember our history. The CMA opposed Justice Hall's report in 1964. The CMA opposed the Canada Health Act in 1984. The CMA intervened in the Supreme Court of Canada in 2006 to have Quebec's health insurance laws struck down. Dr. Day and the CMA want to bring the US model of investor-owned health care to Canada, and convince people that this is the only way to remedy waiting times or other problems in our health care system. They know this is not true.

Every doctor who leaves the public system to work at Day's for-profit clinic makes waiting times longer. Expert research evidence shows this seriously compromises access to care in the public systems by taking badly needed surgeons, nurses, and technicians out of the public hospitals. You either want a single-payer system in this country or you want an American-style system. And don't kid yourself that there's anything in between.

Canadians are proud of and must fight to defend the core principle of medicare: every man, woman, and child should receive care based on need, not on their ability to pay. To ration health care based on ability to pay, rather than need, is a perversion of Canadian values. As Dr. Martin Luther King, Jr. said: "Of all the forms of injustice, inequality in health care is the most shocking and inhumane."

I would invite Dr. Day to set up a not-for-profit clinic so that he could become part of the solution — not the problem. Rather than drive the system South, organized medicine in Canada should commit to changing the way services are delivered and move to what my father called a model of preventive medicine. We know there are problems with wait times, lack of home care, and drug coverage. Let's all work together to fix these problems rather than using the problems as an excuse to go back to the days before medicare when doctors could charge whatever they wanted and care was rationed on the basis of ability to pay.

It is time to build on medicare's success and move forward with the second phase.

★ ★ ★

As part of her opening statement at the SOS Medicare 2 conference, Shirley Douglas showed a film clip of her father, Tommy Douglas, receiving an award at the 1979 SOS Medicare 1 conference. This is a transcript of his brief remarks on receiving the award:

"In expressing my thanks, I just want to say that I'm glad you're having this conference and I congratulate the Canadian Labour Congress for holding it. I am concerned, as many people are, about medicare — not with the fundamental principles, but with the problems we knew would arise after it was put in place. Those of us who talked about the need for public health insurance back in the 1940s, '50s and '60s kept reminding Canadians that there were two phases for medicare.

The first was to remove the financial barrier between those who provide health services and those who need them. We pointed out repeatedly that this first phase was the easiest of the problems we faced. In governmental terms, of course, it means finding the revenue, it means setting up the organizational and administrative structure, it means exercising controls over costs, but in the long term it was the easiest problem to surmount.

Phase 2, however, would be a much more difficult one: altering our delivery system so as to reduce costs by putting the emphasis on preventive medicine rather than treatment and drugs. I think we have to realize now that we have not yet grappled seriously with the second phase. We must now move increasingly toward group practice, whether it be community clinics, cooperative clinics, clinics set up by the doctors themselves. Only through group practice of this kind will it be possible to focus mainly on the prevention of illness instead of the treatment of illness. Only in that way are we going to be able to keep the costs from becoming so excessive that people will be easily convinced that medicare is too expensive to maintain.

It is time that we took a look at the present system to see whether or not we are carrying out the vision that was contained in the report of Mr. Justice Emmett Hall. I am delighted that Mr. Crombie, the minister of national health and welfare, appointed Mr. Justice Hall to conduct this [1979] inquiry into public health care. I have complete confidence in his competence and integrity. I am sure that his report will provide a blueprint on how we can work together, irrespective of political party or region or profession or interest, to make medicare what it was intended to be: a program that would provide in Canada a society which had freedom from fear and freedom from want.

I hope that from time to time we will gather as we are gathering now, to the end that we may be able to build in Canada a program that will provide the maximum amount of good health, enable people to enjoy good health and provide them with remedial services when that good health is no longer present — and do this without fear of the financial burdens which have crippled so many people in other places and other times.

Thank you for inviting me to be here, thank you for your

tribute, and may I wish you well in your deliberations now and in your efforts to preserve and perfect medicare in the future."

Tommy Douglas, 1979 SOS Medicare conference

CHAPTER 2

The Struggle — at Home and in the World — for Health Care as a Human Right

Stephen Lewis

More than fifty years ago, in 1956, I came to Saskatchewan to learn the meaning of democratic socialism. I believed in democratic socialism. I had been told that it was a requirement to believe in it at my various household lunch and dinner conversations, where my father and mother made it clear to me that, if I were not a social democrat, I would be disinherited. But it was important that I knew what it meant, so I came to Saskatchewan in the summer of 1956 and worked at the Saskatchewan Social and Economic Planning Board with that magnificent fellow whose name many of you will know — Tommy Shoyama — and I was fascinated in those days at the amount of time that was directed to questions of health, hospital insurance, and the health insurance that was yet to come. And it taught me a principled and important lesson: that the realities of health were deeply embedded in the cultural and electoral system of Saskatchewan.

Then there was an election called and I had the incredible privilege of travelling around the province with Tommy Douglas as he
engaged in electoral politics in his own absolutely irrepressible
way. Watching him on platform after platform, I loved every
minute of it. I was with Tommy in that memorable encounter in
Weyburn, in the then Weyburn psychiatric hospital, where he
walked up and down the wards, hand outstretched, saying hello to
all the people who were there. One fellow to whom he said,
"Hello, I'm Tommy Douglas, Premier of Saskatchewan," clearly
didn't believe him, and replied, "So glad to meet you, Mr. Premier,
I am Napoleon Bonaparte."

In the process of watching and travelling with Tommy, I learned
again that the reconnoitering of health care on the campaign trail
was absolutely central to the political life of the province and certainly central to the principles that Tommy Douglas so deeply
conveyed. I was so overwhelmed by the experience that I stopped
in the riding of Souris-Estevan and managed the campaign for a
very young candidate, Kim Thorson, who at twenty-one was only
two years older than me at the time. Thorson was elected on that
occasion and went on to serve with distinction in the
Saskatchewan legislature, where he was a leading proponent of the
Saskatchewan Health Insurance Plan.

I left Saskatchewan and went off to Africa, returning in time to
come to Saskatchewan again during the bitter doctors' strike in
1962. My assignment was to invite foreign doctors to come to
Saskatchewan during the strike — doctors who were sympathetic to the position of the government — and to help place them
in various parts of Saskatchewan. Even more fascinating was to
work on the community health centre network which was thriving in Saskatoon and in Regina, and to help set one up in Moose
Jaw. It was, of course, a very difficult and tense environment during the doctors' strike, but enormously encouraging in the way
the province came together and the government prevailed.

In the 1960s and 1970s, I sat in the Ontario legislature, as hospital insurance and health insurance gradually became implanted, even with a government of obdurate and obstinate pre-paleolithic Tories. The adoption of hospital and health insurance was a memorable moment for me because it was perhaps the centrepiece of my experience in the Ontario legislature. It was more than that. As for so many of us across the country, the public health care system that Tommy Douglas had established in Saskatchewan was the ideological centrepiece of our political lives.

Since I departed the political scene in Ontario, much of my life has been spent abroad, and so I have been somewhat but not completely out of touch. I did take notice of the major developments on the Canadian health care front, including the reaffirmation and strengthening of medicare provided first by the Royal Commission headed by Mr. Justice Emmett Hall and then, most recently, by the Royal Commission of Roy Romanow. In the intervening years of constitutional negotiations and debates, it clearly emerged from poll after poll that the defining characteristic of our society for Canadians was their public health care system.

Throughout the same decades, however, and culminating in the last few years, there has been a drum roll of other forces at work — the forces of reaction and the forces of privatization, the forces of greed and ideology combined, determined to strip medicare of its human legitimacy and from it extract a profit. I therefore recite a series of self-evident truths, which all of us, I think, will embrace.

We know that public health insurance works and that public health care works. We know that it is rooted in social justice and the human imperative. We know that it is an absolutely accurate mirror of all the international conventions which have been signed and ratified around the globe, whether it's the Convention on the Rights of the Child, or the Convention on the Elimination of All Forms of Discrimination Against Women, or the

Covenant on Economic, Social and Cultural Rights, or the
Covenant on Civil and Political Rights. Time and time again you
hear the same phrase: that it is a human right to have access to the
highest obtainable standard of health — words that are entrenched
in the annals of the human rights community.

We know that the five principles governing the Canada Health
Act are, or should be, sacrosanct, and that everyone, regardless of
income, must have access to health care. Those rights are guaranteed by the Health Act's principles of universality,
comprehensiveness, and accessibility.

We know that there are large costs involved in a health care system of the kind that we cherish, but that intelligence and
efficiency and equity can keep those costs at reasonable levels.
Whether we are talking about waiting lists or about emergency
rooms or about the introduction of pharmacare, the application of
common sense and reason will make health care a viable commodity for the entire population without the kinds of restrictive
and subversive procedures that exact such a punitive outcome.

Michael Rachlis, in one of his studies, describes how several
hospitals and clinics and laboratories around the country have
developed innovative methods for dealing with waiting lists, testing, and other problems. If we could have these models adopted
on a large scale across the country — which could be done if we
had governments with any common sense — we could swiftly
rescue our health care system from the depredations of the priva-
tizers and philistines.

We know, above all, that the private sector erosion of health
care introduces double standards and two-tier coverage, and ultimately costs that are crippling. If nothing else, the fact that the
cost of public health care in Canada takes 9 to 10 percent of our
GDP, compared to the 16 percent of the US GDP that is the cost
of its largely private system, which incidentally leaves 45 million
Americans without any health coverage — that fact alone should

suffice to preserve and enhance Canadian medicare. As long as the United States maintains its very expensive and inadequate system, Americans will never be able to improve it or make it universally accessible.

The private interests in the United States are so deeply entrenched that it's no longer possible to reform the system, root and branch, as is required. Remember the mortifying humiliation that was experienced by Hillary Clinton and Ira Magaziner at the outset of the Bill Clinton years when they attempted unsuccessfully to reform the health care system. The insurance industry and the doctors' consortiums are even more deeply entrenched now than they were then. A few states have attempted to improve the medicare and medicaid programs in the US, but are having tremendous difficulties as the costs constantly keep accelerating. The amalgam of public and private care is ultimately destructive of a reasonable health care system.

We know that it has been analyzed ad nauseam, and it is frankly irrefutable that the private carriers and the doctors now have a stranglehold on the American system. We know all of this, we understand all of these self-evident truths, and yet the combination of ideology in Alberta and the flawed judicial reasoning that sanctioned privatization in Quebec puts our health care system in peril. There is need for a Herculean political campaign to rescue and reconstitute the original visions of Tommy Douglas.

This is a deeply ideological struggle, not just one of costs and organization. Social democracy for me is a meaningful force, and the whole object of the exercise is to achieve a degree of social justice and equality, without which there is no reasonable prospect for this planet. We are confronting an ideology known as neoliberalism. It is on display every year at the World Economic Forum sessions in Switzerland, attended by all the heads of the major multinational corporations, leading politicians, and prominent academics and media celebrities. They all get together in a celebration of neoliberalism, an orgy of triumphalism for the private sector, always disputing and diminishing the value of the public sector and public services.

We are confronting an ideology that is mirrored in the new acquisitive extravagance of the stock market, so that when I wake up every day I hear of this new apotheosis of capitalism — this morning's takeovers beginning at $4.7 billion and ending with $50 billion, and covering the mining sector and the *Wall Street Journal* and *Reuters*, and the likelihood of Microsoft purchasing Yahoo. It's capitalism quite out of control and it's a kind of intellectual and institutional process that wears away at the foundation and the value of the pubic sector, whether it's health or education or any other public service that is vital to people's lives and livelihood.

We are confronting an ideology that negotiates bilateral trade agreements that increase intellectual property rights even further than they are enshrined in the World Trade Organization's (WTO's) treaties. They extend the life of patents for pharmaceutical companies, enabling them to keep drug prices up and health care costs up. These pharmaceutical companies are becoming ever more aggressive. In Thailand, for example, the pharmaceutical company Abbott holds a drug called Kaletra, a second-line drug for AIDS sufferers. Most of the people who are receiving anti-retro-viral treatment for AIDS are on first-line interventions. But after four or five years, some of these people develop a resistance and need second-line drugs, of which Kaletra is one of the major ones. Abbott, however, refused to lower the price of Kaletra, so the government of Thailand was forced to turn to a generic drug manufacturer and issue a compulsory licence to produce a low-cost version of the drug that its AIDS sufferers could afford. This is entirely legitimate and legal under the WTO's intellectual property clauses. But the pharmaceutical company, in retaliation, threatened to withdraw the other seven drugs it had on the

Thailand market. The dispute finally ended when the company agreed to lower its prices, but only if the government agreed to withdraw the compulsory licence.

These pharmaceutical companies act as if they have the power of nation states, the power to take on governments. Thirty-nine pharmaceutical companies got together in a coalition a few years ago to take the government of South Africa to court when it tried to lower drug prices. The drug companies were subjected to such an extraordinarily effective public protest that they had to retreat with their pharmaceutical tails between their legs, but the setback did little to curb their arrogance. Right now the drug company Novartis is challenging patent law in the major courts of India, and the government of India is very concerned because, if Novartis prevails, then the generic anti-retro-viral drugs to treat AIDS may well dry up — and India is the primary source of those drugs at this time. But Novartis has no intention of withdrawing its court case. It is perfectly willing to protect its patent rights at the expense of people in the developing world, even though those markets are largely inconsequential compared to the overwhelming markets for these drug companies in the West.

Our governments' collective ideological proclivity to defend the profit-obsessed interests of major corporate investors and shareholders is really profoundly unsettling. We are confronting an ideology where expenditures for military buildups, conflict, and war invariably supersede and transcend the expenditures for improving the human condition.

The Congressional Research Service of the United States recently did a careful study of the costs to the United States of the war in Iraq. It found that the war was costing the United States $8 billion a month. When you put the cost of the war in Iraq together with the cost of the war in Afghanistan, we are spending every month in these two conflicts more than we have ever raised in one year to subdue a pandemic that has taken 25 million lives and has 40 million people in its grip. We are confronting an ideology, in other words, that is deeply entrenched and profoundly unsympathetic to the nature of the human condition.

The new book by Naomi Klein, titled *The Shock Doctrine: The Rise of Disaster Capitalism,* has captured in ways I have rarely seen, the forces that have been amassed against the treasured nature of the public benefit. All you have to do is look at the profits that are being made from the war in Iraq by the corporations that now infest that country.

We are confronting an ideology that, over the centuries in the continent I know the best and love, the continent of Africa, has imposed a series of depredations that are almost beyond comprehension. Starting with slavery, moving to colonialism, the voracious alliances of the Cold War, and then the structural adjustment programs imposed on that continent by the World Bank and the International Monetary Fund (IMF), the consequences have been horrendous levels of poverty, hunger, and disease. These are ideological perversions that are deeply destructive of the human condition, even to this day, and for me this is beyond comprehension.

The IMF still imposes on several developing countries what it calls a "macroeconomic framework," which makes it impossible for those countries to improve their social programs — impossible for ministers of health, for example, to pay their health care workers adequately or hire the needed additional nurses and doctors. This callous abuse of countries that are literally struggling for survival should be inconceivable, but it happens all the time. In my own personal experience of the last five years, I have seen the dark underside of an ideology that never adequately responds to any of the moral and human imperatives with which this world is blighted, and so millions of people die unnecessarily.

One of the worst aspects of neoliberalism is that it does not accept or recognize health care as a basic human right. I must admit that I am completely bewildered by the indifference of the international community to this and other basic human needs. I am sixty-nine years old. I have kicked around in politics and in diplomacy and in multilateralism, and I thought I understood the way the world works. But I now realize I don't understand the way the world works. I don't understand the levels of indifference, inertia, passivity, and insensitivity to the plight of the millions of people who are struggling to survive.

The most recent report on HIV/AIDS from the United Nations announced with a note of optimism that there are now two million people being treated for this disease internationally. But the report added that there are another five million people afflicted with AIDS who require treatment but aren't getting the anti-retro-viral drugs they need, over two million of them are children. We have the drugs, but we have yet to repair the infrastructure, to improve the human capacity that has been decimated by the impact of the virus. It would be quite possible to do that, if the world summoned its energies and its focus. The refusal to do so is to me incomprehensible. How is this possible? The pandemic has been raging for more than twenty-five years, and 80 percent of these perfectly lovely and decent kids, if they don't get treatment, will die before the age of five.

You may know that we have what we call a miracle wonder drug named Nevirapine. If you give one tablet to a mother during the birthing process and the liquid equivalent to the infant within seventy-two hours of being born, you reduce the transmission of the infection by over 50 percent — which means that hundreds of thousands of kids who are born HIV-positive and are doomed to an early death would otherwise be born HIV-negative and have the potential for full lives. Why are we losing these children? How is that happening? It's because we are facing the same kind of ideological instincts, the same lack of commitment, and the same indifference to the public sector that ultimately morphs into an indifference to human health itself.

I'm shocked, too, by the behaviour of the G-8 countries because they reflect the way these countries' governments behave around the sustaining of the best and most principled health care system. They gather together for their summits and they make all kinds of public commitments about doubling the foreign aid to Africa by the year 2010 from $25 billion a year to $50 billion a year, and then, no sooner do they end their conference then they start to renege on their commitments. No one is asking these countries for more than they promised. We're merely asking them to keep their promises, but most now lie in tatters. Even with my own cynicism about the world, I was astounded when the Development Assistance Committee of the OECD recently produced its figures showing that, despite the G-8 summit in 2005 and the jamboree and excitement that attended it, foreign aid actually *declined* between 2005 and 2006. Our own country's foreign aid, as a percentage of our GDP, went down and will continue to decline, even though Canada is the only G-8 country with successive government surpluses.

All of this political indifference and betrayal happens while peoples' lives are continually at stake. As a social democrat, as someone who shares Tommy Douglas's view of the world — a profoundly different ideology — I join with all progressive Canadians in striving to preserve and enhance the treasured public health care system that Tommy bequeathed to us. The crucial nature of this struggle is highlighted when we look at the terrible condition of the millions of people in other countries who are denied even the most basic and minimal health care.

I am still reeling from the images burnt into my mind from a recent trip I made to Mozambique. I was in Beira, that country's second largest city and a major port. As I often do when I visit a city in Africa, I dropped in at the local general hospital. I went up to the women's ward on the second floor. There were ninety women in the ward and only fifty-four beds. Women were lying on the concrete floor between beds and under the beds and out in the corridors. Many had their families with them and there was such a contagion of anguish and imminent death. And I stood at the door of the ward and I thought to myself, has the world gone mad? They were all young women, all in their twenties and thirties. Women in Africa are disproportionately infected by the virus because of the reality of gender inequality in which the virus is driven by male sexual behaviour. It's the most ghastly of truths that in international health we are unable to overcome the prevailing ideology of indifference. It manifests itself in Canada by the constant battles over privatization and two-tier medicine, but it manifests itself in the Third World in what amounts to an agony of injustice.

So the struggle for social justice and equality never ends, and for me, whether it's the struggle here, or the struggle there, the struggles are inseparable. For me, the struggle represents the meaning of my own social philosophy, and for me it's the voices of Woodrow Lloyd and Allan Blakeney and Roy Romanow and Lorne Calvert and Woodsworth and Coldwell and Stanley Knowles and Ed Broadbent and Alexa McDonough and David Lewis — and of course, above all, Tommy Douglas. And I'm telling you that we are going to win this momentous struggle — that one day the pendulum will swing and the voices of these champions of medicare will prevail.

CHAPTER 3

The Douglas Legacy and the Future of Medicare

Greg Marchildon

It is in the natural order of things that the reputations of the vast majority of political leaders decline after their lifetime. As human beings, we tend to forget about most of the past — only the most significant events or achievements are remembered. While most leaders hope to leave a legacy that lives beyond their own lives, few do. Tommy Douglas was one of those rare exceptions. In a 2004 CBC poll in which 1.2 million Canadians cast their votes, Tommy Douglas was the people's choice as the "Greatest Canadian of all time." He was one of four political leaders who made it to the top ten; the other three were all prime ministers: Pierre Trudeau, Lester B. Pearson, and Sir John A. Macdonald.[1]

The reason Tommy Douglas was selected over these other notable political leaders was, without a doubt, his path-breaking role in the introduction of universal health care in a country that could have taken a very different road. Universal public health care may be the norm in Western Europe, but it is definitely an exception in the Americas. Before Tommy Douglas came along, Canada was on a trajectory that was far more American than European.[2] He and those he gathered around him defied the gravity of time and place by establishing a beachhead for the first universal health care program anywhere in the Americas. Indeed, they established universal hospital insurance one year before the National Health Service was established in the United Kingdom.

What is the essence of the Douglas legacy? Reviewing the historical record as a scholar and past practitioner of public policy, I would say that it involves three separate but very connected characteristics. The first is idealism — the setting of an objective that, while it may never be perfectly obtained, remains your guiding light throughout the clutter of life. This kind of idealism was so aptly captured by the title in Al Johnson's recent biography of the Douglas government: *Dream No Little Dreams*.[3]

The second characteristic is that he was prepared to work with what he had — the people, the resources — in building this New Jerusalem. Like the farmer who can repair machinery with whatever is at hand in ingenious combinations, he was remarkably flexible in the means employed to achieve his objectives. If I had to invent a phrase for this, I would call it "prairie pragmatism."

The third characteristic is that, irrespective of the means selected, Douglas was absolutely tenacious and persevering in pursuing his objectives. Obstacles and delays only seemed to fortify his determination to attain his end.

Let me expand on each of these characteristics: idealism, prairie pragmatism, and tenacity.

Universally available health care is an essential underpinning for a society in which all citizens are to have the opportunity to live their lives to their fullest potential. To Douglas, this meant a real democracy with the participation of all *and* a just economy with opportunity for all. Tommy Douglas's ultimate objective was to transform health from a commodity that was bought and sold into a basic human right, available to anyone on the basis of need rather than ability to pay. To have anything less, he knew, would act as a constraint on our ability to fulfill our mental and physical potential as human beings. He always remembered his own childhood affliction, in which his leg would have been amputated had not a physician been willing to treat him as a charity case.[4] He never forgot the searing experience of the Great Depression when dust bowl farm families could no longer afford medical assistance.

Douglas's prairie pragmatism meant that he seized opportunities when they appeared and he discarded options when they were no longer viable. He took advantage of his own election in 1944 to become minister of health in addition to premier. When a major federal public health care initiative, which he strongly supported, was rejected by the provinces of Ontario and Quebec, among others, during the Dominion–Provincial Reconstruction Conference of 1945–1946, he simply went home to set up a working model of universal hospital insurance to show Ottawa and the provinces how it could actually be done.

Through it all, Tommy Douglas was tenacious. For almost two decades, his government worked assiduously to create a diversified economy that would be capable of generating the revenues necessary to implement medicare: after all, it took almost fifteen years after hospitalization to find the money to include physician services as part of medicare. Even more important, Douglas, along with his cabinet and his successor, Woodrow Lloyd, refused to be blackmailed in a long and bitter struggle with organized medicine in Saskatchewan, much supported by organized medicine and the insurance industry in the rest of Canada as well as the United States.[5] Allan Blakeney too was at the very centre of the storm during the doctors' strike of 1962. He personally experienced the lengths to which a powerful minority is prepared to go to undermine the democratic will of the majority.

As federal leader of the New Democratic Party, Tommy Douglas consistently used his position in parliament to support the faction within the Pearson cabinet in favour of national medicare. He was helped in this by the Saskatchewan "Mafia," those brilliant civil servants who had left Saskatchewan in 1964 to work in senior levels of the Pearson government. This we know from no less than Tom Kent, Prime Minister Pearson's chief policy advisor at the time. In his autobiography, Kent documented how closely he worked with Al Johnson, Douglas's former deputy provincial treasurer, to arrive at a successful agreement with the provinces, particularly Quebec, on national medicare.[6]

Tommy Douglas remained tenacious even after leaving politics. By the late 1970s, he concluded that medicare was in grave danger. In November 1979, he joined 150 other concerned citizens, including Monique Bégin, Bob Evans, and Michael Rachlis. This was the first SOS Medicare Conference. In its plan of action, the conference participants agreed to establish "an ongoing *Canadian Health Coalition* of concerned organizations for the preservation and improvement of medicare."[7] After resuming her post as minister of health and welfare, Madame Bégin would soon remedy some of the more immediate and pressing threats to medicare in the Canada Health Act.

In my view, these are the three characteristics I think we should be mixing in equal proportions in our efforts to preserve and improve medicare and implement phase two of Tommy Douglas's vision: idealism in terms of ends, a certain "prairie pragmatism" in terms of means, and a tenacious commitment to the fundamental changes that are required to reach this goal. As Douglas stated the problem over a quarter-century ago:

> When we began to plan medicare, we pointed out that
> it would be in two phases. The first phase would be to
> remove the financial barrier between those giving the

> service and those receiving it. The second phase would
> be to reorganize and revamp the whole delivery system
> — and of course, that's the big item. That's the thing we
> haven't done yet.[8]

And that is still the thing that remains undone. At the same time, we face a rising tide of hostility towards what was achieved in the first phase of medicare. The recent conferences sponsored by the Fraser Institute and the Government of Alberta gave considerable voice to anti-medicare advocates. The *Chaoulli* decision by the Supreme Court of Canada gave considerable hope to those who want to tear down the principles of public administration and universality as set out in the Canada Health Act.

None of this should be surprising. A small but very vocal and powerful minority has always been opposed to the Canadian model of medicare. They are opposed precisely because, as a policy, medicare is highly redistributional. Every minute of every day, it redistributes resources from wealthier and healthier Canadians to poorer and sicker Canadians. But they are embarrassed to use this argument directly, even when urging more "patient participation" through user fees or other similar policies.

Those of us who support this redistributional model now have an opportunity to have our arguments heard about the second phase of medicare. We can begin the process of planning the concrete ways in which the principle of universality can be extended beyond hospitals and physician care to other forms of health care and to health more generally. While we may not always agree on the means, we must nonetheless find a way to come to a consensus about the way, or ways, forward to improve, to expand upon, and to go well beyond, the first phase of medicare.

In a very important sense, we are always working in the shadow of Tommy Douglas's idealism. When I was in a used book store about a year ago, I happened to pick up a biography of

Douglas. When I walked to the counter, I found myself behind a seventy-something lady who was buying a number of books. She looked back at me and immediately spotted the biography. "Tommy Douglas," she said, "I don't see any these days, but we sure need a leader like him now."

But, as Tommy would have said to her had he been there: he was just an ordinary person; the people of Saskatchewan were just ordinary people; Canadians, for that matter, are just ordinary people: but sometimes, when they put their minds to it, ordinary people are capable of extraordinary things. Especially when they are also principled, persevering, and "prairie pragmatic" in how they go about achieving the second phase of medicare.

CHAPTER 4

Fulfilling the
Douglas/Lloyd Vision

Allan E. Blakeney

It was my privilege and opportunity to serve in the Saskatchewan legislature with Tommy Douglas and in his cabinet when, in 1961, the Medical Care Insurance Act was passed, and to serve with his successor, Woodrow Lloyd, when the plan was introduced, against fierce opposition, in July of 1962.

I feel sure that Douglas and Lloyd — Tommy and Woodrow — would have said then, and would say now, that this was a solid step forward. They introduced hospital care insurance in 1947, and then had to wait twelve years for the federal government to share part of the costs. With medical care insurance the wait was six years.

Yes, these were solid steps forward. But only steps. They were never meant, at least by Tommy and Woodrow, to be the end. Both the report of the Thompson Committee upon which the Saskatchewan plan was based and the report of the Emmett Hall

Commission upon which the national plan was based had much broader visions: health plans should include prescription drugs, dentistry, and other benefits for citizens.

And if we are to honour the legacies of Tommy and Woodrow, we will: 1) defend what we have, 2) recapture what has been lost, and 3) expand coverage in areas of public need.

Douglas would have seen what we have as a solid start to a national health care plan on a European model but tailored to Canadian conditions. That was a good idea in 1947 when hospital care insurance was initiated. It was a good idea in 1962 when physician care was initiated. It is a good idea in 2007 when both need our support.

My second point deals with how we defend what we have. There will always be problems in controlling costs. We have made medical and hospital care — I'll call it medicare — free at the time of delivery: a "free good," as the economists call it. So there will be shortages. If I gave away potatoes, I could create a shortage — particularly if the providers of potatoes had an interest in the increased consumption of potatoes.

I don't want to be misunderstood. I'm not suggesting that care is being delivered that is not of benefit to the patient. I am suggesting that, in many cases, the care being delivered would not be the top priority for spending public money — not even the top priority for spending public money to improve the health of citizens.

If I am correct, then one area of attention in defence of medicare is to change — if we can, and to the extent we can — the way medicare is delivered. This is a familiar theme in several recent studies and reports. In Saskatchewan, this was a prominent proposal set out in the report by Ken Fyke a few years ago. There is widespread agreement that these changes would be desirable and would lead to better use of health resources and better patient care. There is less agreement on how we get from here to there.

I have some thoughts on this. They focus on whether we could change the way physicians and other health professionals are trained; and on whether we could recruit even more female physicians and create conditions that make it easier for physicians to balance professional and family responsibilities. They also focus on how we pay primary care physicians, and on putting more emphasis on delivering primary care by teams of health practitioners, including physicians — but not only physicians — who are focused on health maintenance as well as treatment: the wellness approach.

My third point is this: it is time to advance medicare, to broaden the coverage of medicare. The figures make very clear that the frontier area of escalating costs in providing medical care is prescription drugs, and that millions of Canadians have little or no drug insurance coverage. The experience in Saskatchewan in the 1970s and early 1980s with a comprehensive prescription drug insurance program shows that, if those conditions can be replicated, there are huge savings to be made in providing prescription drugs to Canadians.

It is clear that a national program can provide the largest savings and the greatest equity among Canadians. There may be a significant "local" element in providing, say, home care. There is next to no such element with respect to prescription drugs. A statin drug is the same world wide. I am daily reminded by television that there is an international language for Viagra. The time for a national prescription drug insurance program has arrived. It should be covered by special legislation, as was hospital insurance and physicians' services insurance.

To the argument that we cannot campaign for an expansion of our system when there are clear deficiencies in existing medicare, I say that I do not agree. Opponents will attack medicare, come what may. Let us advocate an expansion of coverage. This may well focus the attack on expansion rather than on existing medicare. As in so many battles, a good offence is the best defence.

The steady drumbeat of attacks on medicare come from people who simply attack the single-payer model and who do not put forward any alternative model for providing medically necessary services for Canadians.

Most of these opponents purport to argue for a parallel private system paid for by the patient or his or her insurer. Which, they assure us, would not draw resources from the public system. I doubt their sincerity or perhaps their predictions of the results of a private system. For many Canadians, this private system is already available. A short trip to the United States will provide the patient with private care without taking resources from Canada's public system — but remarkably few Canadians use this option. And even if governments in Canada offered to pay travel expenses to the United States, I don't think the numbers would increase greatly. This leads me to believe that what these people want is not a parallel system, but the use of the existing system of publicly provided hospitals and diagnostic equipment, publicly trained physicians and nurses, all in priority to other Canadians for the payment of a small part of the total cost. This is hardly a parallel system — just a bit of queue jumping and social climbing: a latté and cappuccino system.

I conclude by repeating: if we seek to honour Douglas and Lloyd, it should not be a case of SOS Medicare. Medicare needs not so much to be defended as advanced.

Two promising areas for advance are: 1) A national prescription drug plan; and 2) Steps to change the way medical care is delivered, particularly primary care.

I believe these positions are widely accepted. The frontier area is how we bring them about. That is what we need to tackle now. As I see it, these are our challenges. These are the next steps along the road to a fully functional and sustainable national health insurance plan for Canada.

That was the dream of Tommy Douglas.

CHAPTER 5

The Canada Health Act: Lessons for Today and Tomorrow

Monique Bégin

I was in Ottawa for the first SOS Medicare conference, at the Lester B. Pearson Building, just over twenty-five years ago: November 5–6, 1979. At least three of the keynote speakers of those days have left us since: Tommy Douglas, Mr. Justice Emmett Hall, and Dennis McDermott. We all agreed then that medicare was in deep trouble. I was at that time in Opposition in the House of Commons, not knowing that I would be back as minister of national health and welfare soon afterward, following David Crombie who had replaced me during the nine months of Joe Clark's Conservative government.

I had first heard of possible problems with medicare earlier that year, when the Liberals were still in office, both through an odd phone call from Dennis Timbrell, the super-confident minister of health of Ontario, wondering about my reaction if he were to institute a user fee in hospitals for certain types of patients, and through a sudden barrage of questions in the House of Commons from Ed Broadbent to Prime Minister Trudeau and then to me on extra-billing and "massive" withdrawals by doctors from OHIP. I did not know what they were talking about, and my department kept telling me there was no problem. Of course there *was* a problem, and this was the beginning of a five-year-long loud and controversial public policy dossier.

It was still the provincial–federal honeymoon on "block funding," which had replaced, in 1977, the two traditional fifty-fifty cost-sharing agreements for funding of acute hospital care, laboratory, radiological and diagnostic services, and physician care between Ottawa and the provinces.[9] The provinces loved this new tax point transfer to them, plus the regular cheque now sent directly to their treasurers, but the new EPF[10] legislation, for all practical purposes, had no accountability mechanism and no teeth.

Justice Emmett Hall, who was with us at the first SOS Medicare conference, had just started a Health Services Review at Crombie's request. In September 1980, he reported to me that our Canadian medicare system ranked among the best in the world, but warned that extra-billing by doctors and user fees levied by hospitals were creating a two-tiered system that threatened the accessibility of care.[11]

I took note and, after another four long, painful, and often bitter and vicious years, the Canada Health Act (1984) (CHA) was unanimously passed by the House of Commons. Why did it pass? For a very simple reason: the public wanted it. And, thanks also to the support of groups like the Canadian Health Coalition, the Friends of Medicare, and organized nursing.

Because of the new neoconservative economic philosophy already rampant everywhere, we could not open new fronts in the battle. We basically repeated the definitions and five conditions of the old Acts — keeping the same rules of the game — but we gave teeth to the deal with an enforcement mechanism and penalties in case of breaches. So, with regret, I asked Justice to prepare a bill very much "acute care and medical care" oriented, and not at all based on health promotion and primary care. There was no way I could even mention home care or chronic care, let alone pharmacare.

Did it work? Yes, the CHA certainly achieved its immediate goal: banning extra-billing and user fees. It did so within the first three years provided by the Act, and each of the ten provinces complied, some even before the Act was applied.[12] Was medicare then safe from erosion and from the development of a two-tier system once and for all? No. First, the CHA could not foresee what form new attacks against medicare would take, nor the new high-tech medicine developments. We did not know that day surgery was becoming the norm, that drugs would replace many surgical procedures, that diagnostic services and labs could exist on their own as independent private services outside hospitals. Little did we imagine that, twenty years later, the same anti-medicare slogans, the same clichés about how great the private sector is, would reappear regularly, trying to brainwash Canadians.

Am I confident that medicare is surviving and will continue to remain the critical key public program it is? Yes, I am. But not if we, the public, abandon it. Not if we, the public, panic about wait times. Not if we, the public, do not make the effort to learn more about it and about other health care systems in the industrialized world. Not if we, the public, do not know our strengths, our challenges, and the uniqueness of our medicare.

Let me conclude with three lessons from the Canada Health Act.

First, we should relax and understand that the American health care scene, with its patchwork of super-expensive administrative structures, its 45 million uninsured, and the millions more under-insured population, is not the norm, but the exception. In the United States, health is a market commodity. Here, it is a public good. Canada is in the norm and we belong with the European industrialized countries who all have a universal public health care system. But we are not exactly like most of them; that is our uniqueness. Most of them do require some small up-front money for services (user fees, co-payments, etc.), but the range of services covered is much broader than ours, including drugs, rehabilitation services, home care, and more. We pay nothing for doctors and hospitals, but that is all we get. On the whole, European countries have much more equitable accessibility and are much more publicly funded than is our system, with a ratio of 80 to 90 percent public funding to 10 to 20 percent private funding. We are only 70 percent publicly funded, with 30 percent out-of-pocket private spending.[13] So, when new programs are proposed, don't close your mind to some up-front payment for services. Ask yourself instead: How much more do we all gain from the public purse? How much does this or that brings us closer to an 80 to 20 percent ratio?

Secondly, the condition called "public administration" does not mean that some services cannot be privately *delivered*. But to qualify under the CHA, they must be publicly *funded* by each provincial single payer: OHIP, RAMQ, Saskatchewan Ministry of Health, etc. This is not negotiable.

Lastly, we must clarify the rules of the game applying to physicians when they interact with both the public and the private health care systems.

CHAPTER 6

Healthy Children First

Tom Kent

My title comes, of course, from the sayings of Tommy Douglas. The goal of medicare is healthy people, "not just patching them up when they're sick."

Not only is preventing better than curing but it's also essential to the viability of universal public care. Medical science will go on improving treatments for our ills. If we rely on treatments, the costs will become "so excessive" — Douglas's words again — that medicare will lose public support.

The problem is that preventive care reduces the costs of patching people up in the future, not in the present. Immediately, it is an additional expense on top of treating existing sickness. In the battle for attention, for dollars, short-term necessity wins over long-term gain. The consequence is that public policy becomes trapped in a vicious circle. As more and more can be done to treat illness, doing too little to prevent it becomes increasingly too little.

Our task is to break out of that circle. Otherwise we will not counter the trend to excessive costs that Douglas correctly foresaw. Some of the obstacles to breaking out arise from within the organization and procedures of the health care system. How to overcome those is best left to examination by people better qualified than I am. I therefore concentrate on the political obstacle. It certainly is not rooted in public opinion. It arises from our federalism, from the confusion of responsibilities between two orders of government.

We started nation wide medicare by finding one way round that confusion. The Pearson government's legislation stated the principles, and federal taxation reimbursed provincial treasuries for half of the costs of programs conforming to these principles.

That worked as the starter. It could have gone on working. It could have been used to broaden services beyond hospitals and physicians, to invigorate preventive care. But it was not. The reforming zeal of the 1960s was the late expression of public attitudes born from economic depression and war. As it faded, so did the political will behind cost sharing. "The feds" soon came to resent levying taxes for services delivered by the provinces, for which most of the credit therefore went to provincial politicians. Hence the process of reducing federal cash, replacing it by provincial taxes, that began in 1977. The federal contribution was progressively uncoupled from costs, until in 1995 all commitment to fixed shares in provincial programs was scrapped by unilateral action in the federal budget.

In sum, the short history of medicare is that the promise that began it has not been kept. Federal support has not remained a stable base. It comes only in amounts shaped from time to time by political pressures and the state of federal finances. Money so provided may make some of the patching-up of people a little faster. There can be no serious pretence that it will do more. Far from making medicare safe for a generation, the most recent "accord" is not even protecting its principles from erosion.

The Douglas warning therefore remains equally important today. Medicare will be safe only when it is directed as much to wellness as against sickness; when it is about health, not patching-up. That requires investment for tomorrow, not improvisation for today. It will not come from the present confusion of federal–provincial dealings. Nor will it come from the diminution of federal government foreshadowed by present talk of so-called "open" federalism. The principles of medicare will be secure only if they are again accompanied by firm principle for the federal part of its financing.

National medicare was made possible by changing the way our federalism had hitherto worked. Its future depends on further change. Fortunately, the way to that was pointed out three years ago, when the provincial premiers collectively suggested that Ottawa take responsibility for national pharmacare. Unfortunately, the then federal government refused even to discuss the idea. A partial excuse might be that, desirable though it is, universal pharmacare is not the first priority. But that is not the point. What mattered about the premiers' suggestion was their openness to re-thinking responsibilities, to assigning a specific role in health services to the national government. Rarely has an opening for creative reform been more sadly missed.

However, the idea need not be lost. The next "new government" could offer to take it up, not for one branch of health service, but for the people whose health is of greatest national importance. It could offer to take full financial responsibility for the health of all Canadian children.

The well-being of children is not a concern of social justice only. It is an essential part of federal responsibility for the economy. Even business economists have come to recognize that investment in human capital is key to prosperity. And the most productive investment is in childhood. That is where an efficient policy for health, for more than patching-up, must begin.

It means more than physician and hospital services. It calls for comprehensive, preventive care: for nutritional supplements as well as prescribed drugs and inoculations; for physical exercise as well as regular check-ups; for eye and dental care; for pre-natal counselling, baby clinics, early childhood centres. And such services must be backed by income supports to combat family poverty.

Young people are the asset on which the nation depends. They are an increasingly scarce asset. The nation needs for all of them the opportunities now enjoyed by those who are fortunate in the incomes and education of their parents. It is not a need to be met at the provincial level. People are now too mobile for that. Youth brought up with the help of taxes in New Brunswick are very likely to become taxpayers not there but in Alberta.

We have to rely on the equalization principle, now written into the constitution, to offset such fiscal discrepancies for provincial services as established as primary and secondary schooling. But recent controversies have painfully demonstrated the political limits to equalization. It cannot be stretched to enable provinces to provide additional services at comparable levels of provincial taxation.

New federal finance was necessary to start nation wide medicare. Such a federal initiative is just as crucial to our moving on to positive programs for health. In consequence, reformers commonly call for a repetition of the cost sharing that the 1960s made familiar. Unfortunately, it is a broken instrument. It will not work again. Federal politicians know that it does not yield sufficient credit for their money. Provincial politicians know even better that it cannot be relied upon.

Therefore, the needs of our youth can be met only if we again develop a new federal–provincial relationship for a purpose so special and important. Divided finance will not work this time. The initiative that could work is full, 100 percent federal financing.

This runs counter to the conventional wisdom that public money will be carefully spent only if the spenders are the people who have to find the money. In truth, the relation between revenue and expenditure is that simple only on a small scale. In big organizations, private and public, avoidance of waste necessarily depends on firm benchmarks for the control of reasonable costs. That is never simple to devise or easy to enforce. But, with goodwill, it is no more difficult between governments than between departments within one government. And the health of our kids would provide the strongest of pressures for goodwill.

A federal offer of 100 percent financing would, of course, be simply the start for negotiations. The detailed arrangements that emerged would no doubt differ between, say, Manitoba and Quebec. But in all cases the negotiations would be very different from the familiar federal–provincial fights over money and over credit and blame for the outcomes. A Charter for Child Health would be a glorious prize for all involved.

Kids are, increasingly, the most popular of public causes. It is the welfare of our children and grandchildren, far more than of today's adults, that powers current environmental concern. Their health care comes most directly home. Financing it would give Ottawa politicians the clear responsibility, the continuing involvement and recognition, that has hitherto escaped them. Provincial politicians would gain the security in social policy that has hitherto been denied them. Ottawa got away remarkably easily with reneging on its promises to the provinces. It could not let down the kids. To start providing for their health would be to go on providing.

Even so, restoring confidence in federal–provincial relations has another condition. The negotiations must be free from any suggestion that new federal finance for children might be used as an excuse to cut down on finance for adult medicare. The present arrangement is supposed to run to March 2014. That liability must be recognized, whatever the future strains on federal finances.

There will be time to settle on firmer principles for later financing, but it should be clear at once that 100 percent federal financing will not be extended to adults. The commonest suggestion for them is 25 percent cost sharing, which would yield about the same dollar amount as the present elaborate calculations will produce in 2013. Anything more than 25 percent would weaken the objective basis for assessing child costs. Ottawa must know that each province's charges for salaries, supplies, and facilities are at the same rates for children as the province incurs, chiefly on its own account, for adults.

Distinction between children and adults is more, however, than a matter of calculation. It underlines the principle of Canadian federalism, whereby each province and its municipalities provide most of the services wanted by its electorate. The role of the federal government is not to impose uniformity, but to concentrate on the services necessary to our common nationality. In this respect, young people, pre-voters, are different from adults. In contemporary society, in the global economy, their health is an asset vital to us all. It has priority as a national responsibility.

Dedication to that responsibility is, to borrow the title of Al Johnson's book about the Douglas government, "to dream no little dreams." Its fulfillment may have to come, in the spirit of prairie pragmatism, by stages. Federal finance could be introduced for pre-schoolers, move on as quickly as possible to pre-teens, and later to age eighteen.

That, I suggest, is the priority agenda for the defence and development of medicare.

CHAPTER 7

The Collective Action Problem

Robert McMurtry

As Joseph Heath wrote in his book *The Efficient Society*, the provision of health care for a population is a collective action problem.[14] A single-payer system, he contended, is the most efficient mechanism to ensure the provision of health care for all. Perhaps that is why all but one industrialized nation has some form of single-payer coverage.

But Canada's medicare is much more than a single-payer method of insurance. It is also just and equitable, and it contributes in a fundamental way to social inclusion. It is universal: every citizen is covered. It is characterized by inclusive risk pooling, not selective risk adjustment. The latter is an essential feature of private, for-profit insurance coverage and by its nature leaves the most vulnerable to fend for themselves.

Perhaps that is why the Canada Health Act of 1984 has achieved an iconic status in Canada. The principles of universality, comprehensiveness, accessibility, portability, and public

administration resonate with Canadians. The five principles capture Canadian values of justice, the common good, and a shared
responsibility for our collective well-being.

Why, then, is there a constant clamour that medicare is in crisis? Is it a manufactured issue by those few who stand to benefit
by the commodification of health care? Or are there real issues
that urgently need to be addressed to modernize the Canadian
health care system?

The answer to both questions is "yes."

The need for change to deliver better care is not in doubt. Few
defenders of the status quo can be found. However, the real issue
is not whether for-profit private care is the answer, but rather
how we can find a collective answer to achieve the vision of
"Medicare 2."

The Possibility of Social Choice

Amartya Sen titled his Nobel address (1998) "The Possibility of
Social Choice," a captivating title.[15] Since the 1980s, choice — and
most particularly individual choice — has been elevated to a high
virtue. Indeed, some market the concept of small government and
individual choice as the prime virtues of the political process.

The notion of social choice has become a threatened species.
The elimination of social choice is not a defensible perspective,
but nonetheless it is one that is constantly chorused as the righteous and true path by some political parties and much of the
mainstream media.

Consider the impact on any jurisdiction of the absence of social
choice. The consequences are difficult to imagine. What would
become of parks, libraries, schools, police, public health, safe water
and air quality, disaster response, pollution abatement, and pandemic influenza response, among others? All of these and other
challenges demand cooperative action. Can climate change be
solved without collective action?

Social choice and social action are essential for the well-being of a neighbourhood or a nation. Individual rights can and must be protected, but not at the expense of the well-being of others. Examples of this order of thinking can readily be identified. Smoking bans at public gatherings, quarantine of a person with a high-risk infectious disease, and the prohibition of impaired driving are three obvious examples.

The fundamental choice is balancing the "me-self" versus "we-self" as governing principles. A country that fails to achieve the appropriate balance is at risk of losing its coherence as a nation. We cannot afford to forget the wisdom of collective action. Such wisdom created medicare in the first instance.

Medicare — Redefining the Future

While there is variance among jurisdictions, medicare has covered physician services and hospitalization costs of all medically necessary services for the past forty years. It has become the most popular public program in Canada's history.

Yet, from the outset there were many things that were not included that in hindsight were crucial omissions. Among them are pharmacare, home care, palliative care, disease prevention, and health promotion. The latter two can best be accomplished by prioritizing the perspective of public and population health. Their separation from medicare was and is a misdirection that must be overcome. This separation has led many observers, with some justification, to label medicare as an "illness system."

Indeed, the greatest threat to the sustainability of publicly funded health care is not so much the aging of the population and new technologies as it is the failure to move upstream and embrace disease prevention and health promotion.

Just as the progress of a nation cannot solely be measured by economic growth, the health of Canadians cannot be measured only by the robustness of bio-medical or disease-focused care. For both, other determinants have an enormous impact. Such determinants include an educated populace, a healthy environment, safe and resilient neighbourhoods, good housing, social justice, and robust democratic governance structures.

Many, or perhaps most, of the policy directions lie outside of ministries of health. However, in the future, the responsibility for tracking the impact of government policy and economic activity should become a priority of an integrated health care system. Such tracking begins with primary care comprising multidisciplinary teams integrated with their community, and ranges up to regional and national level health surveillance.

One example of effective surveillance is the emerging work of the National Working Group of the Canadian Index of Well-Being. In March of 2007, Labonte, Muhajarine, and Winquist wrote, "Notably, gains in health-adjusted life expectancy made in the 1990s peaked in 1996, and have since started to decline. Canadians are increasingly likely to develop a chronic disease or mental illness during their lifetime."[16] They further noted that there is a "consistent and continuing decline in Canadians' self-rated health status," as well as "a worrisome downward trend in health outcomes for Canada's youth, 12–19 years."

Their observations were echoed in the Health Council of Canada's March 2007 report on type-2 diabetes. The findings of the HCC pointed to Canada's failure to put an effective chronic disease strategy in place. Since about 70 percent of health care costs relate to chronic disease care, it is a serious omission.

Such information is of prime importance for all levels of an integrated health care system as well as government leaders. It appears that, in spite of economic growth, there are increasing disparities of health status, to which the health care system is not responding effectively.

The Path Ahead

There are four principles that should guide us in the path ahead.

The first is to respect the values expressed by Canadians and reflected in the Romanow Report tabled in November 2002. The report described an historic dialogue and consultation with Canadians that confirmed the closely held conviction that we have a shared responsibility for the vulnerable, the ill, and the injured.

The second principle is to embrace the reality that medicare can be renewed and rebuilt. Examples of successful innovation abound in every province. "The status quo is not an option" for medicare, or for any other dynamic human system.

The third is that the new medicare must include not only illness care, but disease prevention and health promotion. The absence of an integration of public and population health with medicare is the greatest threat the publicly funded health care system faces.

The fourth and final principle is that the profit motive cannot have a role in the decision to provide or not to provide care. As Maggie Mahar wrote in *Money-Driven Medicine,* for-profit, investor-owned insurance carriers often deny coverage for necessary care.[17]

There is risk, too, in for-profit delivery. Too often the outcome of for-profit care delivery is a compromise of efficiency, equity, safety, and quality, as Devereaux and others described in 2002.[18,19]

Change can and is happening within the context of the public care system. The Health Council of Canada has reported many examples of success stories of health care renewal across Canada, many of which are inspiring and reproducible.[20] A failure of decision makers at all levels of the publicly funded system is the slow pace of uptake of best practices. That must and can change. It is a crucial part of the vision for renewal of medicare.

Why is the pace of change not as rapid as it could be? With the reinvestment in medicare that emerged from the First Ministers' accords of 2003 and 2004, there is certainly enough money to deliver on this vision as outlined.

Barriers to Change

Why is progress more difficult to achieve than it should be? The answer is that there are formidable barriers to change. System inertia, inadequate information systems, and a need for better health human resource planning are three examples. It must be recognized, however, that any change is discomforting to the incumbents who may benefit more from existing arrangements.

Interdisciplinary teams and provider substitution would help. In addition, it could address the current mismatch between expertise provided and expertise required for high-quality care. Appropriately trained nurses are quite capable of providing services traditionally delivered by physicians. In truth, the capability of health care professionals at all levels is under exploited. Most health care personnel are able to do more than their current scopes of practice. It represents an opportunity for cost-effective enhancement of accessibility.

Conclusion

As Lee Iacocca and Catherine Whitney wrote in *Where Have All the Leaders Gone?*: "We're not just a nation of factions. We're a people. We share common principles and ideals. And we rise and fall together."[21]

Both Americans and Canadians could benefit from listening to that advice. A renewed medicare is about collective action. We need the commitment of all, from first ministers to hands-on care givers. We need strategically distributed leadership to mobilize a national effort to renew medicare.

After all, politics is the art of the possible. There is a possibility of social choice. In the end, it is a choice for democracy.

PART II

The International
Context

CHAPTER 8

Styles of Rationing Health Care: The United States vs. Canada[1]

Uwe E. Reinhardt

For most of the twentieth century, Americans had luxuri-
ated in the unquestioned faith that theirs was the best
health system in the world. That credo was not totally
unfounded. At its best, the system probably is unrivalled
in the world. Few experts would argue that other nations educate
and train physicians better than does the United States. The
nation's hospitals set world standards in terms of technical sophistication and sheer luxury of accommodation, although the entire
US health system now is beginning to lag the world in the use of
information technology. The nation's pharmaceutical, biotech, and
medical device industries remain world leaders in their fields, both
in terms of technological sophistication and the sheer volume of
innovations. Finally, for terminally ill patients around the world
who can afford our expensive system, it often is viewed as their
last hope.

Erosion of the Faith in US Health Care
These many positive aspects of the US health system notwithstanding, Americans are beginning to lose faith in the global
superiority of their health system, as the rapidly rising cost of
American health care has begun to price more and more of them
out of health care and as doubts have arisen about the quality of
American health care.

The Cost of US Health Care
In terms of purchasing power parity (PPP) dollars the relatively
more market-oriented US health system spent almost twice as
much per capita on health care in 2003 ($6,102) than did Cana-
da ($3,165), and Germany ($3,005), and 50 percent more than
Switzerland ($4,077), even though both Germany and Switzer-
land have much older populations than does the United States.
According to the Milliman Medical Index, average annual medical spending for a US family of four, paid for either by insurers
or out of pocket, and averaged over all privately insured Americans under age sixty-five, healthy or not, reached $13,382 in
2006.[2] Yet according to the US Bureau of the Census, about one
third of American families have a family income below $40,000
per year. [3] With average annual per capita health spending rising
at two to three times the rate of increase in average family
incomes, it is merely a matter of arithmetic to realize that more
and more such families will be priced out of American health care
in the decade ahead, unless they are somehow subsidized by higher-
income families, either at their place of work or through
government programs. Thus, it is not surprising that the number
of Americans found without health insurance at any time has risen
inexorably during the past two decades, even during periods of
economic boom. The total stood at $37 million in 1993, at the
beginning of the Clinton administration. It is now $46 million
and expected to exceed $50 million within a few years. In the

Sunbelt states and in California, roughly a quarter of the population is uninsured at any time.

The Quality of US Health Care

Anxiety over costs of health care and health insurance coverage, however, are not the only source of a growing disenchantment with the US health care system. Health services research in the last decade or so has revealed that the US health system has serious operational flaws and fails to deliver adequate value for the huge financial resources it absorbs.

In a stunning report on a large, nation wide research project, Elizabeth McGlynn et al. reported that US adults received on average only about 55 percent of the care generally recommended for their condition.[4] Earlier, in their well known *Dartmouth Atlas of the United States*, John H. Wennberg and his associates at Dartmouth University had published data showing that total medicare spending per beneficiary varied across hospital-market areas in the United States by a factor of close to three even after adjustment for inter-regional differences in fees paid, the age-gender composition of the elderly in the various market areas, and the case-mix severity typical of medicare patients in the market area.[5] The high-cost regions lie primarily in the Sunbelt and the Northeastern states. The Wheat Belt states and Oregon tend to be low-cost areas. More recent work on medicare patients in the last two years or six months of their lives corroborates these findings.[6] Remarkably, subsequent research by the Dartmouth research team indicates that these enormous variations in health spending per capita are not associated with commensurate variations in the quality of care being delivered, in medical outcomes or even patient satisfaction.[7]

Even more remarkable in this regard has been a study by Katherine Baicker and Amitabh Chandra, indicating that there actually appears to be a negative correlation between the medicare

spending per capita in a state and the rank that state has in a quality ranking, based on an earlier study of process measures of
quality.[8] The authors conclude that states with relatively more
general practitioners tend to have more effective health care and
lower health spending and states relying relatively more on medical specialists tend to have higher medical spending but lower
process quality.

Recent cross-national research has indicated that the United
States does not rank consistently high in cross-national studies of
the quality of health care either. In a 2005 cross-national survey of
patients with health problems in six nations, for example, it was
found that 34 percent of American patients reported medical,
medication, or laboratory test errors, versus 30 percent in Canada, 27 percent in Australia, 23 percent in Germany, and 22 percent
in the UK.[9] Earlier, in its *To Err is Human: Building a Safer Health
System*, the prestigious Institute of Medicine (IOM) of the US
National Academy of Science had estimated that between 44,000
to 98,000 Americans annually lose their lives in US hospitals due
to avoidable medical errors.[10]

Smarter use of modern information technology (IT) is thought
to be the most effective way to reduce medical errors in medicine.
Perhaps surprisingly to many Americans, recent research shows
that American primary-care physicians now lag their colleagues in
many European countries considerably in their use of electronic
clinical information systems.[11] A serious underinvestment in IT
had been noted also in the Institute of Medicine's *Crossing the
Quality Chasm*, whose authors concluded that:

> The [US] health care system as currently structured
> does not, as a whole, make the best use of its resources
> ... A highly fragmented delivery system that largely
> lacks even rudimentary clinical information capabilities
> results in poorly designed care processes characterized

by unnecessary duplication of services and long waiting
lines and delays.

It is no small irony that one notable exception in the United
States to a lag in the application of IT is the US Veterans' Administration (VA) health system, the system Americans reserve for
their veterans and, ironically again, the only model of purely
socialized medicine left in the world outside of Cuba. The VA
health system is now widely acknowledged to be the national
leader in the smart use of IT and quality control.[12]

Finally, while Americans tend to look askance at nations that
are more conservative in their adoption and use of high-tech
devices and procedures, the Institute of Medicine notes in its
Crossing the Quality Chasm that "there is substantial evidence documenting overuse of many services — services for which the
potential risk of harm outweighs the potential benefits." A glaring example of this tendency has been the precipitous use of
autologous bone marrow transplantation, or HDC/ABMT,
which had blithely been applied as an acceptable procedure
against breast cancer, even before being subjected to clinical trials to demonstrate its effectiveness. More than 30,000 women
had been made to suffer through that highly risky and painful
procedure before careful studies showed it to be ineffective.[13]
Many American physicians are the first to admit that US health
care ought not to be viewed as the proper standard for the use of
high-tech procedures.

Looking Across the Border
Besieged by the cost squeeze in health care, the rising number of
Americans without health insurance or with shallow coverage,
and the growing evidence of highly varied quality and cost-effec-
tiveness of American health care, Americans have of recent begun
to look across their borders, perchance to draw lessons from how

other nations finance and manage their health systems. In this inquiry, neighbouring Canada is a particularly inviting target, for a number of reasons.

First, the training of physicians and nurses in Canada and the US follow similar professional standards, which greatly facilitates the movement of this type of human capital between the United States and Canada. Second, with the exception of Quebec, Canadians and Americans share many cultural traits that affect behaviour towards the health system. In particular, they share the same language and media. Third, as shown in table 1, in terms of purchasing-power-parity dollars, Canada has consistently spent only about half as much per capita on health care as has the United States, and yet it often ranks above the United States in terms of measurable health outcomes metrics. This is quite an astounding spending differential that invites comparisons of the United States with the Canadian health system.

Finally, opinion surveys over the past decades have suggested that Canadian citizens' certainly are not more dissatisfied with their much more constrained health system than are American citizens with their richly endowed system, as can be inferred from table 1. In those surveys, respondents who would like to see their health system "completely rebuilt" are thought to take the dimmest view of their health system.

A Snapshot of Canada's Health System

Canada's health system consists of thirteen distinct, provincial, tax-financed, single-payer health insurance systems that obey a unifying template laid down in the federal Canada Health Act. That federal Act encourages considerable national uniformity through the mechanism of federal cost sharing, just as does the medicaid system in the United States It is why so many outsiders speak of "Canada's national health system," as if it were one.

The tax-financed provincial insurance systems procure physician

Table 1: Health Systems Views Among Citizens, Canada
and the United States, 2004 and 2005

	System works well, only minor changes are needed	Fundamental changes are needed	System needs to be completely rebuilt
All Adults 2004			
Canada	21%	63%	14%
United States	16%	47%	33%
Patients with health problems, 2005			
Canada	21%	61%	17%
United States	23%	44%	30%

TABLE 1 Source: C. Schoen et al. "Taking the Pulse of Health Care Systems," *Health Affairs* web exclusive (2005), Exhibit 1.

services, hospital services, and sundry other health services from a mixed public–private (for-profit and not-for-profit) health care delivery system that is not drastically different from the American delivery system, although it is much more constrained by the market power and uniform prices characteristic of single-payer systems. For the comprehensive set of services covered under the Canada Health Act, patients typically enjoy first-dollar coverage.

The public insurance systems jointly pay for about 70 percent of total national Canadian health systems. The remainder is paid through private insurance or out of pocket for services not covered under the Canada Health Act. These services include dental and vision care, long-term care, and home care, and prescription drugs for the non-poor and non-elderly. They can be covered through private not-for-profit or commercial insurers, which, until 2005, were not permitted to cover services covered under the Canada Health Act. In June 2005 the Canadian Supreme Court ruled that the prohibition of private insurance for medically necessary services to which access is restricted through queues under the public system infringes on citizens' rights. That ruling has opened the door to the development of a two-tiered health insurance and health-care system in Canada, an issue of heated current debate in Canada at this time.

The Advantages of Single-payer Systems

Although much maligned by free-market devotees, single-payer health insurance systems do have a number of advantages relative to the more pluralistic, more market-oriented systems.

First, by virtue of their administrative simplicity, single-payer systems are the ideal platforms for a uniform information infrastructure, based on common nomenclature and technical processes. The single-payer system of Taiwan, for example, can track health spending by provider and patient on a virtual real-time basis. In the United States, the lag between delivery of service and recognizing its expense can easily exceed one year. Furthermore, Taiwan already employs a smart card for patients and is bound to leapfrog the United States in the use of IT, and Canada as well, for Canada so far does not appear to have exploited this potential nearly as much as it could have.

Second, because the administrative structure of single-payer health insurance tends to be simple, the administrative cost of operating such systems tends to be low. Taiwan's single-payer national health insurance system, for example, devotes less than 2 percent of total spending to administration as, incidentally, does the US single-payer medicare program. By contrast, the highly pluralistic and fragmented health insurance system in the United States carries with it extraordinarily high administrative costs, which constitute a significant part of higher US health spending. Private health insurance carriers in the United States, for example, have medical loss ratios between 75 and 85 percent, which means that they spend between 15 and 25 percent on administration, marketing, and profits.

In a careful, multi-million dollar comparative study of the US health system and several European systems, based on the actual, real-resource use for several tracer medical conditions, the McKinsey Global Institute[14] found that, in 1990, Americans on average used $390 fewer real medical resources per capita than did Germans, but spent $737 more per capita on higher prices, $360 per capita more on administration, and $256 more per capita on "other," some of which may have been administrative overhead as well. In their more recent study of administrative costs of the Canadian and US health system, Steffie Woolhandler et al estimate that in 1999 the US health system entailed $1,059 per capita in administrative costs (about 24 percent of total per-capita health spending, then at $4,335). The comparable administrative expense for Canada was only $307 in purchasing-power-parity dollars (12.7 percent of total per-capita health spending of $2,408). The authors estimated that between 1969 and 1999, the fraction of the total health labour force accounted for by administrative workers grew from 18.2 percent to 27.3 percent in the United States, but only from 16.0 percent to 19.1 percent in Canada.[15]

While one can always quibble at the margin over the estimated administrative costs of health systems, there is little doubt that, whatever the virtues of America's pluralistic and highly complex health insurance system may be, it comes at a very stiff price in terms of real-resource and financial costs. Brookings Institute economist Henry Aaron, for example, although questioning some of Woolhandler et al's numbers, stipulates at the outset of his commentary that the US health system is "an administrative monstrosity, a truly bizarre mélange of thousands of payers with payment systems that differ for no socially beneficial reasons, as well as staggeringly complex public systems with mind-boggling administered prices and other rules expressing distinctions that can only be regarded as weird."[16]

Third, and very importantly, a single-payer system is the ideal platform for the implementation of an egalitarian distributive ethic in health care, if that is what a nation wishes. Canadians seem sincerely to believe that the mantra "all men (and now women, too) are created equal" goes beyond the mere act of conception, to life thereafter. Although Americans mouth that mantra as well, they cannot possibly claim to carry it much beyond the stage of conception — surely not in education, nor in health care, nor even in the administration of justice. In the United States, socio-economic status plays a major role in access to each of these basic human services.

To illustrate, legislators in the State of New Jersey think nothing of paying a pediatrician $30 to see a poor child from the inner city covered by the state-run medicaid program, all the while paying that same pediatrician $100 or more for treating their own children. Similar price differentials exist also in other states of the union. Economists teach their students that relative prices signal relative social valuations to suppliers. In this case, state legislators signal that a pediatrician's professional activities have relatively little value when applied to a poor child covered by medicaid, but double or triple that value when it is applied to other children, including their own. Not surprisingly, large fractions of American physicians fully understand that signal and refuse to treat medicaid patients altogether. To most Canadians, these pricing practices probably would be deemed ethically unacceptable. Canadians express their egalitarian ethic for health care by paying the providers of health care the same fee for the same service, regardless of the socio-economic status of patients.

Similarly, the Canadian public and its legislative representatives would be unlikely to tolerate the common practice among American hospitals and pharmacies to charge uninsured Americans with little or no market power — in most instances members of low-income families — prices that can exceed by a factor of two the prices these same providers charge private health insurers for the same goods or services. Nor have American hospitals blanched at hounding uninsured Americans mercilessly for unpaid bills, often through bill collectors and even the courts, and sometimes to the point of seeing some of the debtors jailed, as was documented in a series of exposes published by the *Wall Street Journal*.[17]

The Disadvantages of Single-payer Systems

It was noted earlier that Canada spends only about half as much per capita on health care as does the United States, in spite of the fact that Canada is part of the high-cost North American market for health professionals and other health care inputs. The provincial plans achieve these low costs through three mechanisms.

First, by virtue of their monopolistic power as buyers they can procure health care at prices set just high enough not to lose out too much to the neighbouring US market. Here it must be recalled that US and Canadian health professionals are trained to similar standards, which means that the two health systems effectively buy health manpower in one North American market. It can also explain why Canada's health system will always be relatively more expensive than European systems with larger real-resource endowments in health care.

Second, the provincial health plans can and do use global budgets for hospitals and physicians to limit the bills these providers can submit for payment. Such budgets may be effective short-run remedies, but over the long run they can trigger undesired financial incentives. They can make it financially advantageous to prolong convalescent stays and force queuing on more acute, more expensive admissions.

Third, the provincial plans constrain the physical capacity of their health care delivery systems through direct, mandated limits on the number of high-tech, high-cost facilities or procedures allowed to bill the provincial plans.

Each of these cost-containment mechanisms carries with it the danger of being applied to excess. The restrictions on the physical capacity, for example, have begotten fairly long queues for elective surgery, for a variety of diagnostic procedures, and for cardiac-care and cancer-care procedures that Americans would consider urgent. If such queues become too long — as they appear to have become in Canada — they can become the Achilles heel of a single-payer system and destroy the egalitarian social contract underlying a single-payer system.

A number of Canadian commissions recently have examined the management of queues in Canada's health system and suggested remedial policies. In June 2006, for example, the Federal Wait Times Advisor proposed evidence-based, normative benchmarks for tolerable queues,[18] and so did the Health Council of Canada in its Annual Report of 2006.[19] Here it must be noted that Canadian health policy experts do not consider some queuing per se as a sign of a health system's shortcomings, if clinical evidence indicates that such queuing does not trigger untoward health effects, besides impatience. As C. David Naylor — noted Canadian health policy analyst and now President of the University of Toronto — lectured Americans on this point over a decade ago: "Queue-based allocation of health services, particularly if it is predicated on explicit and objective criteria with selective delay, is potentially superior to price-based rationing, because the latter will almost invariably lead to implicit and arbitrary denial ... No queues imply excess capacity ... Dismissing health services queues as some inevitable and evil by-product of 'socialized medicine' is fallacious."[20]

Be that as it may, Canadian and American critics of the Canadian health system have seized upon the queues as the platform on which to base their attacks upon the Canadian health system. An illustration of this line of attack is "Looking North for Inspiration," penned by Nadeem Esmail and Michael Walker of Canada's free-market oriented Fraser Institute.[21] Their central proposition is, in their words, that "rationing services by imposing longer waits is inherently inefficient. The very existence of chronic delays in delivering services implies that the system is failing to use prices to equate supply and demand." That proposition invites critical comment.

Styles of Rationing Health Care

The idea that a market approach to health care can avoid rationing is a time-hallowed but fallacious mantra in the American debate on health policy. First-year student of economics know that the price system is just one of many ways to ration scarce resources. To quote Harvard Professor Michael Katz and Princeton Professor Harvey Rosen (who until last year served on President Bush's Council of Economic Advisors) in their textbook *Microeconomics*:

> If bread were free, a huge quantity of it would be demanded. Because the resources used to produce bread are scarce, the actual amount of bread has to be rationed among its potential users. Not everyone can have all the bread that they could possibly want. The bread must be rationed somehow; and the price system accomplishes this in the following way: Everyone who is willing to pay the equilibrium price gets the good, and everyone who is not, does not.[22]

If readers substitute "health care" for "bread" in this passage, they will have an idea about how a price system works in health care.

The effects of price rationing at its extreme can be inferred from *Hidden Cost, Value Lost*, a report by a distinguished panel of health services researchers and other stakeholders convened by the Institute of Medicine. The panel estimated that some 18,000 Americans die each year prematurely for want of health insurance.[23] To be sure, most uninsured Americans eventually do receive needed tertiary health care from their neighbourhood hospitals when they are critically ill. But there is a large empirical literature indicating that the price system rations uninsured Americans out of the timely, early-stage primary and secondary care that might have avoided their serious or fatal illness. For example, far more uninsured children with asthma end up in the hospital in serious condition than do insured children. Yet at this time, some nine million American children remain without insurance coverage.[24]

It is not clear to this author on what ethical or scientific basis anyone could judge this approach to rationing health care more "efficient" than rationing by the queue. Indeed, the word "efficient" cannot ever be meaningfully defined in abstraction of the goal that is to be attained efficiently.[25] Why move efficiently toward a goal one does not wish to reach?

It appears that Canadians posit for their health system the goal of a strictly egalitarian distribution of health care. As already noted, few Canadians would consider it ethically acceptable to pay a pediatrician much less for treating a poor child than for treating a rich child, an idea with which Americans have long been comfortable. Similarly, given their ethical goals, one can understand why so many Canadians look askance at the establishment of an upper-tier, private health care system that can draw professionals and other resources away from the general health systems merely to allow Canadians with superior ability to pay to jump the queue in health care. By contrast, so-called boutique medicine offering a more luxurious, time-intensive health care experience to those willing and able to pay for it is quite acceptable and increasingly common in the United States.

Given the egalitarian ethic Canadians wish their health system to obey, they probably would be aghast also at the latest turn of American health policy, as it was recently promoted by President Bush in his State of the Union Address. The thrust of that policy is to goad Americans into health insurance policies with very high deductibles and coinsurance. To that end, the President would allow Americans to make tax deductible deposits into a personally owned Health Savings Account (HSA) to cover out-of-pocket costs and health insurance premiums, but only if they purchase the high-deductible insurance policy the President favours. With a progressive income-tax structure, however, this tax preference automatically makes health care cheaper for high-income people than for low-income people. At the same time, it is elementary logic that an annual deductible of, say, $5,000 per family is likely to induce a lower income family to self-ration the health care it uses much more drastically than it would a high income family. In effect, then, the President and those who cheer on his proposal would look to the lower income groups to bear the bulk of the brunt of price rationing in health care and shift more of the financial burden of ill health from chronically healthy to chronically sick Americans. Although this approach appears to be acceptable to many Americans, Canadians would probably reject it.

The US website www.eHealthInsurance.com is an electronic market for individually purchased health insurance policies. One enters one's family's demographic composition, the zip code of one's location, and the type of policy (HSA qualified or not), and there appears a menu of customized offerings, four of which can be arrayed in convenient side-by-side comparisons. Most of the policies listed there are medically underwritten, that is, make the premiums vary with the insured's health status. Many of them have deductibles up to $10,000 per year for a family, and most of them have in their fine print sundry limitations and exclusions, the most common of which is maternity care.

To exclude maternity care from health insurance coverage, once again, probably would not occur to Canadians, nor to citizens in any other OECD country. Perhaps it can partially explain statistics such as those in figure 1 below, which illustrates how many more babies and mothers die in the United States than do

Figure 1: Infant and Maternal Death Rates, 2002

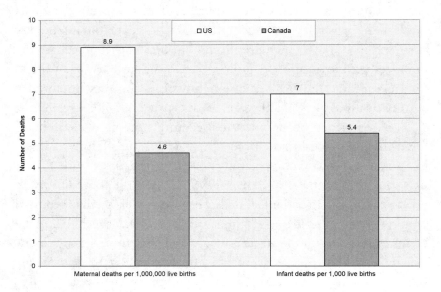

Source: OECD, *OECD Health 2006*. Paris: OECD (2006).

in Canada. That members of the US Congress, who not long ago felt ethically compelled to rush back to Washington, DC to assure the life-support of a brain-dead patient, would passively accept, year after year, troublesome data such as that in figure 1, all the while leaving millions of mothers and children without health insurance, must astound Canadians.

Concluding Remarks

The objective of this paper has not been to advocate the Canadian single-payer health system for the United States, for at least two reasons. First, the highly egalitarian precepts inherent in such systems do not seem compatible with the American social ethic under which it as a violation of individual rights to prohibit the well-to-do from using their own wealth to purchase for themselves a superior experience in education, in health care, and in the administration of justice. Second, single-payer, government-run health systems are not easily administered in clinically and economically sound ways in a nation whose legislative chambers function more and more as bazaars in which the legislators' favours can be as openly purchased by the supply side of the health care system, as they can be in the United States.

At the same time, however, this paper has taken issue with the widely popular but fallacious proposition that government-run, single-payer health systems are inherently less efficient than are more market-oriented health systems. In a previous article, I have argued that such an argument cannot be made at a theoretical level.[26] Furthermore, there is no empirical evidence to support this proposition, as the American health system vividly demonstrates.

In the end, each nation must debate and search its soul which style of rationing — by queue or by price and ability to pay — is most conformable to its dominant social ethic. Simple mantras will not solve that conundrum.

CHAPTER 9

How to Protect a Public
Health Care System

Alan Maynard

Throughout the world there is a continuing debate about the roles of government and the private sector in the financing and delivery of health care. This is unsurprising and is the product of adherents of competing ideologies competing for power, income, and wealth.

The two competing ideologies are the collectivist and the libertarian. The latter puts freedom of the individual from the restraints of government intervention as the primary goal of society. Adherents of this worldview see markets and competition as means of limiting the power of the state and ensuring the freedom of the individual. They hold that goods and services, such as health care, should be funded and provided by private institutions motivated by profit.

The competing collectivist ideology puts equality as the primary goal of social institutions and behaviour. They regard need as the primary determinant of access to health care, where need is defined as a person's capacity to benefit per unit of cost. The collectivists accept that resources are scarce and that health care rationing is unavoidable. They seek to create regulatory institutions that ration resources on the basis of relative cost effectiveness, with care targeted at those who can gain most from selective treatment. Collectivists do not dismiss the importance of freedom, but regard increased equality as the primary goal and the means by which citizens can exercise choice and achieve greater freedom.

Ideologies Competing for Market Share

Health care markets internationally are resource-intensive, inefficient, and inequitable. For instance, the United States has the most expensive health care system in the world, consuming over 16 percent of its GDP. Over forty cents in the US health care dollar are funded by government (for example, medicare for the elderly, medicaid for some of the poor, and the Veterans' Administration for past and present members of the armed forces). The most expensive part of the US health care systems is the private insurance sector. Like counterparts elsewhere (for example, Australia[27]) private insurers fail to contain premium cost inflation and are inefficient in their use of the resources of the insured.[28] Furthermore, as the poor and old are poor risks, over 45 million Americans have no federal or insurance coverage, and consequently face bankruptcy if ill health strikes.

While it is easy to dismiss the United States as a sad case of cost inflation, inefficiency, and inequity, it is essential to recognize that many of the failings of such "private" systems can also be seen in public health care systems. This is particularly true with regard to efficiency. Public health care systems tolerate — just like private insurers — large variations in clinical practice, the failure to deliver proven cost-effective and cheap interventions in areas such as chronic care, and poor measurement of success.

Public and private health care systems fail to encourage and police the translation of evidence into practice internationally. A nice example of this is the poor measurement of success in health care delivery. Some health care systems now publish the relative mortality rates of surgeons in areas such as cardiac surgery. Public access to such data leads practitioners to improve their practices so that the average mortality rates fall and the dispersion of mortality rates around the average falls.

This is welcome and sensible. However, most patients do not die in hospital and hence mortality rates are a very incomplete measure of success. The English nurse Florence Nightingale argued in 1863 that the success of hospitals should be measured in terms of whether patients were dead, relieved, or unrelieved. Nearly 150 years later, we have the means to acquire patient-reported measures of mental and physical functioning, both pre- and post-health care, but we do not use them in either public or private health care systems.[29]

Not only are public systems inefficient, like their private counterparts, but they are also tardy in addressing the issue of health inequalities. In some cases, improving access to care may improve the utilization of the disadvantaged and improve their health. However, access and utilization in "free" public systems may not be equal, and even where it is, may not improve health more cost-effectively than income redistribution, improved education of the poor, and health promotion. Such questions are often asked, but rarely debated with evidence. Furthermore, some health related policies such as health promotion may change the behaviour of the middle classes more than the disadvantaged, and in so doing *increase* inequality.

The ideological debate about health care policy and practice is characterized by the competing parties selecting and criticizing the actual failures of the systems they oppose and comparing them with the theoretical successes of their preferred systems.

Both parties need to accept the similar failures of their preferred systems, particularly in relation to efficiency. Blind advocacy of a particular ideology, which ignores its practical and evidenced problems, undermines the credibility of the advocate and endangers the effectiveness of their preferred system.

It's about Distribution, Stupid!

While collectivists who favour public finance and provision must look to improve the usually poor performance of their preferred system, they must also recognize that their opponents' pursuit of freedom also has significant deleterious distributional consequences. "Marketization" may or may not improve the performance of public health care systems. Any such proposals have to be picked apart carefully.

For instance, libertarians like to chip away at public systems by suggesting — for instance, when the collectivist system is in turmoil due to real and polemically induced problems — the extended use of co-payments and private insurance. This is often advocated by libertarians as a means of "helping" the public system when it is in fact undermining its principles and redistributing income.

Thus the increased use of private insurance is often accompanied by tax subsidies. Since only the more affluent pay taxes, such subsidies benefit the more affluent, diluting the redistributive effects of public health care systems from the affluent to the disadvantaged. Thus, advocacy of private health insurance fails to address efficiency deficiencies in health care delivery, introduces a mechanism that creates expenditure inflation due to the poor cost control of insurers, and is inequitable. The success of ideologues in developing such policies is epitomized by the successes of the Howard government in Australia.[30]

Another favoured policy of libertarians is the use of co-payments. This is advocated as a means of complementing funding and reducing waste. However, user charges are taxes on the user, and the primary users of health care systems are the elderly and the poor. Thus, user charges reduce the redistributive impact of tax-financed health care systems by reducing the tax burdens of the rich and transferring them to poorer, regular users of care.

The efficiency arguments used by advocates of user charges are similarly weak. While the patient is the person who makes the initial decision to use health care, once in the system the principal person who determines demand is the practitioner. Thus, if there is waste, it is not the fault of the patient, but of poor decision making by doctors and nurses. Taxing the patient with user charges is unlikely to reduce the waste produced by such providers.

When libertarians propose changes such as private insurance and user charges, their purpose, conscious and unconscious, is to advantage the more affluent and inflict increased burdens on the disadvantaged who are in need of care. Their advocacy of change may be disguised in the rhetoric of efficiency, but it is essential to beware of lambs in wolves' clothing.

Conclusion
Libertarians also regard collectivists seeking to enhance the public health care sector as wolves disguised as lambs. Collectivists are seeking to redistribute funding and access to care on the basis of need, and this typically benefits the poor, the old, and the chronically ill, who are relatively poor. This is an endless "game" in the political process. Neither side is "right." Choice of the competing perspectives depends on values about what you as a citizen want your health care system to achieve. Defence of what you deem is right requires both modesty about the achievements of your system and clarity about the motives and methods of the wolves seeking to take your lambs to slaughter. Protection of public health care systems requires eternal vigilance.

CHAPTER 10

The Truth about the Drug Companies

Marcia Angell

The pharmaceutical industry is dominated by just ten to twenty giant companies — roughly half European and half American — although they are really global in their reach. They all do business in much the same way, and often act more like an oligopoly than as competitors. And make no mistake: their primary goal is to maximize profits. To keep investors happy, they need to top their performance every quarter, no matter how good it was last quarter. In health care, this imperative has perverse consequences.

As with most investor-owned health businesses, the pharmaceutical industry has a much freer rein in the United States than in other, more regulated economies. In particular, despite the fact that the government pays for many prescription drugs in the United States, there is no public system of price regulation. Drug companies are free to charge whatever they like. The result is that prices in the United States for brand name drugs are roughly twice as high as for the same drugs in Canada and Europe. The United States is thus the major profit centre for virtually all of the big drug companies.

The enormous price disparity between the United States and other countries has proved extremely embarrassing for the industry and for its many friends in Washington, DC. In 1987, Congress, under industry prodding, passed a law forbidding Americans from buying prescription drugs from Canada or any other country. But, by the beginning of this decade, a million or so Americans had essentially decided to become outlaws, purchasing their drugs from Canadian pharmacies. As a result, the price disparity became widely known.

The industry was forced to admit that it was indeed charging Americans much more for their drugs than Canadians, but it had an excuse. It said that the high prices charged in the United States were necessary to cover their high research and development (R&D) costs. Canada and Europe, by regulating prices in various ways, were not doing their fair share of R&D, according to this argument. They were free riders. By default, then, the United States must shoulder the burden. By this line of reasoning, any attempt to moderate US prices would cut into R&D and stifle innovation.

Is any of that true? Are the drug companies *really* strapped to cover their R&D costs? You could make that case only if they spent most of their revenues on R&D, and had enough left over for only modest profits. But, as I show in my book, *The Truth About the Drug Companies*, that's far from the situation. In fact, the major drug companies spend only about half as much on R&D as they do on marketing, and less even than they have left over in profits.

To illustrate, let's look at the top American drug companies — those listed in Fortune's rankings of the 500 biggest companies in the United States. In 2005, these nine companies had sales of $222 billion. According to their annual reports, they spent $32 billion of that on R&D, $71 billion on marketing and administration, and kept $39 billion in profits at the end of the year. So R&D was by far the smallest of the three figures. The profits were huge, as they are every year. That year, they amounted to 16 percent of sales, compared with just 6 percent for all the *Fortune 500* companies. It's hard to make the case, then, that the pharmaceutical industry is straining to cover R&D when they are so profitable and spend so much more on marketing.

It's also hard to make the case that price regulation would stifle innovation when you look closely at the output of the big drug companies. Their major product now consists of trivial variations of top-selling drugs already on the market, like the six statin drugs to lower cholesterol. The fourth of these, Lipitor, is the top selling drug in the world. These are called "me-too" drugs. They're easy to make and very lucrative, because they usually target vague, chronic conditions in essentially healthy people — conditions like social anxiety disorder, the industry term for shyness. Often they target precursors to disease, like high cholesterol, whose definition can be broadened. The market for these conditions is large and easily expanded. After all, there are more healthy people than sick ones. And if a condition is not sharply defined, then it's easy to convince more people (and their doctors) that they have it. Who hasn't been shy at some time? In fact, it's been shown that ads for one "me-too" drug increase the sales of the others in the class. According to the FDA, fully 80 percent of new drugs that entered the market over the past seven years were unlikely to be improvements over existing drugs.

The few innovative drugs that do enter the market are usually based on publicly funded research done in university or government labs all over the world. Sometimes the work is in the public domain, but often it is patented by universities or start-up biotech companies, then licensed to drug companies. Even the first drug in a "me-too" family was usually based on publicly funded research, often dating back to the 1970s and 1980s. The progenitor of Lipitor, for example, came on the market in 1987, the result mainly of publicly funded work in the United States and Japan.

The paradox here is that, while drug companies talk the rhetoric of the free market and innovation, they are not too proud to take government handouts of all sorts, starting with the research on which their drugs are based and government-granted monopoly rights. And they are quite happy to demand protectionist legislation, like the ban on buying drugs from Canada.

This industry has the largest lobby in Washington, and Congress almost always gives it what it wants. One thing it wants now is to lessen the price disparity between the United States and other countries — not by lowering prices in the United States, but by having them rise everywhere else. And it also wants to stop the embarrassing cross-border purchases of cheaper drugs. Washington is now using bilateral trade negotiations to try to achieve those ends. For example, it has induced Canada to crack down on drug sales to Americans, reportedly in exchange for the United States relaxing its barriers on beef and lumber.

Canadians should not be influenced by drug company arguments that price regulation in Canada should be relaxed in order to cover R&D costs and foster innovation. You need not worry about stifling innovative R&D. Drug companies do much less of it than they claim, and what they do they can easily afford. What this industry needs is more, not less, regulation, and I would strongly support national pharmacare in Canada.

CHAPTER 11

Market-based Health Care in the United States and its Lessons for Canada

Arnold S. Relman

Canadians are now debating whether, and to what extent, they should allow their publicly funded provincial insurance systems to pay private for-profit facilities for the delivery of medical services that are covered under the terms of their medicare laws. Those who favour public payment for investor-owned facilities argue that these facilities provide services of equal or better quality, are more efficient, and are more responsive to the needs of consumers than private not-for-profit facilities. Advocates also believe that the private capital invested in the for-profit facilities would relieve the financial burden on the public treasury and would reduce the waiting times for certain elective high-technology services.

In discussing this issue, reference is often made to the United States, which has by far the largest investor-owned health care sector of any country in the world. If Canadians want to see how investor ownership affects a health care system, they should look carefully at what has happened to their southern neighbour.

I have written a book, just published (2007), that deals with this question. It is entitled *A Second Opinion: Rescuing America's Health Care*. It describes how investor-owned businesses became a major influence in the US health care system and with what results. It compares the health care systems of the United States and Canada, and suggests that both countries have a lot to learn from each other. But the most important lesson Canadians should draw from the US experience is that investor ownership of medical facilities has been a resounding failure, and that the attempt to turn our system into a private commercial market is responsible for many of our current problems. The United States has the most expensive health care system in the world, by far, and there is abundant evidence that the public does not get its money's worth.

The superiority of for-profit services is a myth, propagated by those with unquestioning faith in the social value of a health care market and by those who are profiting by investment in that market. But it is a myth, nonetheless, because it is contradicted by the performance of investor-owned facilities and services and by the disastrous history of the investor-dominated US system.

Uwe Reinhardt, one of the most respected and well-known health care economists in the United States, has argued that, in his judgment, the ownership of the delivery of health care is a relatively unimportant issue, and that it is far less important than the question of who controls the insurance side of a health care system. He strongly endorses the egalitarian principles that underlie your medicare insurance plan in Canada, but he apparently doesn't think you need to worry about the public support of private for-profit medical care delivery in Canada.

I strongly disagree with his views about the supply side of health care. I am convinced that investor-owned for-profit medical care and investor-owned medical care facilities are a major cause of the current problems of the US health care system, and that, if permitted to expand in Canada, they would cause similar problems here. They would increase your health expenditures without adding anything of value that could not be provided at less expense by a strengthened and reorganized not-for-profit delivery system under medicare.

The US experience has shown that it is simply not true, as market advocates insist, that for-profit ownership can deliver comparable medical services to comparable patients more efficiently than not-for-profit ownership. In fact, the best and most carefully controlled comparisons in the United States have shown just the opposite: not-for-profit service is usually less expensive for the payers, and any differences in quality that can be demonstrated usually favour the non-profits. Remember, these are comparisons involving similar patients, similar communities, and institutions of similar size that provide similar services. These are the only kinds of comparisons that are reliable.

Let me now consider in a little more detail what we have learned in the United States from a study of investor-owned health care facilities and services as compared with those that are non-profit. The citations can be found in my book.

1. Investor-owned chain hospitals first appeared on the US scene in the middle 1960s, after the enactment of medicare, which is the US public insurance program for the elderly. At first, medicare's "cost-plus" method of payment ensured the net income of any hospital that could fill its beds with insured patients and encourage its physicians to use profitable services. The chains rapidly gained about 20 percent of the non-public hospital market, but then stopped growing two decades later when medicare payment methods changed and became less vulnerable to this kind of exploitation. Investors now turned to out-patient facilities, which were not as strictly regulated, and could still be highly profitable. Not surprisingly, expenditures on ambulatory services increased rapidly. More recently, investors have become interested

in specialty hospitals, which limit themselves to a particular type of service such as cardiologic, orthopedic, or gynecologic elective surgery. Physicians have been important investors in all of these newer kinds of for-profit medical enterprises and have helped to promote their use.

2. Careful comparisons of the performance of the first wave of investor-owned hospitals with their not-for-profit private counterparts revealed higher charges by the for-profits and less charity care. Data on relative quality of service were inadequate for comparison. In the past two decades, since payment methods have changed and much hospital care has shifted to ambulatory and specialized services, there have been relatively few direct controlled comparisons of this kind. However, there are some good data from a statistical study of medicare expenditures to indicate that investor-owned hospitals are still more expensive than not-for-profit private hospitals providing similar services. The new specialty hospitals, which are all investor-owned, "cherry-pick" their patients and are thereby creating problems for the general-service hospitals in their community. A few publicized incidents in specialty hospitals have raised questions about their ability to deal with unexpected complications and emergencies.

3. Some economists, including those at your Fraser Institute, claim that investor-owned hospitals are at least as "efficient" as their not-for-profit counterparts, and that there is consequently no reason to oppose for-profit hospitals on economic grounds. But economists measure "efficiency" by cost *to the hospital* for the production of given services, not costs (or charges) *to the payers*. It seems obvious to me — and I suspect to most of you — that the important question is not the economic efficiency of production, but what society has to pay for its medical services. We already know investor-owned services aren't cheaper, so unless they provide more or better service, they are no bargain for society. There are no credible data to support the claims of market enthusiasts

that for-profit hospitals provide better services than comparable not-for-profit hospitals.

4. Inasmuch as the measurement of the quality of the diverse medical services in hospital or ambulatory facilities is still at an early and unreliable stage, we need to look at comparisons of other kinds of health care services to know what effect for-profit ownership might have on quality of care. In the United States, we have the answer from two kinds of facilities that have a more focused and measurable health care outcome. First, there are the nursing homes, two-thirds of which are investor-owned. Most nursing homes are paid on a per diem basis, so profits depend on keeping production costs down and not on prices or volume of service. Comparative study has shown that serious deficiencies in care were found to be 40 percent more common in investor-owned facilities than in those owned by not-for-profit private organizations. This difference is probably explained by poorer staffing in the for-profits; economists would call this a reduction in production costs.

5. Another informative comparison of quality has been made between the outcomes of treatment in US kidney dialysis units, the majority of which are investor-owned. Like nursing homes, dialysis units are paid a fixed amount, regardless of their expenses, and they have a relatively narrowly defined medical care output. Careful, controlled study has shown a 20 percent higher mortality in investor-owned clinics — a shocking statistic that is probably explained by the provision of less dialysis time by the investor-owned clinics and by their excessive use of a drug that raises the red blood cell count and generates a profit for the dialysis clinic. Evidently, in both examples, there is some trade-off of quality for profits.

6. What are the lessons of the US experience with investor-owned facilities?

First, investor-ownership does *not* save money for the payers of health care. What about saving public money through the capital added to the system by investors? I suppose the answer to this question depends on whether you think this additional private capital exceeds the public costs of the cherry-picking, and the promotion of excessive medical expenditures on high technology by the investor-owned facilities. It seems to me that the bottom-line answer has to be the fact that the rise of investor-ownership in the United States has been associated with rapidly rising health expenditures. This is exactly what one would expect when health care businesses are trying to maximize their income. After all, it is hardly credible that private investors would put their money into the health care system simply to assist communities with their public responsibilities. They obviously want to profit from their investment, and they do this by extracting more payment from the community than they add through their investment.

Second, there is certainly no evidence that for-profit services are usually better than services in not-for-profit facilities — indeed, at least in some cases, they seem to be worse. Overall, the highly commercialized US system produces only mediocre results when compared with other OECD countries or judged by quality guidelines. So investor-ownership by no means guarantees good quality, despite greater expenditures.

Third, what about waiting times? Does Canada need investor-owned facilities to eliminate waiting for certain elective high-technology services? The United States has no waiting times for those who are insured or can pay out of pocket, but that is not primarily because so many of our facilities are for-profit. It is because we spend so much public and private money on technology. In the United States, if you have no insurance or not enough to cover the costs of the expensive high-technology elective treatment you need, you may have to wait a very long time. I believe that, with a modest increase in public funding and appropriate focused expansions of certain facilities, your system could easily eliminate waiting without depending on private investors. I understand that you have already done this in some places, and there is no reason why you could not do more. Waiting times are *not* a necessary accompaniment of a public universal insurance system; it all depends on organization and the appropriate use of resources.

A single-payer universal insurance system, like your medicare, is infinitely better than multiple, competing for-profit plans of the kind that cover some 150 million US citizens, mainly through their employment. I will not repeat the many reasons for this conclusion here. I simply want to say that in the United States we are now witnessing a very worrisome phenomenon: a conservative national administration, stubbornly insistent that private markets can do a better job and should replace publicly administered health insurance, is pursuing policies that are encouraging investor-owned insurance companies to take over coverage of services previously insured by public programs.

Under pressure from the White House, US medicare, the program that covers more than 40 million citizens over the age of sixty-five, is encouraging a growing fraction of its beneficiaries to switch over to a variety of private plans that are paid from the medicare fund, but administered by for-profit investor-owned companies. So far, about 20 percent of US senior citizens have been persuaded to make this switch, but the current administration hopes for more. The private plans are more expensive than the public system and are demanding — and getting — 12 to 19 percent more in premiums from the public purse than the amount medicare spends for coverage in its own program. The private firms claim they provide some extra benefits (which have not been well documented), but in any case they usually charge higher co-payments to beneficiaries. The private insurance lobby is very powerful in the United States and uses its financial clout to persuade Congress and the administration not to ask too many questions about the comparative public benefits of for-profit and government insurance.

I mention this as a warning to Canadians. The for-profit insurance industry is no less hungry for profits and expanding income than the for-profit medical care delivery industry. Once allowed to take public money, both industries will press inexorably for a larger and larger share of tax-supported programs, and your health expenses will soon get out of control, just as they have in the United States.

In conclusion, I remind you that health care is not like other services in the economy. It is not like ordinary commodities traded in a market. The US experience has shown the world that, when you allow investor-owned for-profit businesses to become an important part of your health care system, you end up with the disaster we are now struggling to control. In deciding on *your* future direction in Canada, I hope you will not make the mistakes we did. Do not allow private investors to use your public health care system as a vehicle for generating profits. They will add to your expenses and will take public resources and professional personnel that could better be devoted to improving the services provided through medicare.

CHAPTER 12

Protecting Medicare from Foreign Commercial Interests

Scott Sinclair

A s we reflect on the future of Canada's health care system, we should remember our history lessons. It was only through the determined and tireless efforts of Tommy Douglas and thousands of other dedicated women and men that medicare took root and our health care system flourished. The creation of medicare was not inevitable, and Canadians should not take its continued existence for granted.

Underlining this concern, Jon Johnson, one of Canada's leading trade lawyers, bluntly informed the Romanow Commission that, if the NAFTA expropriation provisions "and the accompanying investor-state dispute settlement mechanism procedures had existed in the 1960s, the pubic health system in its present form would never have come into existence."[31] This sobering reflection stands as a warning that the power of modern trade treaties — whose scope has expanded well beyond traditional trade matters to interfere with the ability of governments to limit and regulate commercial interests — must be contained in order to safeguard the future of Canadian medicare.

As in Tommy Douglas's day, medicare has formidable foes that would profit from its demise and thus seek to undermine it. Our US neighbour has the most highly commercialized health care system in the developed world, with industry lobbies that are among the most powerful in Washington. Current initiatives to deepen continental integration and create a single North American economic space pose obvious risks for medicare in Canada, which differs so markedly from the US system. These are not new threats, but we must guard against our familiarity with them breeding indifference. While foreign commercial interests have to date made only limited inroads in Canada's health care system, if care is not taken this could change quickly.

The principles that underlie Canada's medicare system are at odds with the thrust of modern trade treaties. By establishing a public-sector health insurance monopoly, and by regulating who can provide health care services and on what terms, the Canada Health Act and the medicare system cut against the grain of trade and investment liberalization treaties.[32]

While Canadians have repeatedly been assured that their health care system is beyond the reach of trade treaties, it is, in fact, only partially shielded. Important aspects of health care services are clearly under the domain of the trade treaties.

Under the North American Free Trade Agreement (NAFTA), Canada negotiated two important "reservations," or country-specific exceptions, that shield government measures in the health sector from certain, but not all, of NAFTA's investment and services obligations. The first of these, Annex I, is a general reservation against certain NAFTA provisions that permits the three NAFTA parties to maintain all non-conforming provincial and state government measures that existed when NAFTA came into force on January 1, 1994.[33] The Annex I reservation is "bound."[34] This

means that the "existing, non-conforming measures" are subject
to a legal ratchet; they can only be amended to make them more
NAFTA-consistent. If a measure is eliminated or amended, it cannot later be restored. As health systems change, and especially if
private sector involvement in the health system increases, the protection afforded by Annex I erodes over time.

Canada also negotiated a second reservation that excludes the
Canadian health care sector from certain, but not all, provisions of
NAFTA's investment and services chapters.[35] The Annex II reservation is "unbound." This means that it protects not only existing
non-conforming measures, but allows Canadian governments to
take new measures that would otherwise be NAFTA-inconsistent.
The reservation, however, stipulates that any such measures must
be related to health to the extent that it is "a social service established or maintained for a public purpose." These terms are
undefined and have been subject to sharply differing interpreta-
tions by the US and Canadian governments.[36] While the precise
scope of the protections afforded by Annex II is therefore uncertain, it is again clear that, as private sector involvement in Canada's
health care system increases, the threat of NAFTA challenges
grows.

The General Agreement on Trade in Services (GATS) excludes
services provided in the "exercise of governmental authority." But
these are defined as services provided neither on a commercial nor
a competitive basis (GATS Article 1:3.c). Because the Canadian
health care system is mixed, with significant private financing and
delivery of services, the governmental authority exclusion cannot
be relied upon to protect it fully from GATS rules. Canada's decision not to list direct health services under the GATS provides
more substantial protection. Canada has, however, covered certain
health-related services under the GATS, most notably health
insurance.

Upon scrutiny, the purported safeguards do not fully exclude the Canadian health care system. NAFTA's provisions against "expropriation" without compensation, for example, apply with full force to the health sector. Government measures affecting private health insurance also fall under the financial services rules of the GATS. Where safeguards apply to existing health services, increasing the commercial or competitive element in the financing or delivery of that service narrows the scope of the safeguards and, consequently, increases the exposure of the health service to trade law restrictions.

As trade experts advising the Romanow Commission agreed, the NAFTA investment provisions pose the most significant threat to health policy flexibility.[37] These rules could interfere with the expansion of public health insurance into areas currently insured by private providers. Furthermore, if private insurers or for-profit providers become active in areas now insured or delivered exclusively though the public system, NAFTA compensation claims would make it costly to reverse course and return these services to the public system.

Trade treaty investment challenges are not merely a hypothetical concern. There have already been fifteen NAFTA investment claims against Canada.[38] Just last year, a US investor challenged Canada as a result of the decision of the newly elected Ontario provincial government to block a controversial project to dispose of municipal waste from Toronto in a man-made lake on a former open-pit mine site in northern Ontario. The investor is seeking $100 million in compensation, claiming that this action was "tantamount to expropriation" and deprived the company of the minimum standard of treatment under international law. It is not difficult to imagine parallel scenarios in the health care field where governments, under public pressure, act to halt or reverse experiments in private, for-profit delivery of health care.

Despite such concerns, the message of the trade policy analyses done for the Romanow Commission was generally optimistic and forward-looking. They stressed that the commercializing threats posed by trade treaties, while real, could be navigated around. The report sensibly argued that: "Rather than conclude ... that Canada is hemmed in to the current system and cannot change, the more reasonable conclusion is that, if we want to expand the range of services in the public system, it is better to do it now while there still is very little foreign presence in health care in Canada and the potential costs of [trade] compensation are low."[39] At the same time, however, trade and health experts underlined the need for a precautionary approach to health care reform. Provincial reforms that increase the role of the private sector, particularly foreign commercial interests, in the financing and delivery of health services clearly heighten the risk of trade treaty challenge and of trade treaty obligations limiting future policy flexibility.

These warnings have not been universally heeded. In British Columbia and Quebec, in particular, private, for-profit surgical clinics are proliferating, leading towards the development of parallel private systems. Canada's NAFTA safeguards for health care probably do not apply in such a situation. If a US private clinic wanted to open up on the same terms as the BC private clinics, the NAFTA investment rules protect them. The door is open.

NAFTA arguments could then be employed to expand the private care beachhead. If private clinics are allowed to deliver emergency services, for example, then why should they be barred from providing other medically necessary services? If a US private hospital attempted to set up an intake clinic in BC, it could challenge provincial laws requiring hospitals to operate on a not-for-profit basis as trade barriers. In the event of such challenges, sensitive decisions about our health care system would be made by NAFTA tribunals, not by elected governments. The mere threat of litigation strengthens the leverage and bargaining power of foreign commercial interests.

Once entrenched, foreign investors would enjoy the full protection of NAFTA's expropriation provisions, making it costly for
future governments to dislodge them.[40] The development of a
parallel private system is, in some provinces, approaching the critical mass that could attract significant foreign involvement and
risk locking in the commercialization trend.

On a more positive note, Canada's NAFTA obligations do not
compel governments to provide financial support to foreign, for-
profit providers.[41] Furthermore, medicare's embattled — but
still–intact — ban on private insurance for medically necessary
services significantly curtails the potential growth of the parallel,
private system. The wealthy may pay for faster access to health
services, but, so long as the public system works reasonably well,
most patients will be reluctant to pay out of pocket for health
services that they can get through the tax-funded public system.

The 2005 *Chaoulli* case (in which the BC private clinics intervened) is disquieting. Just as Canada's public health care system has
been built around the public monopoly over health insurance, the
limited protections that Canada negotiated in NAFTA and the
GATS are based on the existing separation between private and
public health insurance "markets." The Supreme Court ruling
could undermine this basic separation by enabling private insurers, including foreign companies, to cover a broader range of
health services. This threatens to neuter Canada's protective trade
treaty exemptions and greatly increase the commercial viability of
two–tier medicine.

These trade treaty risks are not the only, or the most serious,
challenges facing the Canadian health care system. But neither can
they be ignored. Health care systems are dynamic, while the trade
treaty exceptions for health are static. No one should be under any
illusion that, because there have been no health service–related
trade treaty challenges to date, the safeguards are fully effective.

It is the public, not–for–profit character of Canada's health care system that insulates it from trade treaty challenge. If that character is eroded or substantially altered, then trade treaty rules will kick in, tipping the balance further in favour of the forces of commercialization, in general, and foreign commercial interests, in particular. Once foreign investors become established and a process of commercialization is set in motion, it will be difficult to reverse. It is our task, as heirs to the legacy of Tommy Douglas, to ensure that this tipping point is never reached.

CHAPTER 13

Canada's Single-payer Medicare: Role Model for Taiwan

May Tsung-Mei Cheng

In the late 1980s, the government of Taiwan decided to establish full-fledged universal health insurance for the island's 23 million inhabitants. At that time, only 57 percent of Taiwan's population had health insurance through one of over ten insurance schemes. On 1 March, 1995, Taiwan established the universal National Health Insurance, folding in the hitherto uninsured 41 percent of the population. Administered by the central government's Bureau of National Health Insurance (BNHI), Taiwan's NHI covers, since its inception, the entire population for in-patient, out-patient, dental care, drugs, and traditional Chinese medicine.

Taiwan's decision to adopt the single-payer approach — dubbed the "one-pipe model" — began with an international conference held in Taipei in 1989 at which experts from a number of countries described the strengths and shortcomings of their countries' health insurance systems. In the end, the American, market-oriented approach was rejected in favour of Canada's single-payer medicare system and Germany's social insurance system. After further study, including a number of visits abroad by Taiwan policy analysts, a single-payer system modelled closely on Canada's provincial, single-payer health plans carried the day. Several major advantages were seen in that approach.

First, such a system is the ideal platform for implementing the egalitarian ethic Taiwan's leaders sought for Taiwan's health system. Unlike the market-oriented American approach, which segments the population into a myriad of small risk pools with varying degrees of actuarial risk and premiums, a single-payer system forms a single risk pool for the entire population. Citizens contribute to that pool largely on the basis of ability to pay. Providers of health care are paid the same fees for identical services, regardless of the socio-economic status of their patients. By contrast, the state-run medicaid programs in the United States pay providers fees that are only a fraction of those paid by commercial insurance, an economic signaling that is not lost on the many physicians who refuse to treat medicaid patients.

A second major advantage attracting Taiwan's policy makers to the single-payer model is the relatively strong market power it bestows on the demand side of the market. Establishing the NHI did not bankrupt Taiwan's treasury. The average rate of growth of total national health spending in the three years before the NHI was 13.8 percent. Extending coverage to Taiwan's then uninsured population of 41 percent in 1995 led to a one-year surge in growth of 18.1 percent, whereafter the rate of growth continued to decline to the rate of only 3.5 percent in 2005.

Third, a single-payer system is administratively simple and inexpensive. There is one uniform nomenclature for the entire system, which in turn makes it an ideal platform for an electronic information infrastructure. Within the constraints of its administrative budgets (Taiwan's BHNI is allowed to spend only 1.5 percent of its budget on administration), the BNHI has taken full advantage of information technology. All claims processing is electronic, allowing the BNHI to monitor utilization of services and expenditures virtually in real time, by sector, by providers within a sector, and by patient. An integral part of this information system has been, since January 2004, the electronic Smart Card. Issued to every individual in Taiwan, the Smart Card records data on premium payments, co-payments, total spending, diagnosis, prescriptions, major examinations, childhood vaccinations, organ donation, for example. It provides information on where and when the patient was seen, and has the potential for public health applications such as fast tracing of exposure to infectious diseases.

Finally, a single-payer system such as Taiwan's conveys to citizens a sense of community, the notion that in some areas of human endeavour and travail, "we are all in this together." It is a feeling largely absent from market-driven health systems such as the US system. Not surprisingly, polls consistently showed high public satisfaction with the system — 70 percent through 2005 among those surveyed, after which it fell to the 60 percent range.

Unfortunately, like all publicly financed single-payer systems — Canada's included — Taiwan's NHI suffers from a major embedded shortcoming: a tendency of chronic underfunding relative to the claims that citizens and the providers of health care can potentially make on the system.

In the first three years of the NHI's operation (1995–98), the system actually accumulated a sizeable surplus, which obviated the need for a premium rate increase, which the NHI Law permits every two years, based on actuarial calculations. By 1998 the NHI surpluses had been exhausted and a deficit began to develop. Legislators and the public refused a premium rate increase, arguing that the waste and abuse in the NHI should be eliminated first. This stance forced the BNHI to borrow from banks to cover its deficit by spring of 2002. Only in the summer of 2002, largely at the urging of a courageous minister of health, did the legislature approve a small increase in the premium rate, from 4.25 percent to 4.55 percent, which eliminated the NHI's budget deficit through to December 2004. Persistent public and legislative resistance made a planned premium rate increase in 2004 impossible. At the time of writing, the BNHI is once again borrowing from banks to cover its operating deficit.

So far, the budget shortfalls have not led to the long queues one observes in other government-run health systems, notably Canada and the UK National Health Service (NHS). But the continued reluctance of Taiwan's legislature and the public to fund the NHI adequately now imperils the very future of an insurance scheme that has served Taiwan's citizens so well in its twelve-year history. Here it must be noted that, given its GDP per capita (US$16,563), the 6.2 percent of GDP Taiwan currently spends on health care falls short by about 1.0 to 1.5 percentage points of the average benchmark set by OECD countries.

If Taiwan gradually moved its health spending toward the OECD benchmark, with added spending carefully targeted on activities that improve access to care and quality, then this would ensure the NHI's sustainability. Absent such a move, the eventual emergence of a better endowed private tier in Taiwan appears likely, just as might happen in Canada. The potential for public underfunding remains the Achilles heel of all single-payer systems.

PART III

Privatization and the Principles of Medicare

CHAPTER 14

Economic Myths and Political Realities: The Inequality Agenda and the Sustainability of Medicare [1]

Robert G. Evans

Ingenuity: Sustaining Ourselves in an Unfriendly World

In its simplest terms, "sustainability" refers to nothing more than a comparison of rates of change. If a resource stock — a fishery, a forest, an aquifer, a bank account — is being drawn down faster than it is being replenished, then that stock, or better, that pattern of rates is not indefinitely sustainable. Continuous accumulation is equally unsustainable — the trees do not grow to the sky. Human nature being what it is, however, the latter form of unsustainability typically presents as some form of pollution or accumulating "bad" while the former involves running out of "goods."

While the simple arithmetic of trend projection is beyond dispute, its relevance in any particular situation is not. The time horizon is critical. Economists, in particular, tend to be congenitally suspicious of mechanical projections, for reasons well

illustrated in the controversies over the "limits to growth" in the
1970s.[2] Computer models of resource use and pollutant generation used in the study commissioned by the Club of Rome
showed rigorously that the world was approaching, in the relatively near future, absolute limits to economic growth. Worse, even
then-current levels of output and income in rich countries were
unsustainable in the long run. But critics emphasized that the very
definition of a "resource" depends upon the tastes and technology of the day, and that the latter, at least, was endogenous.

Natural resources do not "run out," they simply become
increasingly expensive to locate and extract. But rising prices create powerful incentives to innovate around the tightening
constraint, using an increasingly costly resource more efficiently
and finding substitutes. Accordingly depletion of any one resource
need not constrain the whole complex economic system. Successful innovation will be reflected in a stable (or falling) price for
the commodity that was previously "running out." Long-run
resource price data seem to support this view; the economist
Julian Simon, for example, challenged exponents of "limits" models to find *any* natural resource whose price, over the long run, has
risen in real terms.

More recently students of sustainability have developed a
broader, "neo-Malthusian" perspective. The environments to
which human societies adapt tend to become more hostile over
time, sometimes from natural changes but especially from the
activities of humans themselves — Malthus's point. On the other
hand, human societies have always been ingenious in finding ways
to advance their purposes even in the face of this deterioration.
Successful societies generate a "supply of ingenuity" sufficient to
meet the challenges thrown up by both the external environment
and the consequences of their own (or others') activities.[3] But an
"ingenuity gap" can open up, with potentially serious consequences, if the supply fails to keep pace with the demand.[4]

This concept of ingenuity includes, but goes far beyond, advances in technical capacity, to include most importantly the institutional frameworks within which economic and social activity take place — and which also serve to mobilize ingenuity itself. Fiduciary currency, double-entry bookkeeping, and limited liability corporations were fundamental advances in ingenuity. Price systems and markets are powerful institutional mechanisms, operating automatically to create incentives for technical innovations — or behavioural changes — to relax the constraints of any particular depleting resource. Pollutants become a problem when no institutional framework motivates a corresponding supply of ingenuity to limit their accumulation. "Pollution markets," in which rights to pollute could be traded at varying prices, have been suggested as such a possible framework.

Markets are only one form of social mechanism for mobilizing ingenuity — or indeed for promoting any other social objective. Public regulation, for example, is more typically used for pollution control. The most appropriate institutional choice will depend on the context, and is ultimately an empirical question. There is no one "right" institutional response to every social challenge.[5] Nor, most importantly, is there any God-given guarantee that the supply of ingenuity itself will be sufficient to deal with emerging social problems. In the idealized world of economic theory, automatic self-equilibrating mechanisms always take a society to the "best of all possible worlds" (so long as they are not perturbed by misguided government interventions). But in the real world, societies may not find a satisfactory institutional answer to their problems, becoming more or less "failed" societies with increasing suffering and misery and, in extreme cases, dissolution.

Societies split by deep tribal, ethnic, religious, or economic divisions and having weak or non-existent unifying institutions, are at particular risk. A deteriorating environment may increase internal conflict, both diverting and dissipating the supply of ingenuity.

The incentive to innovate is weakened when there is little security of reward; worse, plundering one's neighbours may become the most profitable application of ingenuity. In the most extreme cases external challenges to deeply divided societies generate a vicious circle of violent internal conflict, deepening divisions and further deterioration. Unable to hang together, the population hang each other separately.

These extreme observations underline heavily the critical importance of *political* ingenuity as an essential basis for other forms of advance, in designing and maintaining institutions for mitigating internal conflict and bridging fissures in the body politic. Absent these, and a whole society can become "unsustainable." Figure 1 provides a compact representation of the dynamics of violent conflict over renewable resources within rather than between states.[6]

Figure 1 Sources and consequences of renewable resource scarcity

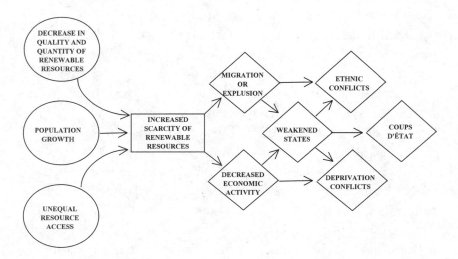

Source: Homer-Dixon et al, "Environmental Change & Violent Conflict," *Scientific American*, 268, no. 2 (Feb. 1993).

States do not generally collapse in high-income countries with highly developed, more or less democratic political systems and massive resources of ingenuity.[7] Conflicts are typically political and legal rather than military; dramatic transfers of power and shifts in priorities take place not through coups d'état but by the election of a Margaret Thatcher or a George W. Bush. Nevertheless the general framework seems to have very broad applicability. Social advance in the most general sense requires a sufficient supply of appropriate ingenuity to meet the challenges of a deteriorating environment. And that supply is threatened by internal divisions that divert ingenuity from promoting collective advantage into escalating political conflicts among competing interests. In particular, this framework seems to provide an interpretation for the seemingly endless conflicts over health care policy in high income countries.[8] In this paper I address the recently reignited debate over the "sustainability" of the current system of universal public health insurance in Canada, showing that certain anomalous features of that debate can be readily understood within the neo-Malthusian framework.

Financing Canadian Health Care through Fat and Lean

To begin, the long-run economic environment in Canada *has* deteriorated significantly since the early 1980s. Figure 2A plots Canadian GDP — gross domestic product — per capita (adjusted for inflation) since the Second World War, fitting a log-linear trend to 1947 to 1981 and projecting it to 2006.[9] Figure 2B shows the ratio of actual to fitted or projected values over this sixty year period.

The closeness of actual experience to this trend prior to 1982 is remarkable. The discrepancy is greater than 5 percent in only four years out of thirty-five, and never reaches 10 percent. Recessions in 1954 and 1957 to 1961 were followed not only by resumption of growth but also by recovery to the previous path — making up the lost ground.

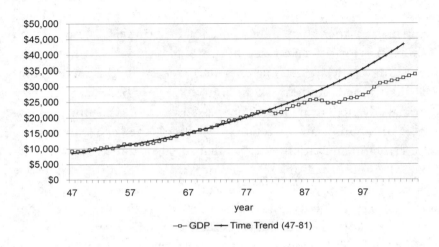

Figure 2A: Canada Real GDP per Capita Compared to
Trend (1947-82) in 1992 constant dollars

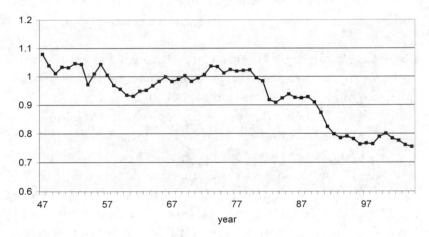

Figure 2B: Canada Real GDP per Capita Compared to
Trend (1947-82) in 1992 constant dollars

The recession of 1982 was different. Real income per capita not only dropped sharply, but failed to recover. Growth resumed in 1983 on a trend line parallel to that of 1947 to 1981, but nearly 10

percent lower. Growth after the even more severe recession of
1989 to 1992 was along a still lower and slightly slower path.
Canadians are not poorer now than in the past; average GDP per
capita (adjusted for inflation) was higher in 2006 than ever before,
and growing (between recessions) at almost the same rate as in
earlier decades. But that average is now about 25 percent below
where it would have been if the last two recessions had been followed by a real recovery. For whatever reasons, the ground lost in
these recessions appears permanently lost, and the amount is huge.

This implies, among other things, a permanent reduction in the
income base from which to meet the demands of an expanding
health care system. Figure 3 displays the ratio to GDP of Canadian expenditure (public and private) on hospitals and physicians'
services from 1947 to 2006, and of total health care expenditure
after 1960. It includes hypothetical lines showing what these ratios
would have been, after 1981, if GDP had continued to grow along
its pre-1982 trend while health spending had evolved as it did.

Figure 3: Hospital and Physician Expenditure (HMD) and
Total Health Expenditure (Hex) over GDP and Trend GDP
(PTGDP), Canada, 1947–2006

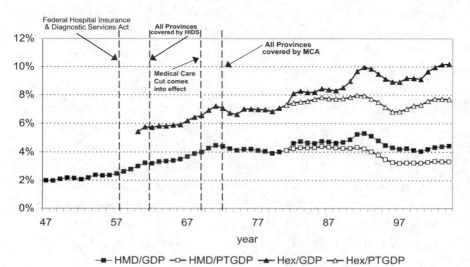

The hospital and physician data are of particular relevance because only these sectors are covered by the federal–provincial public insurance programs — medicare — whose "sustainability" continues to be challenged. Administered by provincial governments, according to federal standards and with federal financial contributions, these provide universal comprehensive coverage without deductibles or coinsurance. Other components of health care, such as drugs, dentistry, and long-term care, are covered through various mixes of out-of-pocket payment, public and private insurance, and direct public delivery.

Perhaps the most striking feature of figure 3 is the remarkable stability of the share of national income devoted to the public insurance programs. Provinces introduced these programs in different years, but coverage for hospital care was nation wide by 1961 and for physicians' services by 1971. The latter date was marked by a sharp break in the previous pattern of continuing cost escalation. Universal, comprehensive coverage was *not* more expensive than the previous fragmented mix of public and private insurance coverage and out-of-pocket payment. Consolidation of expenditures in the hands of a single payer made possible the control of rates of escalation, through a variety of different mechanisms.[10] From 1970 until 1981, the share absorbed by the medicare services fluctuated in a narrow band between about 4 percent and 4.25 percent of GDP.

Nor was the Canadian experience unique. By the 1970s public universal and comprehensive health service or health insurance systems were in place in all the high income countries of the OECD (Organization for Economic Cooperation and Development). All developed, at some time during the 1970s or early 1980s, more or less effective mechanisms of cost control.[11] Figure 4 shows the trends in health care spending relative to GDP for Canada, the United States, and the United Kingdom, and for the average of all OECD countries for which data are available back

Figure 4
National Health Expenditure in Canada, US and UK as Deviation
from OECD Average, 1960-2004

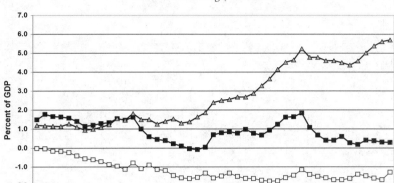

to 1960. The OECD average ratio escalates in parallel with the United States prior to the mid-1970s, rising at an average rate of 3.6 percent per year. From 1975 to 2004 it rises only 1.3 percent per year. The pattern is sufficiently consistent across countries that White referred to it as "the international standard."[12] The one exception, on both costs and coverage, is the United States.

The panels of figure 5 broaden the focus beyond the OECD to address the global picture. These data are drawn from the Statistical Appendix to the World Health Report for 2006.[13] Countries are grouped according to their income levels in GDP per capita measured in "international" dollars (USD adjusted to national purchasing power parities). Countries are unweighted; group averages count each country equally regardless of population size or income.

Health spending is strongly linked to national income, as shown in figure 5A. But only in high income countries does the proportion of income spent on health care rise with rising income. Countries with average incomes below $15,000 (in 2003) spent

Figure 5A: Total Health Expenditures as Percent of GDP (2003) Averaged over Countries grouped by Percent GDP

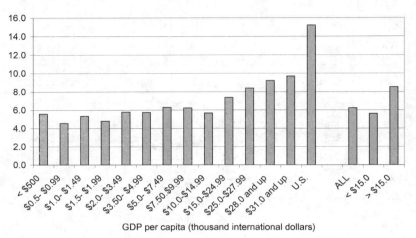

GDP per capita (thousand international dollars)

Figure 5B: Government Health Expenditures as Percent of Total Health Expenditure (2003) averaged over Countries grouped by Percent of GDP

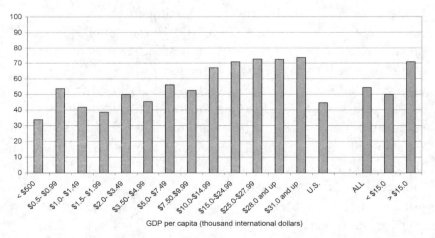

GDP per capita (thousand international dollars)

on average just under 6 percent; those over that level spent over 8 percent.[14] Canada, spending 9.9 percent in 2003, is just above the average (9.7 percent) for its top income group (excluding the United States) — just as figure 4 shows from the OECD data.

High income countries also finance a higher proportion of

their health care through the public sector (figure 5B). Among low income countries, the public share shows an irregular upward trend with income, averaging out at about 50 percent, but in high income countries, other than the United States, it jumps to 70 percent. Canada, at 69.9 percent public coverage, is actually somewhat below the 73.7 percent average for its top income group. Allegations that Canada's public programs to finance health care are fiscally "unsustainable" because they cover an unusually high proportion of health care costs are false.

The distinction between high and low income countries shows up sharply again in figure 5C, displaying the proportions of health care costs met through out-of-pocket payments. There is a strong downtrend; as national incomes rise, the proportion of health care paid out of pocket falls. In the United States, often viewed as a bastion of private payment, out-of-pocket payment actually covers a significantly lower share of costs than in other high income countries — although the costs themselves are, of course, much higher and much more unequally distributed. Moreover the

Figure 5C: Out of Pocket Expenditures as Percent of Total Health Expenditure (2003) averaged over Countries grouped by Percent of GDP

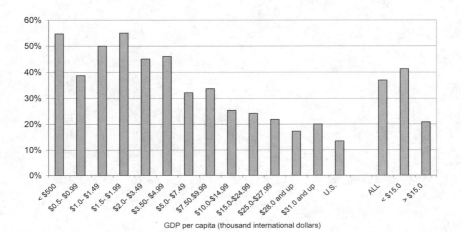

GDP per capita (thousand international dollars)

downtrend across countries begins at relatively low per capita incomes; the (group average) out-of-pocket ratio falls steadily with rising income for incomes over $5,000 per year.[15] Canada, with out-of-pocket payments at 14.9 percent of total health expenditures, is considerably below the 20.1 percent average for its high-income group, but — perhaps surprisingly — slightly above the United States at 13.5 percent.

The missing piece is provided by figure 5D — the share of health expenditures covered by private insurance. On average, countries cover about 5 percent of health care costs through this mechanism, and there is no systematic difference between high and low income countries. But in the United States, 36.5 percent of costs are covered through this mechanism.[16] What makes that country an extreme outlier is not the extent of direct charges to patients, but its heavy reliance on private insurance. This fragmented funding system accounts not only for the very high proportion (for a high income country) of persons with no or seriously inadequate insurance coverage, but also for the unique inability to control cost escalation.

Figure 5D: Pre-paid Insurance as Percent of Total Health
Expenditure (2003) averaged over Countries grouped by Percent of GDP

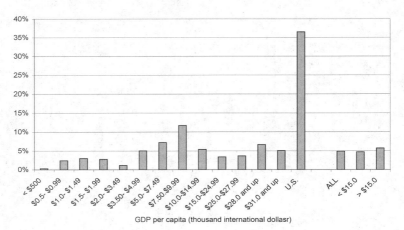

And Canada? Our national medicare system has excluded private insurance coverage (though that may be forced to change following the bizarre Supreme Court decision of 2005). Nevertheless, private insurance, primarily for prescription drugs and dentistry, accounts for 12.7 percent of Canadian health expenditures. This is well over twice the 5.1 percent average among the highest income (non-US) countries. In world terms, Canadians rely unusually heavily on this financing source, ranking fourteenth out of 138 countries (right behind Zimbabwe). Any suggestion that we have a problem of fiscal sustainability because of the minimal role of private insurance simply does not meet the data.

In reality problems of sustainability, or at least of uncontrolled cost escalation, are associated not with public funding but with fragmented public and private funding, as in the United States — or Canada's fragmented payment system for prescription drugs. Single-payer public financing creates an institutional environment encouraging the supply of ingenuity to contain costs; costs are higher in multi-source funding systems where ingenuity is diverted into shifting costs onto other payers.[17,18]

Adapting to Adversity: Public Success, Private Failure

The early 1980s increase in the Canadian share of GDP spent on health care ratio was largely a denominator effect. Health spending stayed on its trend path through the recession, but national income fell. Since the previous income trend was never regained, the share of income spent on hospitals and physicians remained permanently higher. Had there been no recession, or a full recovery, the hospital and medical spending share would have remained in the neighbourhood of 4.25 percent to 4.33 percent for another decade.

The ratio began to follow the same pattern in the next recession, rising sharply to 1992 but again maintaining a constant share

of the pre–1982 GDP trend. This time, however, the fiscal exigen-
cies faced by both provincial and federal governments forced a
quite dramatic response. Public expenditures were frozen or cut
across the board after 1992, including for the first time actual cuts
in hospital spending. By 1997 hospitals and physicians' services
were absorbing the same share of GDP as they had in 1971; if it
were not for the persistent effects of the two recessions that share
would have been back to early 1960s levels.

The pattern for total health care spending is roughly similar, but
with a long-term upward trend. The shares of national income
devoted to total health care expenditure in 1971, 1982, 1992, and
2006 were 7.2 percent, 8.1 percent, 10.0 percent, and 10.3 percent
respectively, while hospital and physicians' services accounted for
4.5 percent, 4.6 percent, 5.3 percent, and 4.4 percent. The year-
to-year movements are strongly influenced by the general business
cycle, but the thirty-five year trend indicates that cost containment has been much more successful in the medicare programs
than in the other health care sectors.

Figure 6: Canadian Health Expenditures as Percent
of GDP, 1975-2006, Selected Components

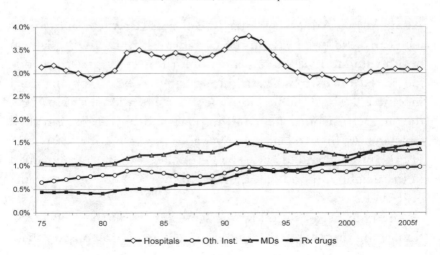

Expenditures on prescription drugs, in particular, which are outside medicare and reimbursed through a combination of public and private insurance and out-of-pocket payment, have been growing very rapidly over the past two decades, more than tripling their share of national income since 1980 (figure 6). This pattern of rapid growth parallels the experience of the whole Canadian health care system prior to 1971 (and the American experience down to the present), again illustrating the link between fragmented funding sources and rapid cost escalation.[19]

The deterioration of the Canadian economic environment after 1982 posed a serious challenge for the financing of health care. That challenge was met initially by allocating a larger share of national income to the health care system. The still larger shock of the early 1990s, however, triggered unprecedented reductions in public funding. Controversy has focused, then and subsequently, on the extent to which this mobilized ingenuity to provide care more efficiently and effectively, or simply reduced the level and standard of care provided and left real needs unmet.

I will bypass this question here, except to note that however one interprets their impact on the health of Canadians, reductions in expenditure must necessarily correspond, as a matter of elementary accounting, to a reduction in total payments to those working in or otherwise supplying resources to the health care system.[20] There is an inevitable conflict of economic interests between those who are paid for providing care and those who pay for it. Mobilizing ingenuity to improve efficiency, if it lowers total expenditure, threatens the financial interests of the former even as it benefits the latter. The deterioration of the overall economic environment since 1981 has tended to sharpen this division, intensifying the political and rhetorical conflict and clouding efforts to determine — and communicate — what actually happened.

For better or worse, however, after 1992 the Canadian public insurance programs did (have to) adapt to the general fiscal circumstances.

Coincidentally, and through different mechanisms, so did American health care. The projection by the American Congressional Budget Office[21] that by 2000 the United States would be spending 18 percent of its GDP on health care was spectacularly falsified; as shown in figure 4 the actual ratio in 2000 was little different from that in 1992.

As with the "limits to growth" modelling of the 1970s, linear projections that fail to take account of the adaptability of complex systems are likely to be misleading. The trick is to create the institutional environments that most effectively mobilize the ingenuity necessary to support that adaptation.

On the other hand, the "managed care revolution" that was widely credited with stabilizing American costs in the 1990s lost its grip after 2000. American expenditures were over 16 percent of GDP by 2005, and are now projected to reach 19.6 percent by 2016.[22] In a similar way, the "limits to growth" arguments largely dismissed in the 1970s have now returned in the form of global warming, and are placing increasing demands upon our collective capacity to mobilize ingenuity — political and institutional as well as technological. Whether human societies can meet those demands is not at this point clear.

Canada's experience at the beginning of the 1970s illustrates the impact of successful mobilization of ingenuity through institutional change. At the end of the 1960s there was growing concern among policymakers (though not, apparently, the public) in both Canada and the United States about the continuing rapid escalation of health costs. The completion of universal public medical coverage in Canada coincided with the immediate flattening of the previous trend; the failure to achieve national health insurance in the United States was associated with a continuation of their previous trend. Considerable ingenuity was applied in Canada, as later in other OECD countries, to achieve this result; even more ingenuity has been expended, in the United States, in frustrating it. But the demand for further ingenuity continues to grow, exactly as Homer-Dixon's framework would suggest.

American opponents of national health insurance (NHI) have claimed for over forty years that NHI would be "unaffordable." The counter evidence, extending from Canada across the OECD world and now to Taiwan,[23] has made no impression on these arguments. Similar concerns were urged in Canada prior to the inception of the medicare programs, though perhaps with more excuse in the 1960s.

Their reactivation in recent years, however, presents us with an obvious anomaly. Why would those alleging the financial unsustainability of Canadian health care focus on the *public* insurance programs, on medicare? Why would any rational person, concerned about cost escalation, advocate transferring costs from government budgets back onto patients, either directly or through increased private insurance contributions? On all the available evidence, accumulated across nations and decades, such a shift would almost certainly lead to *more* rapid escalation.

As the Yale political scientist Ted Marmor reminds us, "Nothing that is regular is stupid." If apparently intelligent and well-informed people (in Canada and the United States) continue, in the teeth of all the evidence, to revive the argument that universal public health insurance is economically "unsustainable" and to advocate diversifying funding sources by increasing private payments, then presumably they have objectives other than cost control.

The Public Fisc: Still Afloat after Heavy Weather

One line of explanation might be that for governments, and especially their treasurers, the GDP or its provincial equivalent is something of an abstraction. What is "real" (subject to the creativity of the public accountants) is the government's own fiscal situation.

GDP patterns strongly affect that situation insofar as they translate into public sector revenues and expenditures. The 1982 recession ushered in a decade of continuing public sector deficits and growing debt and debt charges; the 1989–1991 recession accelerated this fiscal deterioration and raised the spectre of actual bankruptcy for some provincial governments. The harsh public expenditure cuts of the 1992–1997 period, combined with subsequent more rapid economic growth, reversed this situation, generating substantial surpluses at the federal level and a falling aggregate public debt.[24] But important as national income trends may be for the fiscal situation of governments, it is the public accounts for which they are accountable.

In those accounts, provincial government expenditures on health care programs have over the last decade taken up a substantially increased share of total expenditures (figure 7A, right scale).[25] Between 1995/1996 and 2005/2006, health spending by all provincial (and territorial) governments in Canada rose from 34.9 percent of total program spending (net of debt service charges) to 42.4 percent. This trend appears to provide strong evidence that

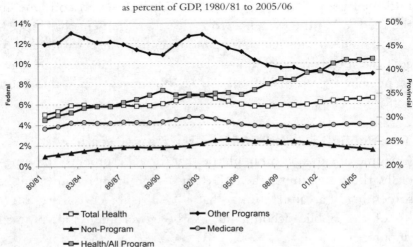

Figure 7A: Federal and Provincial Government Expenditures
as percent of GDP, 1980/81 to 2005/06

escalating health care costs in the public sector are increasingly crowding out other and important forms of public expenditure — clearly an unsustainable situation. Allegedly this problem can be addressed only by transferring costs from public to private budgets.

The story is more complicated, however, and the appearance is deceiving. A closer look at figure 7A shows that there is something unusual about the eight-year period from 1995/1996 to 2003/2004, during which the health share climbed to 42.2 percent. During the seven-year period from 1988/1989 to 1995/1996, by contrast, there was no change at all in the ratio of aggregate provincial health spending to other program spending. Of particular importance, there has been effectively no change in the two years since 2003/2004.

Moreover, if we look at total provincial government health spending relative to national GDP since 1995/1996 (also in 7A) we see a much weaker upward trend. Provincial spending on the medicare programs is in fact flat, taking up the same 4 percent share of national income in 2005/2006 as in 1995/1996. Claims that public medicare is "unsustainable" find no support in these data. (Provincial health spending on programs other than medicare has been growing — we referred above to the escalation of prescription drug costs.)

It follows that provinces must have been cutting back on their non-health program spending, and as figure 7A shows, they were. Provincial government spending on other programs took up a roughly constant share of national income from 1980/1981 to 1995/1996, between 11 percent and 12 percent. It has since fallen steadily, to 8.9 percent in 2003/2004, and appears to have stabilized there. Yet this quite significant reduction was not driven by an "unsustainable" surge in health spending, because no such surge occurred.

A claim that health care is "crowding out" other programs

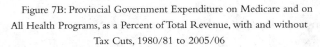

Figure 7B: Provincial Government Expenditure on Medicare and on
All Health Programs, as a Percent of Total Revenue, with and without
Tax Cuts, 1980/81 to 2005/06

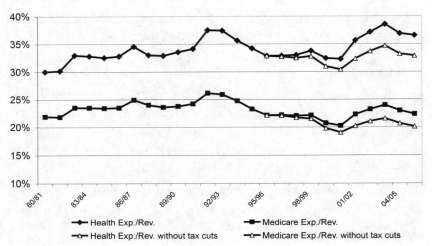

could still be salvaged, if cuts to aggregate spending were being forced by a declining revenue base while political considerations made it difficult or impossible to impose parallel cuts on health. Other programs would then have had to bear more severe cuts because of the inflexibility of the health care programs as present-ly structured. But this would imply that health spending was rising as a share of provincial revenues as well as of program expendi-tures. In fact such an increase did take place, but had little or nothing to do with trends in health spending (figure 7B).

Starting in 1996/1997, several provincial governments intro-duced a variety of fiscal measures, including, in particular, reductions in their rates of personal and corporate income taxa-tion. By 2005/2006 the resulting net revenue foregone amounts to about $28 billion, or nearly 15 percent of aggregate provincial government own-source revenues (excluding federal transfers). Had provincial governments not chosen to use the reviving econ-omy as an opportunity to cut tax rates, the share of aggregate provincial revenues devoted to health care would in 2005/2006 have been very slightly below its level in 1982/1983, over twenty years previously. The proportion taken up by medicare programs would have been below its level in any previous year reported in the Finance Canada Fiscal Reference Tables.

There is thus no basis whatever for a claim that health care is "crowding out" other provincial programs by taking up a grow-ing share of provincial revenue. That impression can be sustained only by ignoring the fact that provincial governments, in aggre-gate, have deliberately lowered their revenue base through tax cuts.

Despite these tax cuts, however, provincial spending on the medicare programs is still a smaller share of provincial revenues than it was in 1982/1983. Total health spending, which includes the costs of public pharmaceutical insurance programs, has risen, but the increase from 30.0 percent to 36.6 percent is not dramat-ic over twenty-five years, just over a quarter of a percentage point per year. And in any case most of that increase is accounted for by the tax cuts; abstracting from those, the up-trend over twenty-five years in the share of provincial revenue devoted to health care is just over one-tenth of a percentage point per year.

Health spending does not appear to be placing an increasing strain, over the long term, on the provincial revenue base. The recessions at the beginning and end of the 1980s certainly reduced that base, and each resulted in, among other things, a jump in the proportion of total revenues going to health care. Since the eco-nomic ground lost in those recessions was never really recovered, that ratio stayed up through the 1980s. In the 1990s, (politically difficult) cuts and rationalizations in the medicare sector brought the ratio back to its long-term level, consistent with the now lower path of economic growth.

But if health spending has been taking a relatively stable share of revenue while increasing its share of program spending, then the ratio of revenue to expenditure must have been rising. And it was, for nearly a decade (figure 8A). Provinces reacted to the recession of the early 1980s by running persistent deficits; the 1989–1991 recession exacerbated their weak fiscal positions. By 1992/1993 aggregate revenues were nearly 20 percent below expenditures (including debt service). This was unsustainable, and serious expenditure cutting began in both the health and non-health sectors. Figure 7A shows the corresponding downturn in both spending components, relative to GDP.

But the persistent deficits that were a hangover from the 1980s are long gone. The Canadian provinces, in total, moved into surplus seven years ago, in 1999/2000. In the absence of the income tax cuts and other fiscal changes that began in 1996/1997, provincial governments budgetary revenues would now be nearly 20 percent above their expenditures. As it is, they are about 5 percent above. Correspondingly, the relative cost of debt servicing has

Figure 8A: Canada, Provincial Governments, Total Revenues over
Total Expenditures, 1980/81 to 2005/06

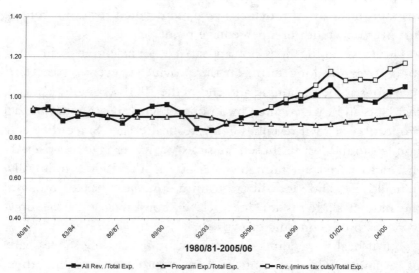

Figure 8B: Canada, Provincial Government Revenue, Total and
Components, as percent of GDP, 1980/81 to 2005/06

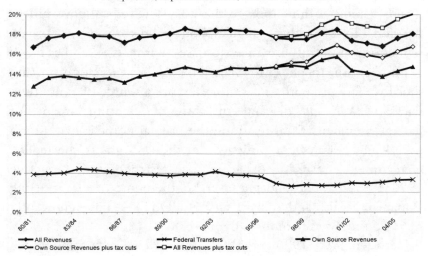

been falling and, as shown in figure 8A, program expenditures are
rising as a share of total expenditures.

As figure 8B shows, however, the tax cuts have in fact served to
stabilize, not to depress, provincial own-source revenues relative to
national GDP. The "income elasticity" of provincial revenue sources
is apparently greater than unity, so that in the absence of the rate
cuts, provincial governments would be taking an increasing share of
national incomes, and a share well above the long-run trend.

These aggregate surpluses, however, are not spread evenly. The
unequal distribution of economic development and particularly of
resource revenues results in very large disparities between so-
called "have" and "have-not" provinces. While wealthier provinces
have been cutting their tax rates, and driving the aggregate data,
fiscally weaker provinces are still struggling to keep their heads
above water. They are also under political pressure to compete in
the "tax cut" game. The much-publicized "fiscal imbalance" in
Canada is among the provinces, not between the provinces and
the federal government.

Federal–Provincial Fiscal Relations — Of Course

There is another dimension to the story. The federal government transfers money to the provinces, both as "tax room" — tax rate reductions to permit provinces to raise their rates — and as block grants of cash, to help provinces support health, education, and social welfare programs. These transfers are a source of continuing friction. Without delving into the fascinating arcana of federal–provincial fiscal relations, the critical point is that after a number of years of chipping away at the cash grants, the federal government introduced a major restructuring, effective 1996/1997, that consolidated several of them into one item — the Canadian Health and Social Transfer (CHST) — but significantly reduced the overall amount (figure 8B).

Between 1995/1996 and 1997/1998, federal cash transfers fell by about $5 billion, or nearly 20 percent, leaving a substantial hole in provincial budgets. Critics argued, with some justification, that the federal government was fighting its own deficit "on the backs of the provinces." That federal fight was outstandingly successful: the Government of Canada has been recording surpluses ever since 1997/1998 and, barring major recession (or major federal tax cuts), seems likely to do so for the indefinite future.

It is hardly surprising, therefore, that provincial governments have for a decade demanded restoration of the cash amounts unilaterally reduced through the introduction of the CHST.[26] Rather than restoring the cash grants to their pre-CHST rate, however, the federal government began in 1998/1999 to cut its own income tax rates. A substantial amount of new federal money has since begun to flow to the provinces, but as figure 8B shows, this has not restored the previous relationship of federal transfers to GDP.

On the other hand, the federal government seems to have taken the (also understandable) view that there was no benefit to either the health care system or its own political fortunes from transferring more revenues to provincial governments whose principal priority was cutting their own income tax rates. The government of Ontario, in particular, (ideologically at odds with the federal government during much of this period) had by 2003/2004 cut a cumulative total of $61.9 billion out of its own revenue base.

The decline in federal transfers — relative to GDP — has meant that total provincial revenues have been a bit below their long-run trend. But by 2005/2006, increases in these transfers, though not quite restoring the 1995/1996 ratio to GDP, had brought total provincial revenues back to baseline.

Amid the continuing inter-governmental wrangling, one fact stands out. Between 1996/1997 and 2003/2004 the federal and provincial governments, between them, cut personal and corporate income tax rates so as to remove an estimated $170.8 billion from public sector revenues. By 2003/2004 the annual public revenue foregone amounted to an estimated $48.9 billion — over 60 percent of public sector expenditure on health care.

In summary, the Canadian federal and provincial governments have over the decade of the 1990s succeeded in restoring fiscal positions undermined by earlier unfavourable developments in the general economy. This process had two distinct phases. Prior to 1996/1997, provincial health and non-health expenditures were both being reduced, relative to GDP. Since then there has been a resumption of the flow of public funds into health care, more or less in proportion to the rise in GDP, while the shrinkage of non-health programs continued into the early 2000s. Hence the rise, after 1996/1997, in the share of health in provincial program spending, a rise that ended in 2003/2004.

But the cuts to non-health programs after the end of the 1990s were no longer being driven by the need to balance provincial budgets. That job, difficult and important, had been done. The tax cuts after 1996/1997 were a fiscal choice by right-wing governments in several of the larger provinces, a choice that then

necessitated continuing expenditure cuts to maintain the fiscal
balance previously achieved. Presumably finding it politically
more difficult to make further cuts in the health care sector, these
governments made deeper cuts to non-health programs. One
could argue that in this way health care was in fact now "crowding out" other programs. But the source of the pressure was no
longer fiscal exigency generated by poor overall economic performance, rather it was the political decision to take advantage of
an improved fiscal situation to cut tax rates rather than to maintain spending on public programs.

Governments are elected to make choices, fiscal and otherwise,
and the provincial governments making these choices were duly
and democratically elected. But it would be erroneous, and misleading, to claim that an unsustainably expensive public health
care system has been the source of the pressure on other public
programs. The argument that the health programs are economically "unsustainable" has no more basis in the public accounts than
it has in the national accounts.

What's the Real Issue? The Inegalitarian Agenda

So the anomaly remains. These data are perfectly well known in
provincial and federal finance ministries; indeed these ministries
are their source. They are not known to most of the public; that
raises a whole other set of issues as to the role of the media during this period. (What politicians are aware of is always an open
question.) So what *are* the real motives behind the claims of
unsustainability?

An important clue lies in the pattern of some of the provincial
tax changes. Figure 9 is calculated directly from the federal and
provincial income tax schedules for single residents of Ontario
and British Columbia. Between 1997 and 2002, individuals in
both provinces with annual taxable incomes of $15,000 and
$25,000 (and no other complications) had their tax liabilities

Figure 9: Income Tax Reductions in Ontario and
British Columbia, 1997-2002, as Percent of Taxable Income,
by Income Level

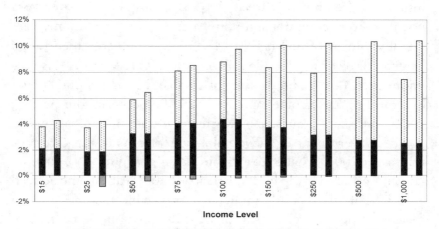

reduced by about 4 percent, with roughly equal reductions in federal and provincial taxes. But the percentage reductions increase
steadily with annual income, reaching nearly 9 percent (Ontario)
and 10 percent (BC) at $100,000. Beyond this point the federal
reductions decline as a share of income, but the provincial reductions continue to increase. In Ontario these increases are quite
small, and do not offset the federal decline. But in BC they do,
reaching nearly 8 percent for a taxable income of $1,000,000. At
that level, after-tax income would be larger in 2002 by $104,097
($78,754 from the province, and $25, 342 from the federal government). After-tax income at the $15,000 level in British
Columbia would rise by $645 ($327 provincial, $317 federal). The
comparable provincial amounts for Ontario are $49,293 and
$255.

Rate changes immediately introduced by the British Columbia
government newly elected in mid-2001 account for most of the
increased inequality of after-tax incomes. Later changes in other

taxes reinforced this effect.[27] British Columbia, like the neighbouring province of Alberta, also levies compulsory health
insurance "premiums" (unrelated to risk status). Public coverage is
not, however, conditional upon payment; the "premiums" are
actually a form of poll tax. In May 2002 they were raised by 50
percent, or $216 for a single individual.[28] Figure 9 shows this pre-
mium increase as a proportion of taxable income; it offsets over
one third of the income tax cut at $25,000 per year, four percent
at $100,000, and a quarter of a percent at one million.

The Government of Alberta also increased its health care premiums in 2001, by about one third, but its approach to income
taxation was even simpler. On January 1, 2001, Alberta introduced
a provincial "flat tax" of 11 percent of taxable income above a
basic exemption level, substituting for the previous percentage of
the (relatively progressive) federal liability. This approach twists the
whole tax schedule above the basic exemption level to decrease
the relative burden on the wealthy and increase it on middle
incomes.

In all three provinces, the higher the income, the greater the
percentage gain from income tax reductions. In addition, the cuts
to public expenditures imposed in these provinces along with a
variety of additional fees for public services were significantly
regressive in their impact.[29]

One has to conclude that these provincial governments were
pursuing, for whatever motive, a quite deliberate agenda of regressive income redistribution.[30] Nor are they alone. Historically,
Canadian governments have significantly mitigated, through taxes
and financial transfers, the degree of income inequality that is
generated in the marketplace.[31] Changes since the mid-1990s
appear to have reduced this buffering effect, and post-government
income inequality is now on the rise.[32] Taxes and transfers are only
part of the process by which governments influence the distribution of economic well-being. Expenditure programs, such as

public education and health care, also play a major role in detaching benefits from ability to pay. In all public health insurance systems (at least in the high income, industrialized countries) people in the upper income brackets subsidize (on average) the care of those lower down, while at the same time, the relatively healthy subsidize the care of the comparatively unhealthy. There is no other way to maintain a modern health care system — at least none is known.

There is, however, considerable variation among national systems in the nature and extent of this subsidization. The Canadian medicare programs, covering hospital and physicians' services, are almost entirely financed from general taxation and provide care "on equal terms and conditions" to the whole resident population. In the United States, in sharp contrast, people of different incomes receive care on very different "terms and conditions" depending upon their employment status, age, and ability to pay. Most European systems make care available on more or less equal terms and conditions to the whole population, but several (unlike Canada) permit providers within the public system to sell, to those willing and able to pay, more timely access to a perceived higher standard of care. Purchasing these advantages for themselves, the better-off are not required to contribute to a similar standard for the rest of the population. The payments go into providers' pockets. These two features underpin all arguments for "two-tier" care.

The distribution of the cost of public health care across the population varies considerably among these national systems.[33] Financing raised through direct taxation tends to distribute the burden more or less proportionate to income, indirect taxation is more regressive, and social insurance programs can be either more or less proportional to income (France) or quite steeply regressive (Germany, the Netherlands) depending upon their structure. But private payment, whether through private insurance or directly out of pocket, is by far the most regressive. Low-, middle-, high-,

and very high-income people pay the same amounts for the same
services, but these payments represent very different shares of their
respective incomes.

Since health is correlated with wealth, on average, lower-
income people would pay an even larger share of their incomes
for health care through private payment — if they were to get
equal service for equal need. But of course they do not. Higher-
income people spend more on health care through private
payments, and get more services, but spend a much smaller share
of their incomes in this way. This pattern is similar for both private insurance and self-payment, because private insurers in a
competitive market must set their premiums in proportion to the
estimated risk of the insured. For equivalent coverage, healthier
people will pay less, regardless of their incomes, and sicker people
will pay more.

The distributional impact of public, tax-based financing of
medicare in Canada is dramatically illustrated in figure 10 drawn
from a unique study in Manitoba.[34] For a sample of about 40,000
Manitobans, individual-level data on the costs of hospital and
physicians services paid by the public programs were linked with

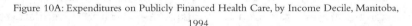

Figure 10A: Expenditures on Publicly Financed Health Care, by Income Decile, Manitoba,
1994

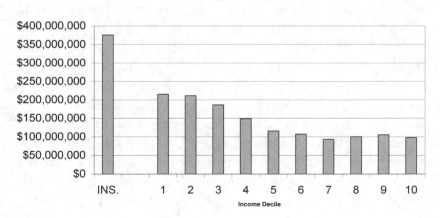

corresponding individual (actually family) income-level data from the Canadian Census. These records were then made anonymous, expanded to represent the entire population of Manitoba, and grouped into income deciles of roughly 105,000 persons each.

Figure 10A shows that total provincial expenditures for the care of persons in the lowest income decile were just over $200 million in 1994. These costs fell, for successively higher income deciles, until the middle of the income distribution. From the fifth decile upwards, public expenditures were roughly $100 million in each decile or in round figures $950 per person — on average. There would of course be a great deal of variation in individual costs among the members of each decile, some generating very high costs and others none. But above the middle of the income spectrum there appears to be no systematic relation between expenditures and income. In the lower half of the income distribution, by contrast, health care needs — or at least use, rise as income falls.

Figure 10B: Tax Contribution to Health Care, by Income Decile,
Manitoba, 1994

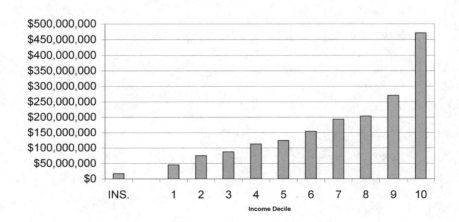

The INS category are persons who are permanently institutionalized. This group — about 18,000 people — accounted for about $375 million in public outlays or roughly eleven times the per capita costs of people in the lowest income decile of the non-institutionalized population.

Figure 10B shows the estimated tax contributions — income and sales, of persons in each decile. These are much more skewed than the utilization of care, with people in the top decile contributing about $470 million to the maintenance of the public health care system while those in the bottom decile contributed less than $50 million. Contributions rise steadily by income decile, as one would expect; the large jump at the top decile, almost doubling from the next highest income band, reflects the extent of concentration of income at the top end.[35] (Since 1994 before-tax incomes in Canada have become considerably more unequal and concentrated among the highest earners.)

Figure 10C shows the obvious calculation, subtracting decile-specific tax contributions from the value — or at least cost — of

Figure 10C: Net Transfer to/from Income Decile, Public Financing of Health Care, Manitoba, 1994

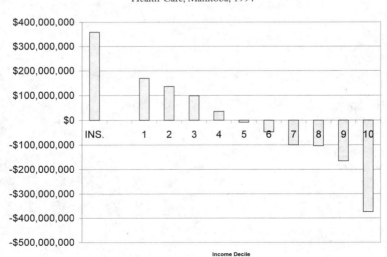

Income Decile

Figure 10D: Net Transfer by Income Decile, as Share of Consumable Income, Manitoba, 1994

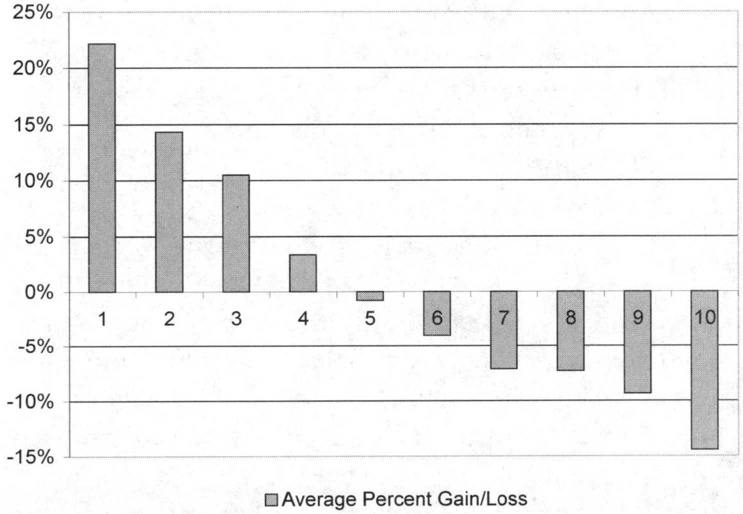

☐ Average Percent Gain/Loss

care received. Figure 10D then converts this net dollar benefit or cost into the proportion of consumable income (net of income and sales taxes) received in each decile. (The INS population are excluded because their incomes are so low that they would blow up the scale.)

In 1994, the roughly 105,000 Manitobans in the top decile contributed about $380 million to the financing of the health care system, or about $3,600 each, over and above the cost of the services they used. Coincidentally, this almost exactly equaled the cost of caring for the permanently institutionalized population. The second-highest decile contributed half as much net, about $1,670 each, and the fifth decile broke even. These net contributions cost those in the top decile just under 15 percent of their consumable incomes, while augmenting the incomes of those at the bottom by about 22 percent.

Whether these financial transfers across the income distribution are fair or unfair is a matter for political or ethical judgment. But, what should be obvious is that they exist, are large, and are a potent source of political debate. In particular, as a matter of simple arithmetic, any shift away from tax finance toward more private insurance or user charges would shrink each of the bars in each of these charts toward the horizontal axis. People in higher income deciles would contribute less, those in lower income deciles would contribute more. (As well, of course, the healthy would gain at the expense of the users of care.)

Thus the "private/public" debate about financing sources is, in all modern health care systems, fundamentally a debate about Who Pays? and Who Gets? The Canadian universal tax-financed system requires higher-income people to contribute more to supporting the health care system, without offering them preferred access or a higher standard of care. Any shift toward proportionately more private financing would reduce the relative burden on people with higher incomes and raise it farther down the spectrum. Insofar as private payments may also limit access by people with lower incomes, private finance also opens better access for those willing and able to pay. Relative to universal, fully tax-financed public insurance, an expansion of private payment would thus enable the wealthy to pay less (in charges, private premiums and taxes) and get more (in volume, quality, and/or timeliness). And conversely for those with lower incomes. This conflict of economic interest is real, unavoidable, and permanent in all systems, which is why the public/private debate is never resolved (and why it is typically so occluded with "econofog" about how more private financing can make everyone better off!).

Cutting across the income spectrum there is a third equally deeply entrenched conflict feeding the endless public/private financing debate — Who Gets Paid? — and how much.

Private insurance systems, for example, incur heavy administrative costs to identify relative risks and set corresponding premiums, to market policies, and to adjudicate and pay individual claims, as well as to reward investors and (sometimes spectacularly) senior executives. These overhead costs absorb between 15 and 20 percent of the revenues of Canadian private insurers. In addition, there are substantial costs imposed on providers of care and beneficiaries or their representatives, in negotiating with insurers and trying to ensure that claims are in fact paid.

In the United States, these overheads were recently estimated at 31.0 percent of total health care expenditure in 1999.[36] In a universal public system most of these costs vanish; the comparable estimate for Canada was 16.7 percent and that includes extensive private insurance for dentistry and drugs. The *excess* administrative costs in the United States were estimated at $209.0 billion or 17.1 percent of total American health expenditures. But all these billions represent income for insurers, benefits managers, and administrative and financial staff in hospitals and clinics. In a universal public insurance system, most of these jobs would not exist.

Payments to care providers raise exactly the same issue. Insofar as public single-payer systems have been relatively more effective in controlling overall costs (particularly prices) of health care, they have to the same extent controlled the incomes of providers. Hence the intense opposition to such coverage in North America from economically motivated providers, most notably the for-profit pharmaceutical industry. Again the conflict of interest is real and fundamental. For a firm whose products have high fixed costs of development and are sold at prices far above variable cost, any reduction in prices comes straight off the bottom line.

Not all providers thrive in a private funding system. Health and wealth are correlated; a high proportion of costs are generated by a relatively small proportion of people with above-average morbidity and below-average incomes. The income base of the provider community as a whole depends on a high proportion of public funding. Even in the "private" United States, about 60 percent of health care expenditure comes directly or indirectly from public funds.[37] But a multi-source financing system, with supplementary private financing and public sources that are indirect and difficult to control, provides the best income opportunities for providers — meaning, higher health care expenditures.

Political Wolves Masquerading as Economic Sheep

These embedded conflicts of economic interest over Who Pays? Who Gets? and Who Gets Paid? play roles in the framework of figure 1 analogous to tribal, ethnic, or religious divisions. They are always present, but tend to flare up into more intense and self-reinforcing political conflict under economic stress. Such conflicts may pose a real threat to the sustainability of Canada's medicare. But it is a threat from private interests pursuing a redistributive agenda, rather than from expenditures outrunning public resources.

The relative deterioration of the economic environment in Canada since 1981, with its particularly powerful impact on the public fiscal situation, has resulted (among many other things) in a number of relatively successful efforts to "do more with less."[38] On the other hand, a number of policy proposals for structural "reform" represent, in reality, the application of ingenuity to redistribute burdens and benefits — to eat the other fellow's lunch. Efforts to promote — and to expose and combat — such "reforms" distract from the very real needs for improved system management and adaptation to a less favourable environment.[39]

The wealthy in the modern world may be increasingly reluctant to accept a single standard of care for the whole population, with no preference for themselves, while contributing a relatively larger share of the cost. Private financing quite genuinely offers them "more, for less," while offering the rest of the population "less, for more." It may lead to a less efficient and more expensive system overall, through increased overhead costs, weaker control over prices, and reduced potential for managing care patterns.

Diversion of care from those with greatest needs to those with greatest resources will result in a less effective distribution of services. But the wealthy still come out ahead.

It also appears that in several countries, including Canada, political systems have become increasingly sensitive to the priorities of the wealthy, for reasons well beyond the scope of this paper. Claims that Canada's medicare is economically or fiscally unsustainable represent part of a broader propaganda campaign to advance those priorities, "softening up" a generally skeptical and unsympathetic public to accept that the current form of public health insurance (which most Canadians still strongly prefer) is simply impossible to maintain. The agenda has been advanced by right-wing governments in the larger provinces, with sympathetic coverage from the country's dominant newspaper chain. In these circumstances the political sustainability of the public system is very much an open question. But the claims of *economic* unsustainability appear from the data to be themselves wholly unsustainable.

That Was Then, This Is Now?
Or are they? Unsustainability is a claim about the future, not the past, and that claim is buttressed by current fiscal projections showing public health care spending growing much faster than provincial revenues. As noted above, the most recent data do show a resumption of more rapid rates of cost escalation. Is there now a real economic wolf at the door?

The future is an uncertain place, and all forecasts will be falsified. But why should the future be different from the quite sustainable past? A standard triad of reasons is typically offered — and has been for decades. They are classic examples of "Zombies" — ideas and arguments that are intellectually dead but will not stay buried.[40] They are repeatedly disinterred to advance interests that are very much alive.

The triad consists of interlinked claims about trends in demography, technology, and public attitudes, each asserted to be generating increasing needs or demands (the distinction is typically fuzzy) for increasingly expensive health care. Aging populations have greater needs; advancing technology creates ever more expensive possibilities for intervention; and "public expectations" of the health care system are ever-increasing. People just want more, and want it now. But (it is further asserted) no government can afford to meet these ever-expanding needs/demands. So we should, indeed must, limit the public liability, and let those who can, buy more for themselves if they wish. There is really no alternative.

When one undoes the packages of these broad generalities and looks at the actual data, a very different picture emerges.

The zombie of the aging population, a.k.a. "apocalyptic demography," has been studied in particular detail. The average age of modern populations *is* rising. And, on average, elderly people *do* have greater health needs and generate greater costs. But it is *not* true that these patterns will place an unsustainable burden on public health care systems. Holding age-specific per capita use and cost rates constant, Canadian population forecasts indicate a rise in per capita costs of about 1 percent per year — well within the range of prevailing rates of economic growth.

And, well below observed rates of growth of expenditures. Use and cost are primarily driven not by changing age structure, but by changing patterns of care use — what is done to and for patients. These patterns obviously respond to the evolution of scientific knowledge and technical capacity, but the link is neither simple nor direct.[41] New technologies may be inherently either cost-enhancing or cost-reducing — there are many examples of each — but it is the way in which they are taken up and applied that determines their impact on costs. That process of up-take and application is primarily controlled by clinicians (subject to available capacity), and the cost-enhancing bias of technology arises *inter alia* from the economic incentives that they face.

There is extensive evidence of the provision of questionable or simply inappropriate services, old and new, at unnecessarily high cost. But efforts to evaluate outcomes, eliminate ineffective or questionable practices, and restrain the exuberant proliferation of interventions have typically met indifference from clinicians, if not active resistance. Apart from issues of professional autonomy and pride (and the urge to "do something"), this reaction has roots in the ineluctable reality that cost containment must always threaten someone's income.[42]

The potential for transferring a large proportion of in-patient care to ambulatory or day care facilities, for example, has been well documented in Canada since the early 1970s. But large-scale uptake was slow until the rigorous budgetary restraints of the 1990s. The transfer eliminated jobs; widespread claims of "under-funding" and threats to patient health have not been substantiated.[43] If substantial additional funds flow into the health care system, the incentives for improved efficiency are relaxed.

The clearest examples of inappropriate and excessively costly choices of intervention can be found in the pharmaceutical sector. The principal driver in Canada of rapid cost escalation is the replacement of older, off-patent drugs with new patented ones at prices that may be ten times higher. These are marketed as superior, but the regulatory process does not require new drugs to be tested against those they will replace, only against placebo. In some major trials high-profile (and high cost) new drugs have shown no additional benefits.[44] Large additional expenditures, stimulated by intense marketing, are in effect buying nothing.

But what about public demand for the newest and the best, at any cost? Again the pharmaceutical experience is instructive. Manufacturers have always engaged in intense and highly sophis-ticated marketing, primarily targeting physicians. American pharmaceutical manufacturers — for whom data are available — now spend twice as much on marketing as on research.[45]

More recently the industry lobbied successfully to eliminate American regulatory restrictions on advertising directly to the public, and is now spending over $4 billion annually to manipulate public expectations. Such advertising does change physician prescribing behaviour[46] — why else would a for-profit industry spend the money? Canada's ban on advertising prescription drugs directly to patients is now facing a constitutional challenge mounted by the communications conglomerate CanWest Global, with an obvious interest in, and only in, the potential advertising revenues. (There is no evidence of a groundswell of supportive public opinion!) In this environment, to speak of "public expectations" as if they represented independent consumer choices is at best dangerously naïve, and at worst deliberately deceptive.

Managing patient expectations has always been a significant part of the professional role. The difference between a physician and a for-profit firm is that the former is responsible for the health of patients, the latter for the earnings of shareholders. In both cases expectations management has very significant effects on trends in health expenditures, but those effects depend on the incentives created by the institutional environment in which the process takes place. That environment is determined by public and private policies and is always politically contested — as the pharmaceutical example makes clear.

Such matters as technology assessment, medical practice guidelines, and efforts to promote the practice of "evidence-based medicine" are highly political, interacting with the economic incentives embodied in the different structures for reimbursing physicians and hospitals. Medical and other professional associations and unions take a very active interest in these matters; advancing the economic interests of their members is one of their principal responsibilities. The recent growth in Canadian health

care costs includes some very successful physician fee bargaining.
To pretend that trends in health care use and costs are determined
by impersonal forces external to the industry itself is just that, a
pretense.[47]

Whether or not the recent rise in Canadian medicare expenditures presages a period of more rapid longer-term escalation is
thus a critical question, but the answer does not depend upon
external forces. Rather it will, as in the past, depend on the outcome of political and administrative contests between those who
pay and those who are paid for delivering or financing care. Projecting cost trends is akin to predicting the outcome of the Stanley
Cup; there is certainly relevant information, but it is not a scientific exercise.

Private Morality, Public Choices — and Consequences

In the end, though it looms large in the public debate, the question of "sustainability" may not be about expenditure trends at all.
Reinhardt argues that it is actually a moral issue, a debate about
what the members of a society owe to each other.[48]

To illustrate, suppose what I have argued is incorrect, and we *are*
in fact entering a new era in which advancing medical technology really does offer dramatic improvements in health — at
dramatically increased expense. Citizens might quite rationally
accept this bargain. Health care spending would then rise as a
share of GDP — why not? (That is exactly what happened in
Canada when universal public hospital insurance was introduced;
there was consensus, right or wrong, that more spending would
produce better health for everyone.) At root, the arguments for
cost containment have always been about seeking value for
money, containing price inflation and paring away waste, not
about foregoing effective care.

But who should pay, and who should get the care? Under public insurance, the burden would fall on taxpayers and the benefits

would go to patients. Government expenditure on health care would rise, as would taxation. The claim that such increases would be "unsustainable" boils down to saying that this pattern of burdens and benefits is morally wrong. People should not get care that they cannot afford. And people who can afford a higher standard of care for themselves, should not have to contribute, through taxation, to support a similar standard for others.

This moral position does not appear to be widely shared by the Canadian public. Nor can its advocates credibly claim that governments "cannot afford" such increased expenditures, while simultaneously advocating and carrying through substantial cuts to income taxes. Considerable ingenuity must therefore be devoted to finding general harms from an expanded public sector.[49] This ingenuity might more constructively be directed toward improving the efficiency and effectiveness of the health care system. But those who allege unsustainability largely ignore the evidence on waste and inappropriate care, and implicitly or explicitly also allege "underfunding" — thus coming into alliance with provider interests.

Reinhardt's comment on the US Congress is worth quoting:

> That no one in the U.S. Congress shows much interest in the glaring inefficiencies that could easily be addressed within the current medicare program [in the US, covering only those 65 and over] speaks volumes about the true, but hidden, agenda that actually drives the quest for privatizing … Crisply put, the objective is to shift responsibility for health spending on older persons from the general taxpayer onto the older people themselves.[50]

Canada's universal system has done a much better job of mobilizing ingenuity to deal with these "glaring inefficiencies," but a much better job than the United States still leaves much to be desired. More significant reforms continue to be stalled by the political struggles over Who Pays? Who Gets? and Who Gets Paid? Claims that the Canadian public system is both economically unsustainable and underfunded seem driven by the same agenda that Reinhardt identifies in the US — containing public outlays while letting private expenditures go where they will. Such a mixed system would be more expensive and less efficient overall, escaping the price restraints imposed by the public single payer and bearing significantly increased administrative overheads. But it would be better for the wealthy.

Hence Reinhardt's assertion that "sustainability" is actually a moral issue, of defining the mutual obligations of the members of a community. Public choices are private morality writ large. There *is* a wolf at the door of the Canadian medicare system. But it is a political wolf dressed in phony economic clothing to deceive the sheep.

CHAPTER 15

Chaoulli's Legacy for the Future of Canadian Health Care Policy[51]

Colleen M. Flood

Introduction

Much has already been written about the *Chaoulli* decision,[52] but its full policy impact is still to be played out. Initially, the importance of the decision was considered by many to be limited given that technically it applied only to Quebec. Moreover, the Quebec government could choose to respond, not by abandoning one-tier medicare, but through reducing wait times to what the court considers a reasonable length.[53] Since the decision was released, however, it has become clear that the legal impact of *Chaoulli* will be dwarfed by its normative impact on policy debates. Prior to *Chaoulli*, advocates of privatization were discounted as either ideologues or speaking from the perspective of their own vested interests — for example, private clinics that would reap financial gains from further privatization of Canadian medicare. Now, these positions have the normative imprimatur of legitimacy (indeed superiority) from no lesser body than the Supreme Court of Canada. The debate has swung widely from when discussion of anything other than public funding was akin to heresy, to now, when the only option on the table is private health insurance.[54]

All of this has brought Canadian medicare to a fork in the road. At the time of writing, critical decisions are about to be taken across the country. Unfortunately, the level of debate about public and private insurance that has been sparked by *Chaoulli* reflects the poor account of public and private insurance dynamics in the *Chaoulli* decision itself. I discuss the majority judges' poor appreciation of the interface between public and private health insurance across different health care systems and how, subsequently, this lack of understanding has been reflected in media discussions of policy options. I then discuss likely future challenges in other provinces, before moving on to the most critical aspect of all of this — governmental response and what the future holds for Canadian medicare.

The Court's Grasp of Health Care Policy

In *Chaoulli*, Deschamps J., writing for a slim majority (it was a 4:3 decision) dismissed the Quebec government's claim that the law prohibiting private health insurance is needed to protect the public health care system. The majority found this law to be in breach of Quebec's Charter of Human Rights and Freedoms.[55] Deschamps J. did not rule on the Canadian Charter of Rights and Freedoms[56] but the other majority judges — McLachlin C.J. and Major J., writing for themselves and Bastarache J. — did. These three judges concluded that, in addition to breaching the Quebec Charter, the law was "arbitrary" and thus in breach of section 7 of the Canadian Charter and could not be saved by section 1. The minority found Quebec's law prohibiting private insurance did not breach either the Quebec or Canadian Charter. Thus, on the critical issue of the Canadian Charter and the application of

Chaoulli to similar laws in other provinces, the court was split 3:3.

The majority did a quick tour of health care systems around the world. Deschamps J.'s judgment glided over the health care systems in Austria, Germany, the Netherlands, the UK, New Zealand, Australia, and Sweden. Drawing on the Kirby report,[57] McLachlin C.J. and Major J. outlined the basics of the Swiss, German, and British systems with passing reference also to Australia, Singapore, and the United States. Their primary purpose was to demonstrate that public and private insurance coexist in a number of jurisdictions. They concluded "that many western democracies that do not impose a monopoly on the delivery of health care have successfully delivered to their citizens medical services that are *superior to* and *more affordable* than the services that are presently available in Canada [emphasis added]."[58] But they provide no discussion of the factors that lead them to such a damning conclusion.[59] Nor do they note the extensive private insurance industry that already exists in Canada.

There are many errors in the majority judgment and many errors in their conclusions vis-à-vis health policy.[60] Here I will focus on three. First, I contest the characterization of Canada as an oddity in having a goal of preventing a flourishing two-tier system. Second, I contest the conclusion that Canada's system is inferior to other health care systems. Third, and most seriously, I discuss the majority's failure to distinguish between countries that allow parallel or duplicate private health insurance (such as would be allowed after *Chaoulli*) and those countries in which private insurance plays a role (as it does in Canada) but *not* for the purposes of enabling those who hold it to jump wait-list queues. In this context, I discuss the failure of the majority to consider *why* many countries take a range of legal measures to protect their respective public systems from a duplicate private tier. The primary goal of countries that take these measures is to protect valuable capacity (the work time of specialists and other medical professionals) in the public system — a goal that the majority judges completely dismiss.

a. Portraying Canada as an oddity

The majority judges characterize Canada as an outlier from the rest of the world in prohibiting private health insurance for essential hospital and physician services. But, they do not note that Canada is tied for third place in the OECD in 2003 with respect to the extent to which private insurance plays a role in funding the health care system.[61] The private sector, both in financing and delivery, plays a very significant role in the Canadian system already. Where Canada differs (and then only in six provinces including Quebec prior to *Chaoulli*) is in explicitly prohibiting private health insurance for "medically necessary" hospital and physician services. But one cannot write off the Canadian health care system on this basis alone as akin to those within Cuba or North Korea.[62]

Where Canada does not differ from other countries is in trying to suppress through legal means a flourishing private sector for essential care. As I discuss, many countries use a range of other indirect methods apart from expressly prohibiting private health insurance to protect their public systems. As a result of the majority misunderstanding the prevalence of this policy objective, the consequences of *Chaoulli* are much worse than originally envisaged in that it provides the basis for some provincial governments to consider removing the prohibition against doctors working at the same time in both the public and private sectors. In my view, this law performs a much more important role in protecting the public system than the laws banning private health insurance that were the subject of the *Chaoulli* decision. Indeed, the latter is almost a red herring as evidenced by the fact that some provinces (New Brunswick, Newfoundland, Nova Scotia, and Saskatchewan) do not ban private insurance and yet still have no flourishing two-tier system. Why is this? Because other regulation limits the extent to which physicians can or are willing to work in the private sector and unless a significant number of doctors work at least part of their time in the private sector then there are no private services to insure.[63]

The majority judgment written by Deschamps J. acknowledged that laws, such as those prohibiting physicians working simultaneously in the public and private sectors, protect the integrity of public insurance systems. This is both heartening and bewildering given that, on the one hand, she appears to endorse these laws and yet, on the other hand, she rejects Quebec's arguments as to why it is necessary to protect the public tier from private insurance. The same arguments justifying the measures she seems to approve of also justify the law banning private health insurance. If she rejects these arguments in the context of a challenge to a law prohibiting private health insurance for essential care, it is at least possible that the courts may also do so in the context of a direct challenge to other laws, such as those preventing doctors working, simultaneously, in both the public and the private insurance sectors.

McLachlin C.J. and Major J., in their analysis of s.7 of the Canadian Charter, fail to mention that other provinces and a number of European countries take measures (short of prohibiting private health insurance) to severely limit the scope of a duplicate private tier. By ignoring this fact, McLachlin C.J. and Major J. are much more readily able to dismiss the Quebec government's claim that it is a legitimate policy objective to protect public medicare from the emergence of a duplicate private tier. They do so by characterizing Canada's aspirations in this regard as odd compared to other countries. If they had acknowledged that a number of other countries take legal measures to protect their public systems from a duplicate private tier, it would have been much more difficult to describe Quebec's law prohibiting private health insurance as "arbitrary."[64]

b. Portraying Canadian medicare as inferior

McLachlin C.J. and Major J. reach the damning conclusion that other jurisdictions that "do not impose a monopoly" have "delivered to their citizens medical services that are superior to and more affordable than the services that are presently available in Canada."[65] For health policy analysts this is a breathtaking conclusion. The intractability of comparing different health systems is well accepted.[66]

First, with regard to "affordability," presumably they are not speaking from an individual perspective. Further privatization must result in more direct costs to individuals either through private insurance premiums or out-of-pocket payments and thus decreased affordability. I assume, therefore, they are referring to the overall affordability of the system as measured by total spending as a percentage of GDP. Here it is true that Canada is clustered in the top ten of the OECD in terms of total health care spending, but it is not out of line with other countries of comparable wealth.[67] As the wealth of a country increases so does the total percentage of its wealth devoted to health care — in this regard Canada is exactly where it should be in terms of total health care spending.

The fact that Canada spends more on health care than some other countries does not necessarily reveal much about efficiency. It is important to know that, setting aside drug spending, the vast majority of total health care spending is for the remuneration paid to health professionals. Canada pays its skilled professionals higher rates than some other jurisdictions. Indeed many feel that we do not pay these professionals enough. Thus the fact that we spend more on health in Canada than, for example, the UK or New Zealand, does not itself mean that the money is wasted (or at least no more than in any other system).[68] All it means is that we remunerate our health professionals at rates consistent with our total level of wealth.

McLachlin C.J. and Major J. also failed to note that countries with higher rates of private spending (and, as pointed out previously, Canada already records high rates of private spending compared to many other countries) record higher levels of overall spending (public and private combined).[69] For example, the US government already pays more *public* funds per capita (that is government dollars per person) than is paid in Canada despite leaving over 14 percent of the US population uninsured.[70] By extrapolation, it is obvious that allowing more privatization of the system will increase, and not reduce, overall spending or "affordability."

McLachlin C.J. and Major J. boldly state that other countries deliver "superior" medical services than are presently delivered in Canada. Again it is hard to know what they really mean by this. One assumes that they do not mean the quality of individual services delivered to patients by clinicians and hospitals because there is no evidence to support this. One must assume that in the context of the facts of *Chaoulli* they are referring to the problem of wait times and that the "superiority" of other jurisdictions relates to the fact that either there is no waiting or their wait times are lower than those recorded in Canada. But in support of this conclusion they make *no reference at all to wait times in other countries*. Had they done so, they would have found that Canada is far from alone in its struggle with waiting times and that many other countries also struggle with this problem — including those that allow private health insurance for essential services.

A recent review of waiting times in OECD countries irrefutably demonstrates that many countries with two-tier systems (in which citizens may purchase private insurance to cover essential hospital and physician services) *also struggle with waiting lists*. Other countries within which waiting lists are a significant policy concern include Australia, Denmark, Finland, Ireland, Italy, the Netherlands, New Zealand, Norway, Spain, Sweden, and the UK.[71] The Deschamps and the McLachlin/Major judgments each

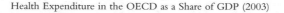

Health Expenditure in the OECD as a Share of GDP (2003)

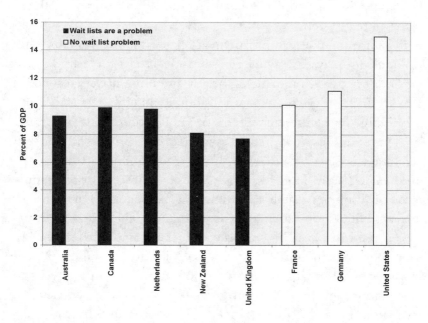

refer favourably to these countries but do not discuss wait times. This oversight is difficult to understand when waiting for care is at the heart of the constitutional challenge before the court. It is also surprising that they did not consider that a number of the countries that do not have wait-list problems have other access problems. The United States for example, does not have a wait-list problem but records 45.8 million people as uninsured.[72] France has very high out-of-pocket payments at the point of service that likely deter those on low incomes from accessing care.[73]

c. *Comparing European apples and oranges*
Another difficulty with both the Deschamps and the McLachlin/Major judgments is that in their summative round-up of the experiences in other health care jurisdictions they fail to distinguish between the different types of systems that combine public and private insurance, assuming that the only purpose of private

insurance is to "top-up" the quality of universal insurance offered in the public system.

The fundamental error is to treat all health care systems, with some role for private insurance, as the same. In fact there are a number of distinct ways of financing health care using private insurance, all with different consequences for equity and efficiency.[74]

I discuss three different systems of public and private insurance. First, I will discuss group-based systems where private insurance is purchased by the wealthy but, in contradistinction to what the *Chaoulli* decision endorses, it is not used primarily for the purposes of jumping wait-list queues, if at all. Second, I will discuss co-payment systems, such as exists in France, where private insurance is used to cover higher out-of-pocket payments imposed in the public system. Third, I will discuss duplicate insurance or two-tier systems where the primary purpose of private insurance is to allow those who hold it to jump wait-list queues. Countries that have these kinds of systems include New Zealand, Ireland, Australia, England, etc., and it is these countries that the court should have closely examined. Here I will also discuss countries, such as Sweden, that ostensibly permit the purchase of private insurance for the purposes of queue jumping, but take other measures — such as preventing physicians working simultaneously in the public and private sectors during working hours — that effectively precludes the development of a two-tier system.

c.1. Solidarity in a group-based system

The court refers favourably to the Netherlands and Germany but these countries are not operating two-tier systems in the sense the majority in *Chaoulli* has in mind, where individuals are allowed to buy parallel or duplicate private coverage to jump queues in the public system. The Netherlands and Germany each have what I would characterize as a group-based system. In group-based systems private insurers *do not* perform a duplicate role as would be allowed by the *Chaoulli* decision, allowing people to jump queues for treatment. Instead private insurance must provide *full* (as opposed to duplicate) coverage for the wealthier segments of the population that buy it.

To elaborate, in the Netherlands, an individual earning less than Euros 33,000 ($48,886CAD) must contribute to and is eligible for social insurance that is similar in its progressive nature to Canadian medicare, although it is not financed primarily out of general taxation revenues but rather out of employer and employee contributions. Dutch citizens earning *more* than Euros 33,000 are not insured by the social insurance scheme but can, if they wish, buy private insurance — most do. The private insurance they purchase, however, does not "top-up" coverage in the public system as allowed by *Chaoulli*: it must cover *all* the needs of those who elect to buy it.[75]

To reiterate and underscore the fact that buying private insurance does not allow queue jumping or preferential treatment, regulation requires that Dutch specialists be paid the same fee by private insurers as by the social insurers.[76] Moreover, it is part of the ethical code of Dutch physicians not to treat patients with social insurance or private insurance differently.[77]

To be clear — and in case you are wondering why anyone would purchase private health insurance — wealthier individuals are not publicly insured. If they do not buy private insurance then they are uninsured. In short, through different means the Dutch system achieves a similarly progressive outcome as Canada medicare; access to essential care is determined on the basis of need and not ability to pay. Private health insurance has a role but it is just a way of funding the system as opposed to enabling those with means to get faster or better care. *Chaoulli*, though, finds that there is effectively a constitutional right on the part of those with means to buy their way to the front of wait-list queues.

c.2. Co-payment systems

Co-payment systems also provide public coverage but impose large co-payments or user charges, and therefore allow the purchase of private health insurance to help defray these out-of-pocket costs. This occurs in the US medicare system (for those over 65) and in France. In France, the co-payments range from 20 percent on hospital care, 35 percent (usually) on prescription drugs and 30 percent for private physician visits (the majority of physicians in France practise privately and provide day treatments or day surgeries). The co-payments are intended to promote patient responsibility in using health care resources, but the extent to which it achieves this goal is limited by the fact that over 90 percent of the French hold some kind of private insurance to help them cover the cost of the co-payment. For those without insurance, the co-payment may have the adverse effect of limiting access to services. So although France does not appear to have a wait-list issue, this may be due to the fact that some people cannot pay the high out-of-pocket costs required to access the system (so, they don't get into the system to wait). In addition to co-payments, access in France is also limited by the requirement that patients pay a health care professional up front for a service and submit the bill twice, once, to their social security insurer for partial reimbursement and a second time to their private insurer to recover the co-payment.[78]

In France, citizens buy private health insurance to cover the cost of co-payments and user-charges imposed in the public sphere. The level of private insurance varies; the best coverage is usually linked to type of employment and income. As a result, the lowest income earners in France have the least private insurance coverage and the highest co-payments.[79] In order to remedy this problem, in part, *public* complementary insurance was put in place for the most poor in 2000.

As in a number of other countries, to prevent the loss of doctors from the public to the private sector,[80] France requires that the fee charged by a doctor in the private sector be set by a government committee (doctors in the public system are paid on salary). From 1980, the rules were modified and any privately practising doctor could become what is known as a *Secteur 2* doctor and bill above the government-set tariff; but concerns about fairness, access, and the failure of price competition to manifest itself resulted in a change in policy in the early 1990s.[81] The new policy dramatically reduced the number of doctors able to qualify to practise in *Secteur 2* (and thus charge whatever private fee they wished to). Currently, about 24 percent of French doctors are in the private *Secteur 2* and are able to bill at fees that are higher than the public tariff, but this percentage will decrease due to the fact that only a very limited number of new doctors can earn the right to be classified as *Secteur 2* each year. [82] Thus France, too, takes measures to protect the integrity of its public system and the loss of doctors from the public to the private sector.

Why would France do this if there are no adverse ramifications in allowing private-pay patients to buy their way to the front of queues?

c.3. The right comparison: Countries with duplicate or "top-up" private insurance

Both the Dutch and German group model and the French co-payment model are very different from the kind of system likely to emerge in Canada post-*Chaoulli*.

In order to mimic the European models touted by the majority as superior to the Canadian system the entire funding base of medicare would have to change, shifting from tax-funded to social insurance premiums. Moreover, the other extensive social welfare programs of Northern European countries would need to be implemented. If we were to follow the French model, large user charges and out-of-pocket payments would need to be introduced at point of service (in France they are about 30 percent of the specialist fee[83]), government subsidies put in place to help the poor cover the cost, and the number of Canadians with private insurance would have to rise to approximately 90 percent of the population. If we are to replicate either the German or Dutch models, wealthier citizens would either be excluded (the Dutch model) or given a once-in-a-lifetime opt-out (Germany) from the public system and would have to pay for insurance covering *all* their health care needs. In contrast to these models the majority judges in *Chaoulli* assumed that all Canadians would retain public insurance, but with an allowance for those with means to spend relatively marginal amounts of money to achieve preferential treatment and to buy their way to the front of queues. This would produce in Canada what is best described as a duplicate or top-up private insurance system.

Post-*Chaoulli* the Canadian system may more likely come to resemble the systems in New Zealand, the UK, Australia, Ireland, Sweden, Spain, Luxembourg, Greece, and Italy. It is these countries that the court should have considered in detail and not countries like the Netherlands, Germany, and France, which are too dissimilar in fundamental respects to be comparable. In the former countries, private insurance *duplicates* coverage of services that are publicly insured. Frequently, countries with duplicate public insurance have problems with waiting lists.[84] For example, an article I wrote with colleagues at the University of Toronto that was quoted by Deschamps J. in support of the different configurations of public and private insurance, also included data showing that reported waiting lists in the UK and New Zealand were, respectively, three and five times longer at this time than waiting lists reported by the Fraser Institute in Canada.[85] This research was not commented on nor was it rebutted. In countries where wait times have been a significant problem — New Zealand, Ireland, UK, etc. — physicians work in both the public and private sectors, with specialists "topping-up" their public sector incomes by private payment.

It is true that, recently, waiting lists in New Zealand and England appear to have been reduced. But there are two critically important factors to consider before leaping to any adverse conclusions about the relative merits of the Canadian system. The first is that reduction in waiting lists in the England is due to the injection of large sums of public funding into the National Health Service and *not* to an expansion of the role for private health insurance. The Blair government tried to ameliorate the effects of allowing duplicate private health insurance in England by new contracts with consultants that limit the amount of time they can spend in the private sector and how many hours of the day they must actually work for their public sector salaries.

In New Zealand wait lists have been reduced by managerial fiat: now an individual cannot be put on a public wait list unless the system is able to meet his or her needs within six months. If the system cannot cope, the patient is sent back to his or her family doctor to "manage" her needs until the public system is able to meet them or the patient pays for the service privately — a de facto queue has formed for the waiting list. But these "waiting lists" for the real waiting lists are not centrally recorded and cannot be readily used to criticize government performance. This latter experience illustrates that it is easier to ration more harshly in a system where the political elites are not subjected to the rationing process because they hold private health insurance — a phenomena discounted by the majority.

c. 4. Measures taken in countries that allow two-tier to limit private insurance
Many countries that prima facie allow top-up or duplicate private health insurance (they do not have a law explicitly prohibiting it) have other laws to stop the deleterious effects of the private tier

on the public system. For example, McLachlin C.J. and Major J. discuss the small amount of private insurance in Sweden, but fail to mention that physicians there are restricted from working inside normal office hours in the private sector. In effect, Swedish physicians must choose one or the other, and the inability to operate primarily in the public system with a top-up from the private sector provides a brake on the extent to which the private sector can develop at the expense of the public system. Similar measures are taken in other two-tier systems, namely Luxembourg, Greece, and Italy.[86] The UK is moving to regulate the amount of time that specialists work in the public hospitals so limiting the amount of time they can spend in private clinics. Why would these countries take these measures, if, as the majority concludes, there is no basis for concern in allowing a private tier? In Canada, similar laws exist in every province except for Newfoundland.[87] Presumably, in Newfoundland the potential private market is insufficient to flourish even in the absence of laws suppressing it.

McLachlin C.J. and Major J. conclude that Quebec's law prohibiting private health insurance fails to accord with the principles of fundamental justice on the basis that it is "arbitrary." They justify this conclusion because, from their cursory review of the dynamics of other jurisdictions, they conclude that public and private insurance coexists in certain countries and infer that the former remains viable. They dismiss arguments about the detrimental effects of a private tier on the public system, merely on the basis that in other countries public and private insurance coexist.

As I have shown, the dynamics of public and private insurance and regulation is far more complex than they allow for, and many jurisdictions take measures to try to achieve the same goal as in Quebec — namely protecting the public system from a private sector.[88]

c.5. The problem of capacity being transferred from the public to the private sectors

Why do countries have laws, for example, preventing physicians from receiving both public insurance and private payment for the delivery of essential services? The key issue is one of capacity: that is, the time specialists and medical professionals spend working in the public system. If specialists are free to work simultaneously in the public and private systems then a disproportionate amount of their time will be spent in the private sector, a problem that will be exacerbated by the differences in fees paid by the respective sectors.[89] In other words, to the extent that prices are higher in the private sector and if specialists are free to do so, they will devote an increasing proportion of their time to private patients who are likely to have less acute or serious needs than those patients left behind in the public system. This is not, as the majority judges variously allege, merely a "theoretical"[90] argument, or one based only on "human reactions,"[91] or one merely grounded in "common sense"[92] as opposed to evidence.

Evidence in support of this includes the fact that many countries have similar laws. Why take these measures if there is no concern about capacity? Apart from this there is more direct evidence. For example, New Zealand has a two-tier system in which specialists are free to work in both the public and private spheres. It has had a chronic problem with waiting lists (although, these are now not reported centrally).[93] The New Zealand Medical Council reports that in 2000, New Zealand specialists spent just 48.9 percent of their time working in public hospitals. Most of the rest of the time was devoted to their private practices.[94] The consequences for public sector wait lists, and the public sector itself in Canada, would be enormous if specialists were allowed to devote just 50 percent of their time to working in public hospitals as is the case in New Zealand's two-tier system, even allowing for significant increases in productivity (as in, physicians working more efficiently or longer hours when allowed to work both in the public and private tier). Inevitably, wait lists in the public system would lengthen. Moreover, there would be profound and lingering effects on, for example, the amount of time that specialists would spend training junior doctors in the public system.

There is also judicial recognition in other countries of the relationship between waiting lists and a duplicate private insurance system. *The Commerce Commission* v. *The Ophthalmological Society of New Zealand*[95] involved a NZ health funding authority that was seeking to reduce long public sector waiting times for cataract surgery by contracting with Australian ophthalmologists to perform 225 operations during January 1997. The court found that the group of NZ ophthalmologists and their Society breached s. 27 of the Commerce Act (New Zealand's competition legislation) by being party to an arrangement designed to hinder entry by Australian doctors into the New Zealand routine cataract surgery market. The judgment includes excerpts from correspondence that make very clear the connection between long waiting times in the public system and surgeons' personal income. In a letter to the funding authority, one of the doctors involved describes the marked reduction in public waiting times for cataract surgery that would occur as a result of the proposed extra surgery and how that would detrimentally affect his private practice:

> Whilst this will have a devastating effect on my private practice with a markedly reduced number of private cataract referrals and cataract operations at Southern Cross Hospital over the new year or more as more people opt for public hospital surgery, my ongoing commitment to the Public Hospital Service now and in the future is however such that I am still prepared to assist just as I did when I performed the extra 66 out-patient clinics seeing 700 extra new patients over the

last 2 years when it would have clearly been financially more advantageous for me not to have done this.[96]

The Court concludes that this particular surgeon knew of the impact that shorter waiting times in the public system would have on his private income and despite his protestations to the contrary had worked actively to thwart efforts to employ Australian surgeons to reduce public sector waiting times.

In the UK too, historically specialists have been free to work simultaneously in the public and private sectors. In recognition of the concern that consultants are spending too much time treating private patients and insufficient time treating hips and knees in the publicly funded system, the UK government has recently tried to introduce productivity measures in the public sector.[97] In its evidence to the Health Select Committee in 2000, the UK Department of Health stated that there was a statistical correlation between those specialties with the longest waiting lists and those specialties where private practice earnings make up a substantial part of consultants' incomes.[98] The UK Select Committee on Health (2000) ultimately recommended that physicians be prohibited from simultaneously working in the public and private sectors.[99]

A recent study (2005) in Australia also clearly demonstrated that the higher the proportion of private activity in any particular sector, the longer the wait in the public system.[100]

Within Canada itself, there is clear evidence about the detrimental impact on public sector waiting lists from allowing a private tier in which physicians can work simultaneously in both the public and private spheres. A 1998 study in Manitoba of cataract surgery which, for a period, was provided by cataract surgeons who were free to work in both sectors, showed that waiting times were, unsurprisingly, lowest of all for private-pay patients (about four weeks). They were higher for services provided by surgeons who practised only in the public sector (ten weeks). But they were *highest of all (twenty-three weeks)* for publicly financed services provided by surgeons who practised simultaneously in both sectors.[101] It is extremely worrying that this evidence was before the majority judges but they nonetheless dismissed the views of expert witnesses on the ground that they did not "present economic studies."[102] One assumes that this evidence was discounted because it did not directly speak to the law banning private health insurance; it does of course speak to the rationale behind the law for banning private health insurance.

McLachlin C.J. and Major J. found that the Quebec government has acted "arbitrarily" in precluding the purchase of private health insurance. If there were really no substance to the concerns of a private tier operating in tandem with a public tier why do the governments of Sweden, Luxembourg, Greece, and Italy (not to mention all provinces in Canada except for Newfoundland) effectively prevent physicians working both sides of the fence — being paid from the public purse and "topping up" their incomes by supplying the same medically necessary care to private-pay patients? Why has the UK government tried to introduce measures into consultants' contracts to make sure they spend more time treating public hips and knees?[103] Are *all* these governments "arbitrary" in their policy choices? This seems unlikely. If one accepts those laws as justifiable because of concerns about capacity then Quebec's law prohibiting private health insurance can be similarly justified.

The Impact of *Chaoulli* on Public Debate and Policy

In the realm of public debate, *Chaoulli* seems to have unleashed the idea that Canadians can have their private insurance cake and medicare too. On the positive side, *Chaoulli* has opened the door for politicians and citizens to discuss openly the possibility of a greater role for private health insurance without the risk of being called heretics. On the negative side *Chaoulli* has enabled those who favour privatization to promote a role for more private financing without having to explain the logistics of such a system.[104] The message of those advocating privatization is that medicare clearly does not work, a private system can only make things better, and the provinces should be free to experiment with combining the two.

a. Supporters of medicare

Those who support a single-payer publicly funded system in Canada have lost credibility by conflating the issues of private *funding* and private *delivery*. Proponents of medicare rail, for example, against P3 hospitals in Ontario, which would be fully publicly funded and thus raise no equity concerns, or private cancer clinics, which too are fully publicly funded. The leader of the NDP, Jack Layton, has clouded the debate further by saying that his party is opposed to any public funding flowing to private clinics.[105] He has however been challenged on the grounds that he himself attended the Shouldice clinic, a private for-profit hospital that specializes in hernia operations that is fully publicly funded.[106]

One has to distinguish between funding and delivery, and then with respect to delivery, between delivery by not-for-profit and delivery by for-profit firms. There are legitimate concerns about the quality of care delivered by private for-profit institutions in some settings but not in all. In my view the issue of not-for-profit *vs.* for-profit *delivery* is not as critical as the issue of access to care as embodied in the distinction between public and private *financing*. Where both financing and delivery become conflated is in the issue of private clinics, for example private MRI clinics, that supply both publicly and privately financed care. That these clinics are condoned is extremely problematic as it raises starkly the problem of physicians having an incentive to build up their more lucrative private practices rather than treating public patients. Similarly, there are concerns with the advent of private clinics that charge annual fees (for example, the Copeman clinic plans to charge $2,300 annually) to patients but argue they are in compliance with provincial laws by billing the public sector for "medically necessary" physician services.[107] The annual fees, ostensibly, are to cover non-insured services but may well be used to indirectly subsidize physicians who work there (treating far fewer patients than usual) in the provision of public health care.

Nonetheless, vocal opposition to *all* things private simply clouds the issues of what really is at stake in *Chaoulli*, and that is the raw prospect of a two-tier system such as exists in New Zealand, Ireland, and the UK, and the prospect that waiting lists in the public system will get worse and not better.

Because the most vocal opponents of privatization in Canada have been fighting the battle of private *delivery*, they have been caught off balance, ill-prepared to fight the battle against private health *insurance*. The opposition to *all* things private makes it easy to discount them as zealots, just as the proponents of privatization used to be written off as zealots. So, for example, Phillipe Couillard, health minister of Quebec, is quoted as saying "I believe there is a place for private health care in our system ... there appears to be a perversion of the debate here in Canada and particularly in Quebec. There are some people who associate any intrusion of private delivery of the health-care system with some kind of social backwardness."[108] But Minister Couillard's remarks are misleading — there is already extensive private delivery in the Canadian health care system. But *Chaoulli* is not about delivery — it is about financing. Notice how Dr. Couillard carefully avoids talking about private insurance, private financing, two-tier systems, or queue jumping — which is actually what *Chaoulli* requires — and speaks in the far more reasonable rhetoric of private delivery, even though at the time he spoke his government was contemplating reform of financing.

b. Newspaper commentary

Media commentary has grossly oversimplified the debates about public and private health insurance. The poor grasp of health policy reflected in the judgment of the Supreme Court has been replicated in the media and particularly in relation to the experiences of other jurisdictions. I will provide three examples here, all from one national newspaper, the *Globe and Mail*. I acknowledge that this limited sampling does not provide a scientific basis for proving the media's poor grasp of health policy and I do not claim to do so. I only hope to demonstrate through a few examples the potential scope of the problem.

The first is a commentary by Lysiane Gagnon who states that in its approach to public funding of health care, "Canada is in a league with Cuba and North Korea."[109] She neglects to note, not only that Canada ranks third in the world for the percentage of total spending paid for by private health insurance, but that the Canadian system allows a significant amount of autonomy and freedom in delivery. By comparison, physicians in the UK, New Zealand, and Ireland, for example, (not to mention Cuba and North Korea) are salaried state employees and hospitals are owned by the state. By effectively dismissing the medicare system as akin to a system in a communist country, she denigrates its larger objective of providing access to necessary care on the basis of need and not wealth, which Canada does through a plurality of funding and delivery mechanisms.

Gagnon goes on in the same piece to point out that the Quebec minister of health has said that Quebec should find inspiration in countries like France, the UK, and Sweden that allow two-tier systems. She notes "only a diehard ideologue, or someone who hasn't traveled much, can argue that countries like France and Sweden, whose institutions were built by a succession of socialist governments, have an unfair system." Ms Gagnon is likely unaware that in Sweden physicians employed in the public system are limited from working in the private sector, and so, as a consequence, the private insurance sector is very small. She is also probably unaware that private health insurance in France is primarily used to pay for large out-of-pocket costs and that many doctors are prevented from billing privately more than a government-set tariff. Ms. Gagnon, whilst travelling in Sweden and France, likely did not explore the complexities of public, private, and social health insurance.

Similarly, Jeffrey Simpson stokes confusion around the sustainability and affordability of medicare. In a number of columns he argues that the rate of spending on the health care system is unsustainable and privatization is the solution.[110] He does not advocate complete privatization but, rather, for medicare to continue with a supplementary role for private health insurance — the New Zealand, UK, Irish (and *Chaoulli*) model. He does not acknowledge a well known truth of health spending, however, namely that 10 percent of patients account for well over 70 percent of total spending costs — they have chronic needs or catastrophic conditions.[111] Supplementary or complementary private insurers will not cover these people and their health care needs unless they are forced to do so by governmental regulation: in other words, the public system must continue to absorb the costs of complex and costly care. Unless Simpson is prepared to advocate complete privatization, either, of certain expensive classes of services, or of health care for certain groups of people (for example, the wealthy), then the introduction of private insurance to allow individuals to jump queues for hip operations and cataract surgery will not improve the sustainability of the public system.

A third and final example is demonstrated in an editorial in the *Globe and Mail* published on December 7, 2005.[112] It was stated that "in two months, Quebec will launch a fierce debate about private care. It has no choice. The Supreme Court of Canada said in June that people are suffering and dying because of waits in the public system, and that Quebec is violating its own rights charter by not letting them buy private health insurance for essential care. The court gave Quebec until June 9 to allow private insurance."

This editorial mischaracterizes what *Chaoulli* requires. Quebec laws are only unconstitutional given unacceptable wait times in the public system. The most obvious solution — and one that would benefit all Quebeckers and not just those able to afford private insurance or qualify for it — is to reduce wait times in the public system.

Uncertainty and Future Litigation

Lamenting *Chaoulli* is to some extent crying over spilt milk; it will likely be many years before the court is able to revisit its conclusions. But in the interim we can expect litigation across the country. Litigation will be instituted by those hoping to break open restrictions on the private sector, for example private clinics.[113]

What we can expect to see are Charter challenges to other laws and not necessarily laws that ban private health insurance. This is because in reality the ban on private health insurance is probably not as important as the other laws across the country suppressing a developing second tier. In an article in 2001 in the *Canadian Medical Association Journal,* Tom Archibald and I documented the myriad pieces of provincial legislation that cumulatively provide disincentives for a flourishing duplicate private tier. We concluded that:

> In Canada, the absence of a private system is not due to the illegality of private health care per se. Private insurance for the kinds of medically necessary hospital and physician services that the public service is meant to cover is illegal in only 6 provinces. However, there has been no development of a significant private sector in New Brunswick, Newfoundland, Nova Scotia or

Saskatchewan, all of which permit private insurance coverage without any restriction on the extent of the coverage, although as noted Nova Scotia is the only province among these 4 that caps the fees of all physicians (whether opted in or out) at the public plan rates. Rather, the lack of a flourishing private sector in Canada is most likely attributable to prohibitions on subsidization of private practice from the public plan, prohibitions that prevent physicians from relying on the public sector for the core of their incomes and turning to the private sector to top up their incomes.[114]

Given this, we are likely to see challenges, not only to laws prohibiting the sale of private insurance for essential services, but to other laws that, in my opinion, are of greater significance in protecting the private tier. For example, we can expect to see challenges to the laws in Ontario that prevent doctors opting out to practice in the private sector, and to laws in Nova Scotia and Manitoba that preclude a physician charging more privately than is paid publicly for a "medically necessary" service. We can also expect to see challenges to the laws in Alberta, British Columbia, New Brunswick, Quebec, Saskatchewan, and Prince Edward Island that effectively prevent the public sector from subsidizing the privately financed sector, for example, by providing that patients who opt to use the services of a private physician receive no public monies to pay for them.

Of course, what is not known is how a court will approach a challenge to laws that more indirectly undercut a private tier than a ban on private health insurance. The difficulty for challengers will be that laws, such as those that provide disincentives to physicians to practise privately, indirectly, rather than directly, achieve the goal of suppressing a private tier. Still, it is conceivable that a court might accept that even these more indirect prohibitions could be considered legitimate targets for challenge. They, prima facie, seem to be about the economic rights of doctors, and given that economic or contractual rights are not protected by s.7, it will be much more difficult to build the nexus to an infringement of life, liberty, and security of the person as was done in *Chaoulli*. But regardless of the merit of these kind of claims and their likelihood of success before the courts, some provincial governments may preempt the needs for such challenges by voluntarily changing these laws using *Chaoulli* as a justification.

Governmental Response

There are a number of possible governmental responses to the Chaoulli decision and we have seen and are seeing different approaches to the question across the country.

a. Reduce wait times

The first (and best) response is to rise to the challenge and improve wait times within the province in question such that, if put to the test, the province in question will be able to demonstrate at trial that the waits are reasonable. Thus any law prohibiting the flourishing of a private tier is not in contravention of s.7 of the Charter. To date, that has been the Ontario government's response, for example through its Wait Time Strategy.[115]

Wait times are beginning to be managed better across the country and if success could be claimed on that ground then the law prohibiting private health insurance would no longer be constitutionally suspect.[116] *Chaoulli* would then have achieved what many claimed to be the ultimate goal of those (including the Canadian Medical Association and members of the Senate) who intervened in support of the constitutional challenge. These interveners supported the *Chaoulli* challenge on the grounds that the court needed to provide the equivalent of a swift kick-in-the-butt to lazy governments by telling them that they are not entitled to preserve a "monopoly" on public health insurance if they don't eliminate wait times.[117] This would certainly be the best and most optimistic interpretation of the *Chaoulli* decision. On the other hand, as I discuss further, it is equally plausible that some governments will be more than happy to give up their "monopoly" on health care.

b. Charter-proof through legal reforms

The other response open to provinces is to improve safety-valve mechanisms — that is, to provide ways for patients who have been waiting for treatment to have their case reviewed and treatment expedited if necessary either within the province, in another province, or in the United States (in essence, a care guarantee). [118] Each member of the Supreme Court agreed that an adequate appeal mechanism was an important determinant as to whether the Quebec laws prohibiting private health insurance were constitutional. In other words, a province may be able to protect its laws from Charter challenge if it provides some sort of timely and independent means to assess when someone has had to wait too long for care and to provide a remedy. This remedy could take the form of ensuring immediate treatment within the province or paying for treatment in another province or country. So far there has been little movement on the part of any province to embed such protections.

The new Conservative government promised a care guarantee.[119] It, however, met a wall of resistance in its attempt to persuade provincial governments to put in place such guarantees and has been hamstrung by its commitment to provincial autonomy. This has precluded more heavy-handed measures to implement a guarantee. The Conservative government response was to announce "patient wait time guarantees' (PWTGs) pilot programs for prenatal care, diabetes, and six surgical areas for children in ten First Nations communities.[120] The idea was that the

Conservative government would implement PWTG where it had constitutional jurisdiction to do so and to benefit a population with very high health needs, thus leading the way for country wide uptake of PWTGS.

There are two problems. First, although it is laudable to improve wait times for First Nations communities, arguably any additional resources would be better employed improving their primary health care and addressing issues like clean water supply, housing, and sanitation. Also, the initiatives seem mostly to be aimed at an area where the specified wait time was already in large part being met; in effect, then, the PWTG is being employed more as a confirmation of a system working well, rather than a method to improve upon the system.

More recently, the federal government in March 2007, launched a Patient Wait Time Guarantees Program,[121] pursuant to which the ten provinces and the three territories agreed (with the carrot of a $612 million federal trust fund) to establish PWTG by 2010.[122] But in what areas and for what standards is largely to be left in the hands of the various provinces leaving one to speculate whether there will be any real substance to the initiative.

c. Capitulate and/or celebrate and allow private health insurance
The third option available to provinces is to celebrate *Chaoulli* and allow the introduction of a supplementary private tier.

In *Chaoulli* the key problem was characterized by the applicant as a government monopoly on health insurance for essential services. Supporters of *Chaoulli*, such as Stanley Hartt, have said that government, as a monopolist, must either improve its performance or "get out of the way" so that people can look after themselves.[123] The characterization of government as monopolist, as opposed to the provider of a unique public good, belies the fact that many governments for fiscal, political, or ideological reasons may be more than happy to give up the on-going battle to maintain one-tier medicare. If the most vocal and politically connected members of the electorate shift to the private insurance sector, this will likely alleviate some of the pressure on provincial governments to perform well. It would likely make it easier for governments to harshly ration services in the public sector, particularly those covered by private insurance (for example, hip and knee surgery).[124] Governments may also be tempted by the idea (even if it is not borne out in practice) that creation of a second tier would reduce the work that has to be done by the public sector. Some governments will be tempted by the idea, not for fiscal reasons but for pure ideological reasons, namely that choice and the market should be allowed to operate freely in health care regardless of merit or consequences.

d. Quebec's choice

These choices in response confront the government of Quebec most directly since it is its laws that were the subject of *Chaoulli*. It asked for an eighteen-month stay in order to be able to better prepare itself or respond to the overturning of the law prohibiting private health insurance. The court granted twelve months.[125]

To understand Quebec's response on this issue some context is important. Quebec has long allowed private clinics to flourish within the province (in contravention of the Canada Health Act (R.S. 1985, c. C-6)), and it appears that in these clinics physicians are providing "medically necessary" services in both the public and private sectors. For example, a *Gazette* article[126] reports that two Westmount medical clinics are charging patients substantial fees for quick access to day surgery and other procedures; the doctors at the Westmount Square Surgical Centre and MD Specialists also bill the Quebec medicare board for those procedures. The federal government, however, has failed to stop this.[127]

To the extent that a supplementary private tier is already tolerated in some measure in Quebec, *Chaoulli* may well be viewed as an opportunity to expand the boundaries of that tier, to legitimize existing practice, and, perhaps, to put some other rules of the game in place. In other words, *Chaoulli* may have been greeted behind closed doors by the Quebec government with relief rather than chagrin.

The initial signs suggest that the Quebec government would use the *Chaoulli* decision as support for further privatization of the Quebec system in ways not required by the terms of the decision. Premier Jean Charest is reported as saying in the National Assembly that he had received an "order" from the Supreme Court of Canada to make room for the private sector in the health care system. It was reported that Quebec is proposing to allow doctors to practice both in the publicly funded system and in a parallel system financed by private funds in which private insurance companies would play a role. As six Quebec law professors point out in an opinion editorial in the *Gazette*, the Supreme Court issued no such order and, of course, it is perfectly open to the Quebec government to respond by reducing wait times for all, rather than opening a private tier.[128]

On February 16, 2006, the Quebec government released its proposed response to *Chaoulli*.[129] The Quebec proposals include a broad range of initiatives, but from the perspective of a direct impact on the wait lists, the most pertinent reform proposal is the implementation of two different types of care guarantee.

The first care guarantee is with regard to radio-oncology, cancer surgery, and advanced cardiac care. The proposal read that the guarantee will provide for a three month maximum wait, then the public sector will pay for your care in a private clinic or outside of Quebec. No private insurance may be purchased to cover this kind of care. The irony is, of course, that in countries with duplicate private insurance, private insurers don't insure this kind of care — it is too expensive and not profitable enough. In other words, even if it were lawful to sell and buy it, the market would not materialize for it in Quebec (or anywhere else).

The second kind of care guarantee covers hip, knee, and cataract surgery — in these cases the guarantee is that after a six month wait, the government will pay for treatment in a private clinic. If a patient is still waiting after nine months, then the government will pay for her care out-of-province. The proposal provides that for these kinds of care — that is hip, knee, and cataract surgery — patients can now buy private insurance for *these services only*. So the impugned law at the heart of the *Chaoulli* decision will be liberalized but only to the extent of allowing the sale of private insurance for hip, knee, and cataract surgery.

The Quebec government's response has, to date, been measured and contains a variety of disincentives for a two-tier system to flourish. The proposals cut across the gambit of possible public/private solutions to the *Chaoulli* decision, which I outlined, with a little bit of this and a little bit of that, they are what I would characterize as a Goldilocks solution — a sophisticated response to the *Chaoulli* decision, balancing the demands of the court with the reality of health policy.

First, the introduction of wait time guarantees within the publicly funded health care system is a public fix to a public problem and the most optimal response one could hope for to the *Chaoulli* decision. However, significant change within the system will be required to get wait times down, change that many players have long been resistant to. For example, the centralization of wait lists — out of doctors' desk drawers and into regional or provincial management, creating more capacity by changing the scope of practice.

Second, the proposals provide for a much more significant kind of reform in terms of public funding and private for-profit delivery. Rather than taking on the difficult political task of changing practices within public medicare — and challenging many vested interests — the easier response is to bring in more capacity by allowing delivery by private for-profit clinics but publicly funded. This is what I'd call the middle ground and follows the response to waiting times by Tony Blair's government in England — the system remains publicly funded but extra capacity is injected into the system by allowing private clinics.

This is, of course, a much preferable option in terms of access than allowing a duplicate private tier as endorsed by the Supreme Court of Canada. It tries to ensure improved access for *all* Quebeckers. Allowing delivery by private clinics might get around some of the embedded stickiness associated with expanding public hospitals (by this I mean, if you expand capacity in a public hospital it is virtually impossible to reduce it later if needs change). But there are still many concerns with this option. The experience in England suggests we need to be attentive to the following possibilities:

a. the bifurcation of responsibility between public hospitals and private clinics with the former getting the tough cases and the latter the easier cases, often at higher rates of remuneration;

b. problems associated with the training offered to junior doctors in hospitals when the easiest kinds of care is no longer performed in public hospitals;

c. the reality that bringing on extra capacity will most likely result in extra public spending and result in additional concerns for provincial governments around sustainability;

d. and, finally, that in the absence of new resources or greater efficiencies, money spent on managing waiting time may well be at the expense of other needs.

The final plank of the Quebec government's proposals that I will discuss is removing the law prohibiting private health insurance. It is interesting that the Quebec government is not proposing to defend this law given its proposals for wait time guarantees. Senator Kirby and the Canadian Medical Association argued before the Supreme Court that wait times guarantees would be the only way for the Quebec government to be able to legitimate the law prohibiting private health insurance. So why liberalize the law given that wait time guarantees are promised?

On a very positive note, the Quebec government appears to have been (at least temporarily) persuaded by those who reacted strongly to early suggestions that the law prohibiting doctors working in both the public and the private sectors should be liberalized. The Quebec government says it will keep this law. Currently, there are only 100 Quebec doctors that choose to opt out of the public system and practise privately — far more than in any other province. We will have to see whether or not the demand for private insurance will significantly increase the extent of the private market and thus the enticement for doctors to move from the public to the private sector or, as I have argued here, that the effect will not be significant unless and until doctors are able to work simultaneously in the public and private sectors. In any event, the Quebec government also stated that it would consider restricting the number of doctors opting out if the numbers become too high and deplete public system resources.

Since the last Quebec election and the rise in prominence of the Action Démocratique party (which included in its platform plans for two-tier Medicine) there have been more disturbing rumblings indicating further privatization plans. In the May 2007 election, the Quebec government announced the appointment of Claude Castonguay to head up a new commission on the future of health care financing in Quebec. He is known as the father of Quebec medicare and his recent conversion to privatization will likely not only impact the report that he provides but also shape public opinion.[130]

Conclusion

Let me conclude, in the spirit of media sound-bites, with the top ten reasons why, despite what their politicians, the media, and a majority of the Supreme Court are telling them, Canadians should not embrace private health insurance for essential hospital and physician services.

10. Countries in which private spending is high spend more in total on health care, not less. The United States already spends more public dollars per capita than Canada does, and leaves 48 million Americans uninsured.

9. We have a shortage of doctors and nurses. Most developed countries do. Wealthier provinces are luring doctors from poorer provinces. This problem will be exacerbated with the introduction of private insurance coverage for services that are presently publicly insured, such as hip operations. Doctors will move their business into the private tier. They will do work that is elective in nature for the not-so-needy, leaving those with greater need to wait even longer for care in the public system.

8. A two-tier system is one in which you can buy private insurance to jump queues and doctors are free to work part of their day in the public system doing public hip operations for public-pay patients and part of the day in the private system doing hip operations for those who pay privately. This is what is being mooted by the Quebec and Alberta governments as a good idea. That it is not a good idea is demonstrated by countries that already have two-tier systems, like the UK, New Zealand, and Ireland, where they have very long public waiting lists. Why copy them?

7. In countries that have two-tier systems often only a relatively small percentage of the population holds private health insurance (for example 11.4 percent of UK citizens); their doing so is closely associated with wealth. In other words, the vast majority of Canadians would not benefit from being able to buy

private health insurance as either they will not qualify for it or they won't be able to afford the premiums.

6. From the perspective of a private insurance company, if you are on a waiting list you do not have an insurable risk. You don't have a risk of disease or illness, you *have* the disease or illness — current needs that must be met. If you can't pay cash, the public system is your only option. Mr. Zeliotis, the patient at the heart of the Supreme Court's decision in *Chaoulli*, exposes the fallacy in the idea that private health insurance will fix our waiting list problems. Mr. Zeliotis, 65 years old and with pre-existing heart and hip conditions simply would not qualify for private health insurance, at least for those conditions.

5. Don't buy the baloney that Canadian medicare is in league with communist states like Cuba and North Korea. We are third in the world in terms of the contribution of private health insurance to the funding of our system. Physicians and hospitals are not respectively employed and owned by the state. We already have a significant level of private financing and private delivery, higher than many other developed countries. The real question is whether privatizing insurance for essential hospital and physician services will make our system better or worse.

4. NAFTA requires that we must compensate US-based private insurers for denying them access to Canadian "markets" if we subsequently change our mind about the benefits of two-tier insurance.[131]

3. Many countries (for example, Sweden) and nearly all provinces protect the public system by way of laws limiting the extent to which doctors employed and paid by the public sector can be employed and paid by the private system. In Canada the relevant laws require that doctors either work wholly in the public sector or wholly in the private sector. These laws are critical to ensure a high standard of access and quality in the public health care system.

2. Governments and health care providers can fix wait lists. Together they have been able to achieve extraordinary improvements, for example, in cardiac care treatments in Ontario and with respect to orthopaedic services in Alberta.[132] There is now little or no waiting for diagnosis and treatment; most of these gains have been achieved as a result of better coordination of existing resources and our talent. We can and will do it in other areas. Victory is within our grasp.

1. **And the top reason why we shouldn't allow private health insurance for essential services?** Access to essential care should be based on need and not ability to pay. If resources are constricted we should revisit what is essential but not allow a two-tier system for what are core services. We should run a health care, not a wealth care system.

CHAPTER 16

Bill 33: The Fallout from the *Chaoulli* Decision in Quebec and its Impact on Equity in Health Care

Marie-Claude Prémont

The *Chaoulli* decision from the Supreme Court of Canada, concerning unreasonable wait times for some services in the Quebec health care system, has forced upon Quebec society a major debate about the future of public health care. Proponents of privatization have been ready and quick to react. Let's not forget that the Liberal government of Quebec, elected in April 2003 with a call to reengineer the public sector, is lead by Jean Charest, ex-leader of the Conservative Party of Canada. It is therefore not surprising that the proposed program be mostly in line with a conservative agenda, under the guise of giving voice to the concerns of Canada's highest tribunal through a benign tuning of the public system.

The Government of Quebec waited for the results of the federal elections in January 2006 before making public on February 16, 2006, its white paper *Guaranteeing Access: Meeting the Challenges of Equity, Efficiency and Quality*. We can be sure that the election of a Conservative government in Ottawa, although a minority one, was factored into the proposal. The policy paper was followed by a far-reaching nineteen-day Parliamentary Commission where citizens, experts, and numerous stakeholders came to testify. This was followed by the introduction of Bill 33 on June 15, and its enactment at the end of the fall parliamentary session on December 13, 2006.

Bill 33 is the government's response to the *Chaoulli* decision of the Supreme Court of Canada. Beneath a benign façade, the Bill sets up fundamental changes to core principles of the Quebec health care system, which up until now, have assured that maximum financial and human resources be channelled towards a health care system devoted to the whole of the population. It is these same core principles, now jeopardized by Bill 33, that have minimized public support for a private system that caters to only a small portion of the population.

Bill 33 does include some positive changes with the introduction of centralized waiting lists for specialized and overspecialized services, and the management of service corridors inside the health care network. Other features of the Bill are far less reassuring for the future of public health care. Here are four main contentious aspects laid down in Bill 33.

First, Bill 33 will legalize "private hospitals," or "Specialized Medical Centres," in the jargon of the Bill. These centres will be able to offer services (or focus on some of them) that are today delivered by Ambulatory Care Centres (for authorized one-day surgeries), hospitals (for authorized services with overnight stay), and private clinics as we know them across the country. These new private hospitals could be of two types. The first type, where services are paid for with public money, will become a sort of "private extension" of the current hospital with which renewable, exclusive, five-year contracts can be signed. The centre then becomes what the Bill calls an "Associated Medical Clinic." Private laboratories and private doctors' offices can also sign such exclusive contracts with hospitals. This delegates by contract the provision of public services to for-profit private capital corporations. This is not benign.

The second type of "private hospital" envisioned by the Bill is also a private corporation, but one where services will mainly have to be paid for by private money. This second type of private hospital will be staffed by opted-out physicians who, from then on, will be able to offer (legally) authorized surgical services including overnight bed stay.

Other aspects of Bill 33 establish conditions that can facilitate market growth for these private hospitals. First is the provision that the list of authorized surgical services that may be carried out in Specialized Medical Centres (restricted in the Bill to knee and hip replacement and cataract surgery), can be extended in the future by simple regulatory changes from the minister of health and social services. The easy and flexible expansion of public services delegation to for-profit corporations on long-term contracts is therefore at the very core of the program.[133]

Next, Bill 33 will make private insurance available for services carried out in the second type of Specialized Medical Centres (with opted-out physicians). The list of such services could be extended beyond the three acts to cover some or all of the authorized surgeries in the private hospitals by simple regulation of the government, after discussion at the appropriate committee of the National Assembly. It is important here to understand that the private insurance contract must cover both physicians' costs and "hospital" costs associated with overnight bed stay. This is a major departure from current public policy. Contrary to what Minister Couillard was uttering in public, to the effect that the total private hospital insurance prohibition would be reenacted, Bill 33 actually allows both medical and hospital private insurance for surgeries covered by Specialized Medical Centres for opted-out physicians.

Not calling *hospitals* the units where patients are operated on and stay overnight in is nothing but a hoax. Hospital insurance is available in Type 2 Specialized Medical Centres.

Finally, Bill 33 opens up the possibility that compliance with the wait time guarantee will result in publicly insured patients being sent to private hospitals staffed with opted-out physicians. A Type 2 Specialized Medical Centre is basically a cover name for private for-profit hospitals which would just as well benefit from public funding to cover part of their operating costs. The public-private wait time guarantee offers, to an emerging private health care system (the private sector), a client guarantee and a funding assurance.

The Government of Quebec would like to stress those aspects of the Bill that limit, for the time being, the extent of the introduction of private health insurance and the extent of cross-subsidization of public and private health care systems. No one will be fooled by this. Such drastic changes in the course of health care delivery and financing could only be done in incremental steps anyhow. The structure set in place by Bill 33 lays the cornerstone on which two-tier health care can gradually but surely grow. Finally, we must bear in mind that the argument that Quebec has no other option following the *Chaoulli* decision is highly arguable. This argument profoundly confuses the roles of the judiciary and of parliaments. This, like Bill 33, should be a matter of serious concern to every citizen, in every Canadian province.

The *Chaoulli* decision did not need to translate into a proposal like Bill 33, which favours private industry interests over public interest. This means that, although one may feel protected by the fact that the *Chaoulli* decision, strictly speaking, only applies to Quebec, other Canadian provinces need not be faced with a *Chaoulli*-type decision to implement a similarly conservative agenda. Current action plans from conservative-minded provincial governments go to the core of provincial jurisdiction over public health care, like the prohibition of duplicate private insurance, the prohibition of dual medical practice (double-dipping), and physicians' tariff regulation. Emergency calls to the federal government or scrambling to make use of the Canada Health Act may prove insufficient to face the current crisis of propaganda against public health care in Canada and Quebec.

CHAPTER 17

P3 Hospitals and the
Principles of Medicare

Steven Shrybman

The development of "Public–Private Partnership" (P3) hospitals in Ontario, British Columbia, and most recently Quebec, has attracted considerable notoriety.[134] Much of this criticism has focused on the potential for these hospital projects to be more costly, deliver inferior care, and be less accountable than hospitals that are publicly financed, owned, and operated.[135]

Considerably less attention has been paid to the potential for P3 hospitals to undermine the principles and objectives of the Canada Health Act with respect to the delivery of hospital services. While Canada's health care policy elite is fully engaged with the issue of allowing private payment for insured health services, the risks of privatizing *the delivery* of such services have been largely ignored. Yet introducing private investment into the public hospital setting raises obvious questions about the potential for conflicts to arise between the inherently disparate goals of private investors, and those of a not-for-profit hospital board with a universal service mandate.[136]

The essential conclusion of my assessment is that P3 hospitals provide an ideal environment for multi-tiered health care to flourish because the model allows private investors to integrate, within the public hospital setting, a parallel and privately funded health services regime. Moreover, by allowing investors significant control over the design and use of hospital facilities, and over the deployment of hospital staff, P3 hospitals create significant opportunities to stream hospital patients according to their ability or willingness to pay for hospital services.

Certainly, the issues of extra-billing, user charges and queue jumping are not unique to the P3 hospital setting. However, a P3 hospital provides both opportunity and incentive to create a tiered system of hospital care geared to a patient's ability to pay. The lack of transparency surrounding P3 schemes, and the absence of regulations designed to contend with the particular problems they present, will make such practices difficult to detect.

This chapter provides an overview of a P3 hospital model as it has been implemented by Ontario, and assesses the potential effects of this scheme on access to publicly funded hospital services. The focus here is on two related aspects of the P3 model. The first has to do with its impact on the management prerogatives and priorities of the public hospital board. The second concerns the opportunity the model provides for integrating privately funded health care services within the P3 hospital facilities.

The General Structure of P3 Hospitals
There are currently several major P3 hospital projects underway in Canada. This analysis focuses on one of the first and largest — the William Osler Health Centre (WOHC) expansion in Brampton, Ontario. Under the P3 scheme, a private consortium was contracted to design, construct, finance, operate, property manage,

and maintain a hospital facility, and to provide certain non-clinical hospital services.[137] That consortium is comprised of developers, pension plans, private investors, and hospital services and management companies.

The P3 scheme is described by a Project Agreement and numerous related contracts, leases, security instruments, and shareholder agreements.[138] The term of the WOHC P3 contract is for twenty-five years from the date on which the hospital facilities go into service.[139]

In accordance with the Project Agreement, the land upon which the hospital facility is to be situated is leased by the public hospital to the consortium for a period of twenty-five plus years. The consortium then subleases the hospital facility it constructs on that land back to the public hospital for essentially the same period. Ownership of the land and buildings remains with WOHC, but subject to complex leasehold and contractual agreements between the public hospital and the consortium.

In addition to financing and building the hospital facility, the consortium is also contracted to provide an array of non-clinical services, including: building maintenance, materials management, food, housekeeping, laundry, and portering. The private consortium is also contracted to manage the services it has contracted to provide.

Under the Project Agreement the private consortium is entitled to develop, or serve as a conduit for, proposals to provide facilities and/or ancillary services that may include any type of health care or other business, subject only to exclusions for gambling, sexually themed entertainment, or the sale of tobacco and alcoholic products.[140] While the public hospital board must approve such business ventures, its consent may not be withheld unreasonably. Moreover, under the Project Agreement the hospital has the option of entering into a profit-sharing arrangement with the P3 partner with respect to these "ancillary" businesses.[141]

The services component of the P3 scheme is bundled together with the lease for the hospital facilities in a manner that precludes the hospital from extricating itself from the services regime unless it is prepared and able to terminate the *entire* P3 contract. To do so, the hospital must buy out the consortium and this may, in the first several years of the scheme, involve capital outlays in excess of those required to build the hospital in the first place.

The P3 Scheme as a Constraint on Hospital Management and Priorities

By contracting the consortium to manage the services it has contracted to provide, the administration of the hospital is bifurcated; clinical services providers report to the CEO and the board of the public hospital, and non-clinical staff and subcontractors report to an administrator working for the consortium. While contracting out certain hospital services is not an uncommon practice, the scale, terms, and duration of the services component of the P3 scheme are entirely unprecedented.

Under the Project Agreement, the private consortium subcontracts for the specific services, such as food, housekeeping, and materials management, which it is obliged to deliver. This means the hospital has no direct relationship with the companies hired to actually perform many of the services provided under the Project Agreement. Conversely, the obligations of a food or laundry service subcontractor, for example, would be to the consortium, not the public hospital board, and the priorities of these respective entities are quite distinct and may even be competing.

In these ways, the P3 scheme represents a fundamental departure from the conventional management model for a public hospital where authority is vested in a not-for-profit board with a mandate to ensure universal access to insured health hospital services. Public hospitals are accountable to patients, their communities, and to the provincial Ministry of Health, not shareholders or private investors. Under the P3 regime, the authority of the board is significantly moderated by having to work in close collaboration with a private consortium that has a very different mission.

To assess what impacts this model will have on the management and control of the public hospital, it is important to appreciate that to function effectively, the delivery of support and clinical hospital services must be effectively integrated. While team building and collegiality are vital, they are often difficult to achieve and sustain given the complexities of modern hospital care, and the commonplace stresses of underfunding and staffing constraints.

According to a senior and respected hospital CEO, the WOHC P3 model will make the task of managing the public hospital much more difficult because delegating management of support staff and infrastructure services to a for-profit corporation will create an institutional barrier to the collaborative team approach that is essential to the delivery of high quality care.[142]

The ability of the hospital to function well in this environment will depend upon the hospital administrators, working respectively for the public hospital and the private consortium, to forge an effective working relationship in spite of these institutional barriers and the distinct corporate missions they must serve. While such close collaboration can occur, it is by no means likely, and will need to be reforged whenever either administrator retires or is replaced during the twenty-five year term of P3.

The Bargaining Leverage of the Private Partner
In addition to attenuating the management prerogatives of the public hospital board, the P3 scheme accords the private consortium significant bargaining leverage in its relationship with the board for several reasons.

First, the P3 service contract is for the same term as the lease — much longer than the two- to five-year term that is the norm

for hospital service contracts. Under a conventional services contract, where the contractor fails to perform, the hospital may
typically provide notice of the breach, which the contractor has
sixty days to remedy. If that fails, the hospital may then simply terminate the contract. In contrast, the P3 scheme is for a term of
twenty-five years, and while provisions are made for discharging a
particular subcontractor in favour of another, the dispute procedures for addressing performance problems are complex, time
consuming, and expensive.

Second, the typical services subcontract is simple and short.
This is because, in conventional arrangements, both parties have
an interest in making the relationship work. For the contractor,
there is a clear incentive to perform at a high level to achieve
renewal of the arrangement, avoid premature termination, and
protect its reputation in the marketplace. The scope and duration
of P3 schemes entirely transform this dynamic and substitutes an
elaborate and complex contractual regime for the informal agreements that typify conventional contracting-out of hospital
services.

Finally, and as noted, the services and real estate aspects of the
P3 scheme can not be severed. This means even where the services component of the scheme fails and the public hospital is
entitled to terminate the P3 contract, it may only do so by buying out the leasehold portion of the scheme. This may entail
substantial payments to the consortium, its debt holders, and equity investors.[143] For the hospital the procedural complexity and
cost of extricating itself from the P3 scheme may simply be too
onerous.

In these ways, the P3 model fundamentally transforms the typical relationship and power balance between a public hospital and
subcontractors hired to provide discrete support services under
short term contracts. The result shifts the balance of power decid-
edly in favour of the private consortium and its subcontractors.

These companies are obliged to maximize returns to owners and investors, not to provide high quality patient care, nor to ensure universal access to care in accordance with the principles of medicare.

Third Party Arbitration

The P3 scheme also imposes another and more formal constraint on the management prerogatives of the hospital board, which arises from the dispute procedures provided for by the Project Agreement. The entrenched nature of the P3 scheme requires a mechanism for resolving disputes that arise between the hospital and the consortium. Many management and administrative matters will involve questions of resource allocation, cost, and quality of service, which may be contentious between the P3 partners. Under the Project Agreement these disputes are assigned to independent arbitrators or the courts. By this means, key decisions involving the delivery of hospital services will now be made by independent adjudicators and not the hospital board.

Third party arbitration is, of course, a feature of the collective agreements many hospitals have with their unionized workers, but in terms of complexity, scope, and duration, P3 schemes present much greater potential constraints of the management prerogatives of the public hospital board. Dispute procedures are also cumbersome, time consuming, and costly, and create a strong incentive for the partners to settle their differences.

Given the considerable leverage the consortium will have in such negotiations, the service priorities of the hospital may increasingly come to reflect those of its private, and profit-seeking, partner. Each negotiation will also provide an opportunity for the consortium to further its broader interests, including to gain support from the hospital for the expansion of privately funded services, a problem that is considered next.

The P3 Hospital as a Platform for Multi-tiered Care

Private Clinics and other Business Opportunities in the P3 Hospital
In a P3 hospital the allocation of space and support services within the hospital is no longer the prerogative of the public hospital board. Instead, changes in the use of hospital facilities must be negotiated with the consortium, or when that fails, determined by arbitration.[144]

The right to establish privately funded clinics in the hospital allows the consortium to integrate such clinics with publicly funded hospital services in a much more seamless way than is possible when stand-alone for-profit clinics are physically and institutionally isolated from the hospital itself. Physical proximity to both patients and health care professionals significantly increases the likelihood of cream-skimming and other strategies for diverting patients from the public to the privately funded health care stream.

It is also likely to exacerbate the problem of having scarce health care human resources diverted from the publicly funded system. Typically this has occurred when health care professionals are offered a premium for providing services that are funded privately. However, in the P3 hospital setting, the private consortium has another and more direct way to ensure that private clinics are properly staffed, even at the expense of the public hospital's needs. It is simply to direct support staff services to the private clinics it may establish, so long as this occurs in accordance with the provisions of the Project Agreement.

The complexity and opaqueness of P3 schemes will allow the diversion of patients and staff from the publicly funded system, to one that depends upon private payment, to go on with little notoriety.

Uncertain Revenues and Fixed Expenditures

There is considerable evidence to show that P3 hospitals are significantly more costly than the public sector alternatives they replace.[145] But, quite apart from their relative cost, the structure of the WOHC P3 scheme may create new and significant pressures for the hospital board to contain clinical care costs. These may arise because the long-term funding obligations of the Ministry of Health and Long-term Care are limited under P3 scheme to paying for the infrastructure component of the scheme.

Thus, under its funding agreement with the WOHC, the ministry is obliged, subject to the appropriations authority of the provincial parliament, to make annual payments to the hospital over the twenty-five year term of the P3 scheme, but only to cover the costs of the leasehold component of the P3 scheme.[146]

However, only about 60 percent of the annual base charge of $94 plus million that WOHC is obliged to pay annually under the scheme is on account of leasehold charges.[147] The ministry is under no obligation to provide funding to cover the $42 million base charge for the services component of the scheme, even though the services and leasehold components of the scheme cannot be severed. For these service costs, the hospital must depend on annual funding from the ministry, which is vulnerable to the fiscal and political vicissitudes of the day, and which may or may not keep pace with the hospitals' obligations under the P3 scheme. This leaves the hospital in the precarious position of potentially being squeezed between fixed costs, and uncertain revenues.

Any shortfall in ministry funding will require the hospital to raise money from other sources, or reduce expenditures on services, perhaps both. Where expenditure reductions limit the availability of publicly funded services, patients will increasingly look to those that can be purchased privately. For its part, the hospital may also look to additional joint ventures with its private partner for profits to augment any shortfalls in public funding. In this environment, privately funded hospital services may flourish as those dependent on public funding decline.

Adding to these financial pressures may be the loss of conventional revenues from services provided to third parties, such as private insurers or workers compensation plans, which often provide a significant revenue stream to subsidize publicly funded services. Under the P3 scheme, these revenues may be shared with the private consortium, which may also lead the public hospital to support additional private projects to compensate for its diminished share of the revenues from such sources.

In these ways the financial dynamics of the P3 hospital begin to mirror those of a physician who is free to work in the publicly funded health care system, but also to bill patients privately for required health services. In the case of an individual doctor, the motivation is likely to be personal and pecuniary. In the case of a public hospital board, the incentive to allow the development of parallel and privately funded hospital services may simply be driven by the need to meet its financial obligations under the P3 scheme.

Finally in this regard, in addition to these structural financial pressures, the hospital board may face additional pressure from hospital staff to facilitate the development of private services within, or as an adjunct to publicly funded hospital services. This may occur where staff are free to work on both the publicly and privately funded sides of the hospital corridor — often being paid a premium for the latter.

Straddling the Public Funding and Private Payment Divide

Because physicians and private clinics have an incentive to

increase income, and profits, they may engage in practices to augment public funding by billing patients privately — the clearest
examples would be extra-billing or user charges for insured health
services. As we know, both practices are proscribed by the Canada Health Act and banned under provincial health care insurance
plans. Other practices, such as charging block fees, paying kickbacks, self-referring, or simply selling health care services
privately, are regulated in a less consistent manner by the
provinces.[148] Moreover, there appears to be growing non-compli-
ance with these prohibitions, in part because of lax enforcement
by the federal government and some provinces.

It is only necessary to briefly describe the more common practices for private billing to expose how readily these might arise in
the P3 hospital setting, and how difficult they will be to detect
should that occur.

Definitional drift

Under the Canada Health Act, only medically "necessary" or
"required" services need be covered by provincial health care
insurance plans. This has led to the growing practice of selling certain health services to patients under the rubric that they are not,
strictly speaking, necessary. For example, a full body MRI scan is
probably not necessary for a patient suffering pain in a lower limb.
However, by purchasing such a scan a patient suspecting the need
for a hip replacement may jump the queue for both diagnosis and
follow-up surgery. Physicians willing to make such referrals may
also benefit from avoiding billing and fee constraints that apply to
insured services.

This problem of "definitional drift" — the dubious characterization of health services as "unnecessary" — arises most often
when physicians and clinics are permitted to provide both insured
and uninsured services.[149] As we have seen, this co-mingling of
insured and privately paid for services is inherent to the structure

of the P3 scheme, which explicitly authorizes the establishment of private businesses in the hospital setting.

Kickbacks and self-referrals

Private clinics depend on physician referrals for patients. Where referring physicians have a direct or indirect financial stake in the clinic's business, the situation is rife with the potential for conflicts of interest to result in unnecessary referrals. These in turn lengthen wait times for those who actually do need care.

The potential for such abuses has prompted some provinces to regulate the financial relationships doctors may have with the clinics and other entities to or from which such referrals are made.[150] These regulations address the payment of kickbacks and the practice of self-referral. Saskatchewan, for example, prohibits referrals to private clinics owned by the physician or her or his family members.[151] The province also defines "conflict of interest" broadly to preclude various indirect kick-back payments, such as providing rent and equipment subsidies to referring physicians.

Nothing in the P3 scheme itself precludes investment by WOHC staff or directors in the private businesses that the consortium may establish in or as an adjunct to the hospital. Even where regulations proscribe such investments, and are monitored and enforced, there are other ways in which hospital physicians may be rewarded for referrals, such as being accorded preferential access to clinic facilities.

It would seem that the opportunity for such quid pro quo arrangements will be far greater given the scale of P3 hospitals and the number of medical staff working under the scheme. And, the economic self-interest that may influence a physician to refer patients for particular procedures may, in the P3 hospital setting, resonate at an institutional level for reasons already described.

Cream-skimming

Cream-skimming is another problem that arises when for-profit clinics are allowed to provide insured health care services. As the Romanow Commission explained, private clinics have an incentive to:

> "cream-off" those services that can be easily and more inexpensively provided on a volume basis, such as cataract surgery or hernia repair. This leaves the public system to provide the more complicated and expensive services from which it is more difficult to control cost per case.[152]

As the Commission also pointed out, when something goes wrong with a patient at a private clinic, that patient will likely be returned to a public hospital for treatment. Because of the physical proximity of private clinics in the P3 hospital setting, and the ability of the private consortium to integrate privately and publicly funded care, the P3 environment would appear to be ideal for this practice to flourish.

Double-dipping

By and large, provincial health care laws maintain a strict separation between doctors operating within the publicly funded system and those who have opted out. This restriction prevents doctors from "double dipping" by using public health funding to subsidize the costs of providing elite care to those who can pay.

The evidence clearly shows that two-tiered care is not financially viable in Canada if it is required to operate independently of the publicly funded system. Where such cross-subsidies are permitted, the result is a health care system that is fundamentally inequitable, not only because it provides better or more timely care to a wealthy few, but also because it obliges most of us to subsidize services we cannot personally afford.

Where private clinics and other health care businesses are established in the P3 hospital, it would be difficult, and in many cases impossible, to maintain a separation of staff providing publicly funded services from those working in or for private clinics. By assuring the private consortium a steady stream of public funding, while permitting it to establish clinics and other privately funded businesses as part of the P3 hospital, the P3 scheme creates an economic environment that allows publicly funded facilities and services to provide a platform for multi-tiered care based on the patient's ability to pay.

The regulatory vacuum

While Ontario regulates private clinics, it has no legislation to address the more complex challenges posed by P3 hospitals. Rather, the province appears to be relying upon the capacity of the public hospital board to ensure that its private partner operates in accordance with principles of medicare. But as we have seen, the hospital board may have little bargaining leverage under the P3 scheme. To the extent that doctors, nurses, and other health care professionals are able to augment their incomes by working on the private side of the public hospital corridor, there may be little incentive to get tough with the private partner.

Finally, the complexity of P3 schemes makes it very difficult to monitor or ensure compliance with provincial law. For instance, the P3 hospital contractual scheme for the William Osler Hospital complex in Ontario is composed of more than two thousand pages of complex legal documents. Claims to business confidentiality have prevented key elements of the P3 scheme from being made public, and even the ministry is precluded from sharing this information with the taxpayers who will pay for it.

For these reasons, P3 hospital schemes confound notions of transparency or accountability. The regulatory vacuum within which such schemes are being established seriously exacerbates this problem.

Summary

The P3 scheme superimposes on the hospital a highly complex commercial and contractual regime that will substantially moderate the authority of the not-for-profit hospital board to govern and manage the hospital in accordance with its priorities. Under such schemes, decisions about the use of hospital space and the allocation of health care personnel will often have to accommodate the interests and priorities of the private investors who will have a stake in and influence over such decisions.

The opportunities provided by the P3 model to integrate private services into the institutional framework of the hospital will provide new opportunities to facilitate the development of a multi-tiered service model where the quality and timeliness of care depends upon one's ability to pay.

CHAPTER 18

Changing the Landscape in the Health Care Affordability Debate

Diana Gibson

Sustainability eclipses all other issues when talking of public health care these days — a variety of statistics are being misused to claim the sky is falling in. It isn't. Governments often use statistics on health spending without accounting for population growth, inflation, or income growth. Of course they can show costs are rising — with more people and inflation, there are higher health costs. That line looks very different if it is measured on a per capita basis and controlled for inflation. There is also more tax income available to the government with higher population numbers. That potential tax revenue is too often left out of the health affordability picture.

Total health care expenditures run in the range of 10 to 11 percent of national income as measured by gross domestic product. However it is important to look at what that is measuring. According to the Canadian Institute for Health Information (CIHI), in 2005, on average, public health expenditures accounted for seven out of every ten dollars spent on health care. The remaining three out of every ten dollars came from private sources (individuals through direct payment or indirect payment through workplace-based insurance programs) and covered the costs of supplementary services such as drugs, dental care, and vision care.[153] Those out-of-pocket individual expenses have been one of the fast growing areas of health care costs.

Even within that portion that is defined as public health expenditures, it is important to keep a critical eye on what is being measured. The way public health care dollars are spent has been changing significantly. Again, according to CIHI, the share of total health expenditures paid to hospitals and physicians declined, while spending on prescription drugs has greatly increased. Thus, though initial figures on health care indicate that costs are increasing even as a portion of the economy (GDP), this does not apply to spending on hospitals and physicians. The areas to look to for skyrocketing costs are individual out-of-pocket expenses and drug costs, both areas driven by for-profit involvement.

It is for-profit involvement in health care that is the biggest cost driver. I also show that removing services from medicare is driving up overall costs by ensuring greater for-profit involvement in those areas.

This brings us to Tommy Douglas's vision for health care. At the time medicare was introduced, it was also the result of compromise — dental and long-term care were not included and there was no national pharmaceutical program. Preventive care and wellness programs were also lacking. When public health care was introduced nationally it was seen as a first step. The second step was to focus health care on wellness and preventive care. What would it take to make all of these priorities a reality for all Canadians?

It is consistent with Canadian values and the Canadian way of life to ensure that all seniors have full access to high quality

long-term and continuing care regardless of income. The same
applies to dental care and pharmaceuticals as well as wellness and
preventive care — it is consistent with Canadian values and the
Canadian way of life to ensure that all Canadians have equal access
regardless of ability to pay.

Private financing cannot deliver on these goals.[154] For example,
the current patchwork of seniors care facilities does not deliver on
affordability, equity, or access.[155] Acute care beds in many hospitals
are backed up with seniors on waiting lists for beds in long-term
or continuing care. Quality and service delivery have been found
wanting.

On the more general goal of full access regardless of ability to
pay, the private health insurance side receives a worse than failing
grade, it gets a zero — if you can't pay, you don't have access. Subsidy programs do not work. In Australia private insurance has
ended up costing the public system more than if they had stayed
with public insurance due to the incredibly high level of subsidy
required to ensure adequate registration for the private program.
And still only 33 percent of low-income Australians have coverage.[156] In Alberta the experience was the same in the pre-medicare
days. Under Premier Ernest Manning's program for private insurance, less than half of those eligible applied for the subsidy because
the insurance was still too expensive even with the subsidy.

Private health insurance is not a new concept in Canada. We
can look back to pre-medicare when Alberta experimented with
private health insurance. Of course, it is also illustrative to look
south of the border. The leading cause of bankruptcy in the United States is not the crash of the real estate market, nor is it loss of
employment or economic recession; it is medical costs. This was
also the case in Canada pre-medicare. Another striking fact is that
in the US three quarters of those bankrupted families or individuals had private health insurance at the time they fell ill. Private
insurance is not enough — it is full of loopholes such as denied

coverage for people with pre-existing conditions, maximum pay-ments, co-payments, and deductibles that offer little real protection from bankruptcy, much less for health.

Workplace-based or supplementary health insurance gives another good indication of the inadequacies of private insurance. This is the coverage many get through their work for health care costs not covered by the public system such as ambulance fees, health care premiums, pharmaceuticals, and dental. Looking to workplace-based health insurance here in Canada also shows us that private insurance does not deliver on access. This system offers limited access at best. Almost half of Canadians do not have access to workplace health benefits. Women, youth, and visible minorities fare the worst.

The workplace-based health insurance market also shows that private insurance will not deliver on affordability. Private health insurance premiums are skyrocketing; they are growing at double digit rates. When health care services are removed from the pub-lic plan (de-listed or de-insured), costs jump. Vision care is an excellent example. After it was de-insured in Alberta, costs went up 17 percent in one year alone. Because of the number of health care services being removed from medicare, as well as user fees and deductibles, out-of-pocket individual expenses are growing at rates faster than inflation.[157]

Whether it is a public system or a private system for health care, individuals pay. The evidence clearly shows that it is cheaper to have those services funded by the public system. The evidence also shows that private insurance cannot deliver on the Canadian val-ues of affordability, access, or equity. If Canadians want private health insurance, health outcomes will have to be sacrificed to pay the higher costs and profits.

Because of the well known failures of the US example, gov-ernments across Canada point to Europe for examples of a public private mix. But, Canada already has more private involvement in health care than most European countries. Only France and the United States have more. In fact, emulating Europe fits perfectly with Tommy Douglas's vision for health care — Canada could look to emulate the high percentage of services covered by the public system, including dental and long-term care. Canada could also look to emulate the national pharmaceuticals programs that limit patents and reduce pharmaceutical costs. Europe's social programs, poverty alleviation, and inequality rates are also part of their good health outcomes and provide excellent models for Canada. Proportional representation is another key part of the low levels of inequality and high health outcomes of those countries that Canada should look to.

Based on these examples, Canada should be looking not to further privatization but to limiting costs through measures that control the level of profit being made from health care and investing in the social determinants of health. Spending smarter will certainly need to be a large part of any effective health care strategy. Distinctions will need to be made in all health affordability debates between that spent on pharmaceuticals and private out-of-pocket costs verses other public health care costs.

We must shift away from a debate that hinges on a manufactured affordability crisis. Given that public health care is the single most important issue for taxpayers, how much of our national income is too much to spend on the public system? Instead of fighting over how to spend limited and shrinking health care dollars within the public system, it is time to look to expanding that system.

Canadians consistently rate public health care above tax cuts but governments across the country have instead focused on tax cuts at the expense of health care affordability. Health care spending and staffing decisions are regularly made on the basis of arbitrary short term budget changes and politicking. The results are critical staffing shortages in the health care sector and shortages of hospital beds. Politicians speak of either cutting health spending or increasing health spending instead of talking of the outcomes such as cancer incidences or infant mortality rates in indigenous communities.

To change this dynamic would require a paradigm shift, a reframing of the policy debate, away from arbitrary budget numbers and towards meaningful outcomes. And, it is critical that this new vision not be limited by arbitrary and ideological definitions of affordability, but by real projections of demographic and health trends, as well as quality and service standards.

PART IV

*Health Care
Reforms:
Pharmacare, Home,
Community, and
Primary Care*

CHAPTER 19

Completing the Vision: Achieving the Second Stage of Medicare

Michael Rachlis

Today all Canadians are concerned about the state of medicare. Recent international surveys show that Canadians wait longer than most others for family doctor appointments, emergency room service, specialist appointments, and elective surgery.[1] The 20 to 30 percent of Canadians who never wanted medicare now say, "We told you so. This government health plan wasn't ever going to work."

Few Canadians know that the original vision of medicare went well beyond public payment for the old system. The original vision of medicare included new ways of delivering care. But, as Tommy Douglas reminded us in the SOS Medicare Conference in November 1979, this vision would have to be implemented in two stages — the first stage was to remove money as a barrier to access but the second, more difficult, stage would be "to alter our deliver system" in order "to reduce costs and put an emphasis on preventative medicine."

Medicare's Original Vision in Saskatchewan

Saskatchewan led the rest of the country and the continent with its health policy.[2] Before Tommy Douglas became premier in 1944, the province already had a thriving municipal doctor program, provided universal care for patients with tuberculosis, and had established Canada's first cancer control agency. Just months after Douglas was elected premier, the province became the first jurisdiction in North America to cover all cancer diagnosis and treatment.

After his victory in 1944, Douglas appointed Dr. Henry Sigerist, an internationally known Johns Hopkins professor of medicine, to review the province's health system.[3] Sigerist recommended the establishment of district health regions to focus on preventive medicine. The district would include hospital and medical care, diagnostics, public health, and home care. To ensure the focus was on prevention, Sigerist recommended that the medical officer of health head up the health region.

Saskatchewan established the Health Services Planning Commission to continue planning and facilitate implementation of the Sigerist report's conclusions. Southwestern Saskatchewan was keen to move, and on January 1, 1946, the Swift Current Health Region was established. On July 1 of that year, it began providing universal hospital and medical care.[4]

The Swift Current Region financed and provided hospital and physicians' care, laboratory and radiology services, home care, public health, and children's dental services. Its efforts drew broad praise from local citizens and leading physicians in Saskatchewan.[5] The Swift Current region went from having a high level of infant mortality to the lowest in the province by 1965.[6] Even Dr. Arthur Kelly, deputy secretary of the Canadian Medical Association, was effusive with praise in a 1948 Canadian Medical Association article, characterizing the region as:

a successful experiment in the large scale provision of medical care, courageously applied, efficiently managed and remarkably free of attempts to make the facts fit preconceived ideas, financial or otherwise.[7]

The key factors associated with the Swift Current Region's success were:

- **Improved coordination of health care delivery focused on prevention through a local integrated health region:** The region funded and organized a comprehensive package of services including hospital and physician care, diagnostic services, home care, public health, and children's dental services.
- **Prepaid funding:** Services were available to the public on a universal basis, with little or no charge to users.
- **Group medical practice:** The doctors were in private practice, but the regional medical leadership, including the medical officer of health, exerted significant influence in standards of practice and utilization. The medical office of health and public health nurses worked in tandem with the physicians to deliver preventive services.
- **Democratic community governance of health care delivery by a locally elected board:** The twelve Swift Current board members represented the region's eighty-seven municipalities. Community governance would ensure health care remained responsive and customized to the priority needs of the local population.

The Swift Current Region Model Doesn't Spread
However, despite the popularity of the plan with local doctors and the initial positive reviews from Canadian organized medicine, opposition from doctors in other parts of the province and country prevented the spread of the Swift Current model.[8] Organized medicine's biggest concern was that the profession did not want to negotiate with local boards, but rather the province.[9]

Eventually the Saskatchewan provincial government, led by Premier Douglas, moved ahead with medicare's first stage: providing insurance to people when they got sick. In 1947, Saskatchewan implemented universal hospital insurance. When Saskatchewan launched its medical insurance plan on July 1, 1962, over 90 percent of the province's doctors went on strike, refusing to see patients even in an emergency.[10] Eventually, Saskatchewan's doctors essentially settled for what the government had been offering. The settlement of the 1962 Saskatchewan physicians' strike is generally seen as a victory for the government and the birth of medicare in Canada. However, events belie this interpretation.

In the longer term, Canadian governments were collectively shaken by the bitter 1962 doctors's strike and were loath to have a repeat. The federal government did implement a national hospital insurance plan in 1957 and a national medical insurance plan in 1968. In 1969, the country's deputy ministers of health asked the University of Toronto's Dr. John Hastings to write a report on the reorganization of medical practice and primary health care as it moved to public payment. Hastings's 1972 report recommended a similar system to that suggested by Sigerist twenty-seven years earlier: group medical practice, non-fee-for-service payment, and integration with public health and social services.

Despite a positive reception from nursing groups, public health associations, and several provinces, there was firm opposition from the medical profession. The health system stayed pretty much the same for twenty-five years after Dr. Hastings's report. Canadians had first-dollar coverage for hospital and physicians' services, but the delivery system still looked like the 1950s. Almost all physicians are in private practice, billing the provincial medicare plans on a fee-for-service basis. There is little group practice or the use of inter-disciplinary teams.

But the Model Does Work Where it is Implemented

There were some new models of care developed. In Saskatchewan, the 1962 battle for medicare led to the establishment of several cooperative community clinics. The Saskatoon Community Clinic now employs 150 staff and provides medical services to 20,000 patients and community-based preventive services to thousands of others.[11] The clinic has pioneered improvements in access and chronic disease management that are being implemented province wide through the Saskatchewan Health Quality Council. A 1981 study of the Saskatoon Community Clinic found that the community clinic patients had 17 percent lower overall costs and 31 percent fewer days in hospital.[12]

In 1964, a Sault Ste. Marie community group led by the United Steelworkers of America opened the Group Health Centre.[13] The centre now has over 60,000 patients, nearly 70 doctors, 110 nurses, and 50 other health professionals. Group Health, as it is called, has been a font of innovation for over 40 years. Group Health has had a comprehensive electronic medical record since 1997[14] and has been cited for its innovative care in access and chronic disease management.[14] Studies from the 1960s and 1970s found that the Sault Ste Marie Group Health Association Clinic had lower overall health care costs because patients spent 20 to 25 percent fewer days in hospital.[15,16,17]

In the United States and Canada, remote mining and forestry companies have typically provided their own medical services. In the United States, "prepaid group practice," as the plans were called, grew in a major fashion during the 1930s. Studies over the years have concluded that prepaid group practices such as the Group Health Cooperative of Puget Sound and Kaiser-Permanente set standards of excellence for health care system performance. In the most expensive health services research project ever funded, the Rand health insurance study found the costs for Group Health Cooperative patients were 25 percent less than those seeing fee-for-service doctors — due almost entirely to the fact that Group Health patients spent 40 percent fewer days in hospital.[18, 19]

The First Stage of Medicare has been Good for Canadians

The first stage of medicare has been very good to Canadians. Up until the late 1950s, Canadians and Americans had similar health status and similar health care systems, with similar costs. Now Canadians live 2.5 years longer and our infant mortality rate is 23 percent lower.[20] In 2004, the United States spent 15.3 percent of its gross domestic product (GDP) on health care, and Canada spent 9.9 percent. Half of the difference in expenditures is because of the much higher administrative burden of the mainly private US system.[21] Despite having the world's highest health care spending, nearly 60 million Americans either have no insurance or live with someone who lacks coverage,[22] and tens of millions have such bad coverage that health care bills bankrupt half a million Americans every year.[23]

And medicare has been good for business in Canada by picking up the tab for most health care costs. Our manufacturers have an $8 per hour per employee advantage over their American competitors.[24] Medicare keeps hundreds of thousands of our best-paying jobs in this country. By any standard we have done well by adopting Tommy Douglas's first stage of medicare. But, as Douglas predicted, our health system has developed problems.

Failure to Implement the Second Stage of Medicare

Medicare's founders foresaw two-fold benefits when they prescribed more prevention in the second stage of medicare. First, the second stage of medicare would promote better health and well-being among Canadians. Second, it would ensure the long-term sustainability of the health care system. In 1982, Tommy Douglas told a Montreal audience:

> All these programs should be designed to keep people well — because in the long run it's cheaper to keep people well than to be patching them up after they are sick.[25]

Why Completing Medicare's Original Vision is Urgent and Imperative

It is urgent and imperative to correct this situation. The dangers of not moving to the second stage of medicare are becoming more and more apparent. When Canadians first started debating medicare a hundred years ago, we were a young country and most health problems were acute. Today, our main health problems are chronic diseases in an aging population. Almost 80 percent of Canadians over the age of sixty-five suffer from a chronic condition. Of those, about 70 percent suffer from two or more chronic conditions.[26] At least 60 percent of health care costs are due to chronic diseases.[27] And, compared with other countries, our health system does a poor job of keeping people with chronic disease healthy.[28]

Most chronic diseases could be prevented altogether. We could prevent over 80 percent of cases of coronary heart disease[29] and type-2 diabetes,[30] and over 85 percent of cases of lung cancer and chronic obstructive lung disease (such as emphysema).[31] If the potential for prevention could be translated into reality for these four conditions, approximately 2,900 hospital beds could be freed up in Ontario alone.[32]

Financial factors are another driving force for change. Tommy Douglas always said that focusing on prevention would make medicare more sustainable. And a growing body of evidence indicates Douglas was right.[33] For example, a recent Alberta after-care program for congestive heart failure patients leaving hospital reduced future hospital use by 60 percent, with $2,500 in overall net cost savings per participant.[34] Home care nurses ensured that patients were taking their medications, were eating properly, and making other lifestyle changes. And the regular follow-up ensured that corrective measures were taken quickly if a patient began to deteriorate.

Medicare's Achilles' Heel: Long Waits for Care
Compared with other wealthy countries, Canada has some of the longest waits for primary health care, medical specialists, hospital emergency rooms, and elective surgery.[35] Douglas noted in his day that needless "ping-ponging" between different specialists and diagnostic tests caused many delays.

> I have a good doctor and we're good friends. And we both laugh when we look at the system. He sends me off to see somebody to get some tests at the other end of town. I go over there and then come back, and they send the reports to him and he looks at them and sends me off some place else for some tests and they come back. Then he says that I had better see a specialist. And before I'm finished I've spent, within a month, six days going to six different people and another six days going to have six different kinds of tests, all of which I could have had in a single clinic.[36]

Now the waits are longer because there are more specialties, more tests available, and because modern practices won't allow patients into hospital just to have all their tests and consultations at once.[37] All these reasons demonstrate the urgent need to swiftly shift to the second stage of medicare. If we don't do a better job preventing the preventable, the system will collapse from the strain — and many Canadians will suffer needlessly in the process.

Interpreting the Second Stage of Medicare for the Twenty-first Century

Tommy Douglas and the history of medicare in Saskatchewan has given us inspiration for the second stage of medicare, but how do we translate that into a vision of medicare for the twenty-first century? Looking back, it seems that he was decades ahead of his time in calling for what we now call the "Quality Agenda" in health care. For example, the Health Council of Canada noted in its 2006 report:

> Are we providing the safest, most suitable care? Are we investing enough in prevention? Are we reducing inequalities in health? The answer to these questions is no, not yet. But we could. It is the Council's belief that we already have strong evidence and enough experience to pursue a quality agenda.[38]

Over the last fifteen years, reports from many countries on hospital complications have spurred interest in the quality of care.[39] A 2004 Canadian study showed similar results to those in other countries. One Canadian in fourteen suffers a complication while in hospital, and over one-third of these could be prevented.[40] Somewhere between 9,000 and 24,000 Canadians die annually from preventable complications of their hospital care. That's 5 to 10 percent of all deaths.

And thousands of Canadians die every year because of poor quality health care outside of hospital, especially from medication complications and inadequate chronic disease management and prevention. For example, about one-quarter of older women are being prescribed sedatives, contrary to clinical practice guidelines.[41]

Of course, this isn't the fault of any one professional, one profession, or one organization. Most countries face similar problems, although some do better and some do worse. Many jurisdictions have developed quality initiatives. There are health quality councils in Saskatchewan, Alberta, and Ontario. Each of these councils, as well as others in other countries, have developed principles for health system renewal.[42,43,44,45] Their work was used as the basis for the list of principles for the second stage of medicare (see below). The principles are divided into essential ones, which are what we want, and the instrumental ones, which help us get there. This chapter addresses the essential principles. Other speakers at the meeting dealt with instrumental ones.

The Principles for the Second Stage of Medicare

Essential Principles — What We Want

1. Population Health Focus: There should be a determined effort to continuously improve the overall health of the population.

2. Equitable: There should be continuing efforts to reduce disparities in the health of those groups who may be disadvantaged by social or economic status, age, gender, ethnicity, geography, or language.

3. Client-centred: Client-centred care respects individuality, ethnicity, dignity, privacy, and information needs of each clients and the client's family. That respect should pervade the health system. Clients should be in control of their own care.

4. Effective: The best science and evidence should be used to ensure care is the best, most appropriate possible. Innovations should also be based on best evidence, whether they are new ways of coordinating care, preventing disease, delivering service, or using technology.

5. Accessible: Clients in need should get timely care in the most appropriate setting. The system should continuously reduce waits and delays.

6. Safe: People should not be harmed by the care that is intended to help them. The system should monitor and continuously reduce adverse events.

Instrumental Principles — How We Will Get There

1. Efficient: There should be continuing efforts to reduce waste, including waste of supplies, equipment, time, ideas, and health information.

2. Accountable: The system should be highly accountable to clients, their families, and funders. There should be clear quality objectives for all health service providers. The objectives and funding should be aligned at the provincial, regional, and local levels to ensure clients and families experience fully integrated care.

3. Appropriately Resourced: The health system should plan for appropriately trained human resources; provide a safe and satisfying environment for their work and provide sufficient facilities, instruments, and technology to support productive and effective care.

4. Non-profit Developer: Health care is fundamentally different from commercial goods and services. Markets simply are not designed to deal effectively with health care, which is a social function. Health care providers provide the best care when they work in teams, not as competitors.

What Would the Second Stage of Medicare Look Like?

Essential Principles — What We Want

1. Focused on population health

What's wrong with our current approach?
Our current approach to health care and health policy is based upon treating illness after it occurs. We miss opportunities for prevention. Implementing the second stage of medicare could avert thousands of premature deaths a year and the suffering of tens of thousands of others.

Why do we have this problem?
Our health system was largely designed to treat acute illness. Federal legislation only requires the provinces to cover hospitals' and physicians' services. Our system offers increasingly expensive treatments, but our major health problems continue to be chronic diseases, which cannot be cured but often can be prevented.

Most health problems are related to social, environmental, occupational, economic, and other factors. Governments tend to deal with these health determinants in an uncoordinated fashion. Our country has little in the way of planning for health or social goals as compared with economic ones. If the health system is going to help make Canada a healthier place, it will need to work with other sectors on the non-medical determinants of health.

How do we fix the problem?

We need national and provincial health plans to guide the redesign of the health care system and the way governments make decisions that affect our health. For example, Quebec has coordinated its social policy around a series of health goals since 1987. Since 1998, Quebec has had a National Institute of Public Health, which, among other tasks, is responsible for developing a provincial health plan based upon these goals.[46]

Saskatchewan developed the Human Services Integration Forum to coordinate health and social planning across government departments. It is led by a steering committee, with senior officials representing seven provincial government departments and the Cabinet Office.

The provinces need to help health regions work with other sectors at regional and local levels. For example, Saskatchewan's Human Services Integration Forum integrates its work with ten Regional Inter-sectoral Committees (RICs). The committees include representatives from various provincial and federal government departments, municipalities, regional health authorities, housing authorities, educational institutions, tribal councils, police, and Métis organizations.

Finally, we need health organizations to engage their communities to improve the determinants of health. For example, the Toronto Regent Park Community Health Centre wanted to ensure that the community's children had the opportunity to become the health centre's future administrators, doctors, and nurses. But the community's high school drop-out rate was very high and few children went on to university. In response, the Community Health Centre keyed the development of an award-winning Pathways to Education program which has reduced the community's drop-out rate from 56 percent to 14 percent, considerably lower than the city average.[47]

2. Equitable

What's wrong with our current approach?
Our health system is largely focused on treating people who walk
in the door, not on ensuring that people get the care they need.
Unfortunately, the people least likely to get the regular health care
they need are the most likely to be sick. As a result, there are very
significant disparities in health among different Canadians.[48]

Health disparities have an important impact on the health system. For example, lower-income Canadians are substantially sicker
than upper-income Canadians and consequently use twice the
number of health care services.[49] In 2004, the Federal/Provin-
cial/Territorial Health Disparities Task Group noted that
approximately 20 percent of health care spending was due to disparities among different income groups.[50]

Why do we have this problem?
Certain groups are more susceptible to illness because of their non-
medical determinants of health.[51,52,53] However, disparities in access
to the health care system do play a role in disparities in health. In
general, the health care system and the non-medical determinants
of health interweave with each other to form a complex web of
causation.[54] But the Federal/Provincial/Territorial Health Disparities Task Group noted that "the health sector has an important role
to play in mitigating the causes and effects of other determinants
of health through interventions with disadvantaged individuals,
populations and communities."[55]

How do we fix the problem?
We need to ensure that we are continuously monitoring and
reducing disparities in health and health care. Given that disparities in health arise from a complicated interplay of factors, most of
which are not under the control of the health care system, we

need to clarify what the system can do itself and where it needs to recruit help.

The Saskatoon Health Region has identified significant disparities in health and health care access within its catchment area.[56] For example, there are sixteen times as many suicide attempts in the poorest neighbourhoods as in the wealthiest, but only twice as many physician visits for mental health problems.

The Saskatoon Regional Inter-sectoral Committee (RIC) is co-chaired by the Health Region's vice-president for primary health care and the city's director of parks and recreation. In response to the health disparities research, the health region is working in concert with its RIC partners to develop innovative programs to tackle the disparities.[57] In March 2007, the province announced $8 million in new spending targeted to the city neighbourhoods with the poorest health.[58]

3. Client-centred

What's wrong with our current approach?
Clients should be in control of their own care to ensure that their health care journey meets their own values and expectations. However, clients don't even usually have the information they require to make decisions. The average client requires ninety seconds[59] to explain his problem, but the average doctor interrupts the average client in only about twenty seconds.[60, 61] As a result, physicians often do not have the complete information to assess their clients' problems, and clients are capable of fully informed decision making in less than 10 percent of physician visits.[62] These problems are much worse for people with formal communications barriers, such as physical disabilities, cultural barriers, or lack of English language skills.[63, 64, 65]

Why do we have this problem?
Our health system is based around providers, not clients. Up until recently there has been little provider training devoted to communication skills or to the concept of clients and families as partners in care. Some of these problems could be ameliorated if clients had access to a high-functioning team of professionals instead of the more typical focus on one doctor. Too much of our doctors' time is spent dealing with problems with which they have little training or expertise. Canadian family physicians are less likely to work in teams than those in other countries.[66]

How do we fix the problem?
We need to involve clients in all aspects of their care and in health services planning. We need to ensure that we build in sensitivity and tolerance to Canada's growing ethnic, racial, and religious diversity as we re-design our health system.

During the 1990s, the London Intercommunity Health Centre developed a highly effective program to deal with diabetes in London's large Latin American population.[67] The centre has found that most of the time, when a client's diabetes is out of control, it's due to non-medical factors. So they have a social worker and two community health workers who are part of their team. They help their clients deal with a myriad of problems, from illiteracy to landlord–tenant problems.

Helping clients with their underlying determinants of health has dramatically improved their diabetes results. As of June 2006, the centre's Latino diabetes self-management clinic showed a 22 percent improvement after program intervention, indicating excellent diabetes control.[68]

4. Effective

What's wrong with our current approach?
Poor quality outcomes are a result of care that isn't based on the best scientific evidence. It often takes fifteen to twenty years after an innovation's development before it becomes routine practice. A number of studies have shown that the management of chronic disease is contrary to professionally endorsed clinical practice guidelines.[69,70]

Why do we have this problem?
We're not using the best evidence to inform practice because:
- The evidence doesn't get to where it needs to go. The doctor doesn't have the information at the bedside. The nurse doesn't have it at the client's home.
- The health providers know the evidence, but there is a system barrier that prevents them from using it. Family doctors know they should be doing a better job with chronic disease; but few family doctors work with other professionals like nurses, therapists, and others, and fewer have electronic health records.

How do we fix the problem?
We have to follow the evidence to develop services, and we need to implement electronic health records. We also have to implement high-functioning interdisciplinary teams, especially in primary health care. For example, Ontario has developed an internationally recognized strategy for dealing with stroke, which straddles the spectrum of services all the way from prevention to rehabilitation. It is based on evidence each step of the way. As a result, Ontarians have the world's best access to thrombolytic or

clot-busting therapy for stroke. Eleven percent of Ontario stroke patients get clot-busting drugs versus 3 percent in the United States and most other parts of the world.[71]

5. Accessible

What's wrong with our current approach?
Canadians are more likely than those in most other countries to report long waits for family doctors, emergency rooms, specialist appointments, and elective surgery.[72]

Why do we have this problem?
Canada has fewer doctors per population than almost any other wealthy country, and we are at the low end for hospital beds and diagnostic equipment.[73] However, health systems with fewer resources than ours can run smoothly with few waits and delays. One of the big problems in primary health care is the lack of interdisciplinary care compared with other jurisdictions. Doctors are seeing a lot of patients who would be better off seeing other professionals or managing their own care.

One of the reasons many Canadians face long waits for specialist visits is that the main format hasn't changed in over a hundred years. In most of Canada, specialists schedule their clients for one-hour appointments, after the family doctor has made the referral. But sometimes the visit could have been replaced by a five-minute phone call between the family doctor and the specialist. In other cases, the client and family might need a half-day assessment from a multidisciplinary specialist team.

How do we fix the problem?
We need to focus on clients' needs and use some queuing techniques to ensure timely access. Toronto's Access Alliance Community Health Centre[74] improved the access to its maternal

child programs for new immigrants and refugees by literally taking services to clients. The centre works closely with settlement agencies to identify the Toronto neighbourhoods into which new immigrants and refugees are moving. Then Access Alliance uses existing community ethno-cultural networks to recruit and hire peer outreach workers. The outreach workers and staff from the CHC deliver up to twenty education programs, including six on parenting. They also facilitate well child and women clinics conducted by the CHC's nurse practitioners and dietitians in community settings.

The Saskatoon Community Clinic, Toronto's Rexdale and Lawrence Heights Community Health Centres, and Cambridge's Grandview Medical Centre have implemented "Advanced Access" to eliminate waits and delays.[75] The Saskatchewan Health Quality Council has taken this innovation to 25 percent of the province's primary health care practices.[76]

And we could get needed specialty care quickly, as well. In Hamilton, the HSO Mental Health Program integrates 145 family doctors, 17 psychiatrists, 80 counsellors who are based with the family doctors (most of whom are social workers), and over 300,000 clients.[77,78] As a result of the program, 1,100 percent more clients have been seen with mental health problems in primary health care, while referrals to the psychiatry specialty clinic have simultaneously dropped by 70 percent. All clients are given standardized assessments, and the program has documented improvements in depression scores, as well as general health and functioning.

Finally, we could get faster access to elective surgery. For example, the Alberta Bone and Joint Institute Pilot Project[79] reduced wait times for artificial joints from nineteen months to less than eleven weeks, all the way from family doctor referral right through to surgery.

When you put it all together, we shouldn't have to spend a lot more money in Canada to get same day access to primary health care, routine specialty care within one week, and elective surgery in a month.

6. Safe

What's wrong with our current approach?
One in fourteen Canadian hospital clients suffers a complication while in hospital, resulting in up to 24,000 deaths every year from preventable complications. Thousands more die because of poor-quality health care outside of hospital, especially from medication complications.[80,81]

Why do we have this problem?
The health care system has an outdated view of safety.[82] Other sectors such as transportation have updated their culture to include encouraging disclosure of accidents and near-accidents by offering immunity if the reporting is done promptly. Accidents are investigated to identify systemic factors, not to single out and punish individuals.[83]

The lack of electronic information systems is a key risk factor for clients. To quote the US Institute of Medicine, "In a safe system, clients need to tell care-givers something once." One of the major complaints by Canadian clients is that they repeatedly have to tell the same stories to many different providers. And if clients are incapable of giving this information, the care team won't have it. This risky situation becomes even more dangerous when a client moves from one health care setting to another, for example, from the operating room to the intensive care unit, or from hospital to home.

How do we fix the problem?
We need to ensure that we are using effective services and that

there are safeguards in place when things do go wrong. Information systems are a key facilitator for safety. Dr. David Chan and other McMaster University colleagues developed OSCAR, Open Source Clinical Application Resource, an open-source, electronic health record.[84,85] Dr. Chan has recently assisted a group of Toronto agencies that deal with the homeless establish an integrated record that will be available online to whatever provider requires the information.

The Client Access to Integrated Services and Information (CAISI) Project aims to reduce the risks of chronic homelessness by enhancing the integration of care between agencies at the individual and population levels, using an electronic information system.[86] Providers will not have to search through paper charts or telephone a dozen other agencies to get key information and keep their clients safe.

The Second Stage of Medicare is Coming, But Can We Wait?

We have known the broad brush strokes for the second stage of medicare since at least 1945. The development of the quality agenda in health care has added a lot of detail to the sketch. And there are more and more Canadian examples of these second stage programs with their attendant benefits to health and the health care system. If we could implement the second stage of medicare, we could significantly improve the health of Canadians, including the health of the people who provide care. While medicare has problems, it's pretty clear that we can fix them all without charging clients or contracting-out care to the lowest bidder.[87]

But, while there have been many improvements in medicare, the pace is slow and our public discourse is plagued by the endless debate about privatization. The media have a strong bias against "good news," so they provide almost no coverage of second stage reforms. Google records 300 times as many "hits" for

Vancouver orthopedic surgeon Dr. Brian Day than for the Alberta Bone and Joint Institute. Dr. Day offers quicker artificial joint implants for cash on the barrel. But he would have no customers if the Alberta Institute's pilot project were spread across the country.

Canada needs to complete medicare's first stage by providing public coverage for pharmaceuticals, home care, and preventive dental services. But if we don't refocus our health services on keeping people well, we will never be able to afford the first stage. To quote Tommy Douglas:

> Only through the practice of preventive medicine will we keep the costs from becoming so excessive that the public will decide that Medicare is not in the best interests of the people of the country.

CHAPTER 20

Health Human Resources —
A Nurse's Perspective

Linda Silas

Health care is like hockey — it's all about teamwork.
                                                  –Anonymous

First, let me be very clear. I am a nurse. We don't speak for doctors, but I am sure doctors will agree with the following statement: nurses and doctors don't do it alone and we can't do it alone. The crisis in health human resources is about the whole health care team.

As the years go by, alarm bells sound louder in health work environments, especially in nursing practice environments. The December 2006 release of a comprehensive study of the nursing workforce, the *2005 National Survey on the Work and Health of Nurses*, brought the complete nursing picture into focus.[88]

This survey was undertaken by Statistics Canada, in partnership with Health Canada and the Canadian Institute for Health Information. Researchers interviewed a total of 18,676 nurses,

representing registered nurses, licensed practical nurses, and registered psychiatric nurses, in all provinces and territories.

The impressive response rate of 80 percent indicated the enthu-
siasm and support of nurses for this study. Nurses want the public
and the government to know what it is like to work as a nurse
today, and want to assist in pointing the way forward for employers and governments.

The survey reported:

- Nurses working full-time had a 58 percent rate of
  absence due to illness or injury — higher than the
  rate among the overall full-time employed labour
  force, second only to assisting occupations in support of health services.
- Both overtime hours and illness and injury-related
  absenteeism are higher than a decade ago.

The survey found that nurses face a broad range of physical and
emotional challenges in demanding, often hectic, workplaces:

- The proportion of nurses reporting a high level of
  work stress was higher than that for employed
  people overall.
- Four out of ten nurses did not have a full-time
  job.
- Nearly half of nurses reported that their employer
  expected them to work overtime.
- Fifty percent of nurses regularly work unpaid
  overtime, averaging four hours per week.
- Almost one in five female nurses had more than
  one job. This is double the proportion among
  employed females in the general population.
- Nurses were more likely than the average worker
  to have experienced depression.
- Nearly half of all nurses in direct patient care
  reported that, at some point in their career, they

had a needle stick or sharp injury.

- Almost three in ten nurses who provide direct care
  said they had been physically assaulted by a patient
  in the previous year.
- More than three in ten had experienced pain serious enough to prevent them from carrying out
  their normal daily activities.

Add this to the equivalent of 10,054 full-time jobs (approximately 18 million hours) worked in overtime in 2005, as reported
by researchers Jenssen & McCracken. The cost of nurse absenteeism and overtime is estimated at over $1 billion.[89]

The survey paints a national picture of a workforce needing
care. The great majority (88 percent) of nurses reported satisfaction with their jobs, but still want to see immediate improvements
in their working conditions. In spite of highly stressful and difficult working conditions, nurses continue to tell us they love being
nurses.

Closer to Home

Let me paint the picture of the working conditions for nurses in
Manitoba and Saskatchewan.

The survey said:

- Nurses in Saskatchewan have worked longer in
  nursing than nurses elsewhere in Canada.
- Saskatchewan nurses are most likely to have at
  least one other job, and are most likely to work
  more than forty hours per week, than nurses elsewhere in the country.
- Saskatchewan nurses are most likely to report
  emotional abuse from a patient or a physician,
  and most likely to report high job strain. They are
  also most likely to have missed work due to
  physical illness.

- Nurses in Saskatchewan are more concerned about the availability and effectiveness of personal protective equipment than nurses elsewhere.
- On a positive note, Saskatchewan nurses are most likely to report access to mechanical lifting devices.

The survey said:

- Manitoba has the highest percentage of nurses in Canada who say their mental health has made it difficult to handle work. Surpassed only by British Columbia, Manitoba's nurses report the second highest rate of nurses who have missed work due to mental health.
- Manitoba nurses are more likely to report physical assault than nurses elsewhere, with the exception of Newfoundland and Labrador.
- Manitoba has the highest percentage of nurses in Canada with arthritis and second most likely, after Saskatchewan nurses, to have at least one musculoskeletal condition.
- Nurses in Manitoba are second only to Alberta in having the lowest number of full-time jobs.
- On a positive note, more nurses in Manitoba than elsewhere would agree that they make important patient care and work decisions.
- Child care is also more available to nurses in Manitoba than to those in the rest of Canada, with the exception of Quebec.

We must ask why there are approximately 600 nurse vacancies in Saskatchewan. We must also ask why we don't see free, expedited nursing education programs.

If tomorrow the Harper government realized that Canada is short at least 16,000 police officers, it is likely that action would

be taken to reverse this situation. Why is it not the same for nurses? Post-secondary education costs for nursing students can be up
to $40,000 and up to $100,000 for doctors. Free, expedited education programs would make it easy and attractive for young
Canadians to become nurses and doctors. That's what we need in
Canada.

We need more action, lots more. This means we need more staff
— lots more! Why isn't the nursing shortage an election issue
everywhere, like it is in Manitoba?

There has been some movement at the front lines recently in
protecting the health and safety of nurses:

- Nurses in British Columbia, Alberta,
  Saskatchewan, Nova Scotia, and Manitoba are
  using safety-engineered devices as a result of regulatory change.
- British Columbia and Ontario have purchased
  new beds and lifts to prevent back injuries among
  staff, and Nova Scotia is testing lift teams.
- There are pilot projects at spotlight organizations
  around Ontario through the Healthy Workplace
  Best Practice Guidelines Project.
- In British Columbia, the new 2006 collective
  agreement includes major initiatives to enhance
  health and safety, particularly to reduce and eliminate violence in the workplace.
- In a March 2007 arbitration award, Ontario nurses
  were awarded language ensuring that, in the event
  of the emergence of a pandemic, adequate stocks
  of N-95 respirators will be made available by hospital employers.

But, compared to what we need to keep nurses safe on the job,
these are drops in the bucket.

Three kinds of actions are needed: system, organizational, and individual. At the core of the issue of healthy workplaces is work-load. Addressing workload means addressing retention and recruitment plans.

At a system level, this means the implementation of a pan-Canadian health human resources (HHR) strategy to coordinate dialogue and action on HHR education, retention and recruit-ment — not a race for provinces to poach nurses from one another.

What might a pan-Canadian HHR Strategy look like? National observatories for human resources for health were set up in twenty-two countries in 1998 as part of an initiative by the Pan American Health Organization (PAHO) — the World Health Organization's Regional Office for the Americas — to counter-act the neglect of health workforce issues in Latin America during the 1980s and early 1990s. These observatories have helped to raise the profile of the health workforce agenda, improve the information base, and strengthen health sector stewardship. This is what we need in Canada.

PAHO's common characteristic is multiple stakeholder partici-pation involving universities, ministries of health, professional associations, corporate providers, unions, and user representatives. They help to strengthen strategic intelligence. In all too many cases, the health workforce information available to national deci-sion makers is extremely poor. We need national information, tools and measures, shared standards, technical frameworks, and research methodologies.

Canada needs its own version of an Observatory on Health Human Resources, a pan-Canadian HHR Strategy to facilitate multi-stakeholder participation, strengthen health sector steward-ship, and gather and disseminate strategic intelligence.

In the workplace, at the organizational level, we need innovation. We need to learn from micro-level innovations in the health work-force, encouraging what works and discouraging what does not.

Making these assessments requires specific skills, as well as the system approach mentioned earlier that involves inventory keeping, monitoring, evaluation, documentation and exchange. We need a practical evaluation tool to decide which actions merit further study and implementation. We need to:

- pilot,
- evaluate,
- disseminate, and
- replicate.

Sounds like a nursing process!

At the individual level, it is one word: commitment. We need to cultivate more and stronger partnerships in support of innovation among employers and employees. We need to ensure a strong role for unions, professional associations, governments, and employers.

We need macro resources to support micro innovations; that's where the two levels of government fit in. And last, but in no way least, we need real political will and not just empty promises that conclude in shallow partnerships.

Finally, on medicare: let's be real. We need to commit. We know what is going on out there. Tommy Douglas's vision for the full scope of medicare and the realities of Monique Bégin and Roy Romanow are almost ghosts in the health care debate. As medicare defenders, we need to be loud and in politicians' faces to protect, and yes, enhance and expand medicare to include pharmacare, long-term care, and home care services, and full access for children to health services, including dentistry.

CHAPTER 21

The Electronic Health Record: The Neglected Key to Saving Medicare

Steven Lewis

Medicare has enemies from without and enemies from within. The external threat is the unrelenting attack on its principles from shills who have learned their gift-giving from Troy and their language from Orwell. Tommy Douglas identified the threat from within. Always the fiscal conservative and ever attuned to the temptations of human nature, Douglas knew that providing medical care irrespective of ability to pay was a triumph of social justice that risked its own undoing if it became an end in itself rather than the pathway to the greater goal of a healthy population where more was prevented and less needed cure.

Health care, both public and private, is big business. Many Canadians prosper from the seemingly perpetual orgy of diagnosis and repair. When we are sick, there is an ever-expanding array of tools, techniques, and potions. Absent sickness, we are encouraged to become the worried well. Our logic tells us to keep ourselves healthy and prevent illness; our fears preoccupy us with health care. In this sense, the medicare victory has been too decisive — in becoming an icon of national identity and the major incarnation of social solidarity, it has largely ossified, its reform hobbled by politics, vetoed by powerful interests, and largely ignored by a weary public that just wants its hips replaced fast and well.

The dirty little secret of medicare is that it isn't very good. International surveys continue to show that Canada trails most high-income countries in providing accessible, high quality, timely care. (Often we escape the basement only because the United States is in the league.) Our fragmented, cottage industry medical care system does a poor job of managing people with chronic diseases, pumps the frail elderly full of drugs that often land them in the hospital, and makes people wait unconscionable lengths of time to be seen by a specialist. Our hospitals — like hospitals everywhere — are error-prone risk factories that kill up to 10,000 Canadians a year, a third of the deaths avoidable. Health spending is up $70 billion a year from only a decade ago, and still no great leap forward. Privatizers lick their chops as they survey the damage and enlist the Supreme Court to do their bidding.

Not that there hasn't been change. We now have health regions to govern huge swaths of the system (though notably, not physicians and drugs) and pursue the long, painful path to service integration. There are beacons of excellence, like the Sault Ste. Marie clinic and preventive mental health care in Hamilton. But the triumphs remain the exceptions. The whole is invariably less than the sum of the parts. The primary health care revolution, central to improvement, has failed to catch fire. Hard won victories give way to new threats. Smoking rates are down, obesity rates are skyrocketing. What is to be done?

Medicare needs to preserve its principles, improve its quality and timeliness, and abandon ineffective, costly practices. It needs twenty-first century tools to do a twenty-first century job. Information technology and a culture of quality improvement, far more than another round of restructuring, finger-pointing, or budget-raising, are the building blocks of excellence. The electronic health record (EHR) is essential to effectiveness, efficiency, and accountability. Medicare supporters should embrace it, promote it, demand it, and support governments that invest in it.

An EHR is an electronic compilation of all of a person's relevant demographic, diagnostic, and treatment information, including visits to the doctor, laboratory tests, hospitalizations, home care, drug utilization, and long-term care. It is your health and health care biography: over time, it creates a portrait of an individual's journey through health and illness. It is permanent, portable, transferable, and accessible to you, and any provider, anywhere, but only on a need-to-know basis. You own it, and strict ethical, privacy, and security rules govern its use.

An EHR benefits both the individual and system. Among its payoffs:

- It eliminates the need for endlessly repeated explanations, histories, and cautions. Patients do not have to tell their stories or explain their symptoms anew each time they are seen by a new provider. Providers don't have to waste precious time extracting critical information that may get lost in translation.

- It eliminates errors and risks. The emergency room nurse in Victoria instantly learns the allergies and medication profiles of the unconscious traffic accident patient from Fredericton. Software flags contraindicated prescriptions and potential errors in dosage. Electronic prescribing eliminates errors resulting from illegible handwriting on prescription pads.

- It allows people to be active partners in their own health care. In Denmark, patients have Internet access to their own EHRs. They can add or question data, follow their own treatment histories, and learn more about their own risks and how to prevent them. They also can see who has had access to their records, which powerfully discourages unauthorized use.

- It improves quality. The data can be analyzed in real time, and the results fed back to providers, clinics, and institutions. Doctors can identify diabetics whose blood sugars and blood pressure are poorly managed, which patients need to be seen regularly and which can manage their own conditions, and devise new strategies to improve adherence to recommended lifestyle regimens. It can alert hospitals to emerging problems with post-operative care resulting in readmissions. It allows for comparisons so that all organizations are aware of the best practices and can learn how to achieve these levels.

- It saves money. Tests are done once and the results are available to all who need them. Specialists with instant access to up-to-date histories and test results save valuable consultation time. Reduced medication error and hospital infection rates prevent health breakdown, readmissions, and costly repairs.

- It improves accountability. Governments, boards, and managers have updated information not only on what the system does (activities and inputs), but what it accomplishes (health outcomes). They can set benchmarks and develop policies and incentives that promote excellence and discourage waste and harm. The public has a clearer idea of what it gets for its taxes.

- It improves equity. Aggregated information reveals the distribution of health and health care in the population. Analyses can pinpoint inequities in access and quality by geographic area, by socio-economic status, gender, and ethnicity. The data can create new awareness of neglected and poorly served populations such as those with mental health problems, leading to a rebalancing of budgets and a truly needs-based approach to health improvement.

- It improves timeliness. Bottlenecks, gridlock, and their causes can be identified. Time-stamped requests for appointments and referrals can be analyzed to assess need, forecast trends, and add or shift capacity. Managers and clinicians can reallocate their time and resources to address surges in need.

Large scale, sustained improvements in access, equity, timeliness, and efficiency are possible. The NHS in the UK, the Veterans' Administration system in the United States, Intermountain Health headquartered in Utah, and Brigham and Women's Hospital in Boston — all have documented the achievement of excellence. All have invested in information technology and built its use into the culture of their organizations. Health care is perhaps the most information-intensive of all human services, and it cannot succeed if buried under an avalanche of paper records and unmeasured performance.

A pan-Canadian EHR built on common standards and designed to meet the needs of patients, practitioners, managers, and governments will not come cheap. While Ottawa, through

Canada Health Infoway, and the provinces are all investing more than they used to, the pace of implementation is too slow, the efforts too fragmented, there are too many vendors in the field, and there is not enough money. It will take $10 to $20 billion to do this right. Inevitably, there will be glitches and outright failures along the way: this, alas, is the nature of IT.

The champions of medicare typically rally to the cries of more money, more doctors and nurses, and more beds, causes hung around their necks like garlic to ward off the privatization devil. There has been, and will be, more money; there will be more doctors and nurses; and in some jurisdictions, there will be more beds. More is not the problem; Tommy Douglas rightly saw medicare as a transitional stage on the way to *less*.

History has shown that medicare's viability and effectiveness demands more than more. It requires faster, smarter, better. Medicare's friends rightly chide critics captured by particular interests and hostage to obsolete practices. But we, too, are vulnerable to seduction by the wrong causes and defending the indefensible. Triumphs of principle do not guarantee effective implementation. A national pharmacare program without an information-based revolution in prescribing would be a costly quagmire whose main beneficiary would be industry.

Individuals, health care workers, managers, and governments are variously vulnerable to mishap in the absence of a full-fledged, pan-Canadian EHR. The system is fraught with error, harm, inequity, and waste. The EHR will not make the system perfect, and its development will at times be rocky. It is a necessary but not sufficient tool for improvement. That Canadian doctors are in last position in a survey of seven countries in terms of EHR uptake[90] is a genuine crisis and an unsustainable shortcoming. Unless it is soon remedied, the public system risks internal collapse under the weight of its failures.

Medicare's supporters should therefore fight on two fronts: the battleground of principles, and the trench warfare of system reform. The enemy within is to accept the system's failings and overlook the root causes of sub-par performance. Your bank and your insurance company would fail without modern information technology. Medicare is similarly at risk. Medicare, Tommy Douglas knew, must be a permanent revolution. The EHR is central to the realization of what every Canadian deserves: first-rate, safe, efficient, and just health care.

CHAPTER 22

Health Care Reform As If Women Mattered

Pat Armstrong

In looking forward, we need to make care the objective rather than the problem. And instead of seeing expenditures on health care as the primary issue, we should look at the contributions health care makes, not only to the overall economy and corporations, but also to employment and communities. To do so in ways that are equitable and effective, and thus efficient, we need to recognize that gender matters and understand the ways gender matters in health and care.

Women account for 80 percent of the health care labour force and provide the overwhelming majority of the unpaid personal care. They are also the majority of those who use the health care system, in part because they have the babies and because they live longer than men, and in part because of the ways they are treated as workers and patients in health care. They are also the majority of those who take others for care, although they are a minority of those making the major decisions about health services and about the other factors that shape our health. Integrating gender into our care strategies thus means beginning with a focus on women and ensuring that they are not missing from the plans for care. It means recognizing differences among women as well. This understanding must be fundamental to research, policy, and practices.

Attending to women's health goes far beyond boobs and babies to understanding that the lives of women and men, boys and girls are shaped and experienced in different and usually unequal ways. In planning for timely access to care for hips and knees, for example, we need more research into why women are twice as likely as men to need new hips and into how we can ensure that they get access to care in proportion to their need, taking their responsibilities for unpaid care into account.[91] Only then can we work to reduce the need for new hips and organize services in ways that allocate care where it is needed most and that are appropriate to these needs.

We must start by asking what services are required and where, for which women and men, and why. For example, we know from research by the Aboriginal Women's Health and Healing Research Group that AIDS cases are almost three times higher among Aboriginal women compared to non-Aboriginal women. First Nations and Inuit women have a diabetes rate nearly five times that of other women, with higher relative rates than men. We need to investigate the factors contributing to these differences and inequities, examining the daily conditions of their lives, as well as ideas about these women and their bodies, and the ways they are treated in care. This means establishing not only what services are needed for them but also what kinds of services are available and where they are located, all critical to understanding questions of timely access, efficiency, and equity. Without culturally appropriate services near where they live and without services provided in ways that address causes, relationships, and confidentiality, women cannot receive timely, effective access and they, along with the entire health system, will pay more in the long run. In short, we would begin long before these women reach the health service and evaluate the services with different criteria in mind.

Attending to women's health care work means re-examining the structures and relations in health care work and integrating a gender analysis into our plans for care services. Let me give you some examples.

First, consider the concern over nursing shortages and the aging labour force. It is no accident that the bulk of the nursing labour force is, for the first time, over age fifty. This never happened before because we made many nurses quit when they were young. Initially, they were forced to leave when they got married. Later, married women could stay but they had to leave when they became pregnant. Older nurses tended to be single women who worked as supervisors and often lived in a residence that provided them with food and clean clothes. Yet we not only organize nursing as if they were all as young as they were in the past; we have also intensified the work, speeding up the pace and increasing the demands. It is not surprising, then, that health care work is now the most dangerous occupation in terms of illness and injury, especially given that the women who provide care feel responsible and are held responsible for the care deficit, often putting in unpaid extra hours to provide the necessary care. We cannot understand and address these problems without understanding that nurses are women.

This takes me to my second example of why gender matters and why we should begin with women. Nurses do not make up the majority of those who work in health services, even though they are the focus of much current concern. Indeed, the largest proportion of those employed in health and social services are those usually described as ancillary workers, the mainly women who cook, clean, do laundry, do clerical work, and provide personal care. Their work is often dismissed as unskilled and, increasingly, is not even counted as health care work.

Yet these workers do work once done by nurses and work that is so critical to care that nurses must do it if the ancillary workers are not there. Think *C-difficile* and SARS. Cleaning, as well as laundry, have proven to be critical components in preventing transmission of infectious diseases. And think how crucial accurate records are to care. Drug reactions and tainted blood are just two examples. The costs of poor cleaning, bad food, faulty records, and bad personal care can be enormous, not only to the individuals who need care but also to those who provide care and to the economy as a whole.

To understand the dismissal of such work as unskilled, and thus easy to privatize to contractors, it is necessary to understand how the skills traditionally associated with women's work are rendered invisible and undervalued. And with these workers, the dismissal of women's skills is often combined with the dismissal of the skills immigrants and those from racialized groups bring to the job. We also need to understand the ways women's power is limited by the structures of care and care work, and by defining care as a "labour of love."

The majority of these ancillary workers are personal care providers. In long-term care and home care, they make up the majority of health care workers. And most of those they care for are women. This female majority may help explain why long-term care and home care have received so little attention and support, placing Canada well below Norway and Sweden in public spending on such care; that is, below countries that have placed a high value on gender equity and women's rights.[92] As is the case with nursing, the conditions of their labour are the conditions for care. Within health care, they are among those with the highest risk of illness and injury, suggesting that care itself is at risk.

Like cooking and cleaning, laundry and clerical work, personal care work is associated with women's work in the home and with women's natural capacities. As we send people home "quicker and sicker," and keep more people at home with more complicated care needs, where we expect mainly women to provide the care with little formal training and support, we reinforce the notion that this is unskilled work that can be done by any woman. The work and the skills become hidden in the household. So do the risks to providers and to those with care needs. Indeed, in spite of our talk about accountability, we have very little information on the health hazards faced in the home by either providers or by those with care needs.

Unless we recognize and value this work, and make these workers members of the public health care team, we may well face more pandemics and personal tragedies for patients, as well as growing injury and illness rates for the women doing the work. This means supporting unpaid care work as well, through training and through the provision of alternatives. And to do so means understanding that this is women's work. In addition, it means understanding what makes women sick or injured, how they experience these problems, and the ways they are treated during and after care. It also means understanding differences among women in relation to their health, their care, and their care work. As resources become increasingly unequal, so do differences not only between women and men but also among women.

In sum, planning for care means planning with women in mind, not only for the sake of the women, but also for the sake of the system as a whole. Such planning could make care more efficient as well as more effective.

CHAPTER 23

Pharmacare: Equity, Efficiency, and Effectiveness — We've Waited Long Enough

Joel Lexchin

Canadians have been waiting for pharmacare since the early 1960s when it was proposed by the Royal Commission on Health Care. However, despite repeated promises in the ensuing decades from the National Forum on Health and even the Liberal Party itself during the 1997 election, pharmacare still remains beyond our grasp. As a result, we have the situation where 3 percent of Canadians, or about one million people, are considered uninsured because they pay more than 4.5 percent of their gross family income for prescription drugs, and an additional 3.3 million who pay 2.5 to 4.5 percent of their income are labelled underinsured.[93] The Ontario government estimates that 19 percent of the population or nearly 2.5 million people lack insurance.[94] According to a recently published study out of Toronto's Hospital for Sick Children, a significant number of children lack timely access to necessary medications because of economic problems.[95]

The poorest fifth of the Canadian population spends more money out of pocket on prescription drugs than the richest fifth.[96] For people over sixty-five, it makes a significant difference which province you live in when it comes to drug therapy. A low-income senior in Saskatchewan with average drug use in 1998 would have paid $500 out of pocket, but the same person with the same drug use in Ontario would pay less than one-tenth that amount.[97]

Internationally, Canadian public spending on drugs as a percent of total drug costs or on a per capita basis ranks near the bottom of the list of industrialized countries. The only place that consistently has a worse record than Canada is the United States.[98]

Proposals from Kirby[99] and Romanow[100] have abandoned the idea of first-dollar universal drug coverage in favour of some form of catastrophic coverage. In the case of Kirby, coverage would start once people had spent 3 percent of their annual income on prescription medication; Romanow suggests a $1,500 deductible. In 2003, provincial first ministers pledged "by the end of 2005/06, to ensure that Canadians, wherever they live, have reasonable access to catastrophic drug coverage." However, that pledge has now been superseded by the National Pharmaceutical Strategy, and in its June 2006 report all that it could offer was a set of principles that had been developed for coverage and a recommendation for further study.[101]

Catastrophic drug coverage, while better than nothing for those currently without any insurance, would still leave low-income people vulnerable to high drug costs. In Ontario, the minimum wage of $8 an hour translates into an annual income of $16,000. If Canada adopted the Kirby proposal, that minimum-wage person would be spending about $480 per year on drugs — a considerable portion of her disposable income after accounting for shelter and food.

On equity grounds alone, there is a strong argument for pharma-

MEDICARE

care, but, beyond equity, pharmacare will help Canada control rising prescription drug costs. Retail prescription drug costs are rising at about 8 to 10 percent per annum after controlling for inflation, and since the late 1990s Canada has been paying more for medications than for doctors. One of the main factors accounting for this continual inflation is the use of newer and more expensive drugs in place of older, less expensive products. For example, by 1998/1999 over half of the $1.9 billion being spent by the Ontario Drug Benefit Program was on drugs introduced since 1992/1993.[102] A 2002 analysis done by Green Shield, a non-profit insurance company, found that the price of a prescription for generic drugs barely changed from 1997 while the price for one that contained new patented medications went up by 9 percent per annum.

Provincial drug plans have been largely attempting to deal with rising drug expenditures by shifting costs onto users of the system. This was the approach that Quebec used when it decided to expand its drug insurance system without increasing government expenditures. Prior to the change in the Quebec system, people on social assistance were exempt from any co-payments and seniors paid $2 per prescription. After the change, those on welfare had to pay up to $50 per quarter and the elderly were subject to deductibles and co-payments that ranged from $200 to $925 per year. These charges meant a drop in essential drug use of more than 9 percent for welfare recipients and just under 15 percent for the elderly, with corresponding increases in hospitalizations, physician visits, and trips to emergency departments.[103] (Quebec has recently eliminated the co-payments for those on welfare.)

Encouraging the use of private drug insurance will also do little to either control costs or improve equity. Most private drug plans in Canada are much less aggressive in cost control measures than public plans,[104] and administrative costs in private plans run around 8 percent compared to 2 to 3 percent in large provincial plans.[105] Moreover, private insurance through the workplace is a regressive way of providing benefits. Currently, the portion of insurance received through the workplace that is paid for by the employer is exempt from personal income tax. According to Stabile, the value of the subsidy that an individual receives through private insurance is based on his/her marginal tax rate.[106] In a progressive tax system, like the one that exists in Canada, that translates into higher subsidies for those earning higher incomes. In fact, people in the highest 20 percent income bracket receive a benefit more than three times greater than those in the lowest 20 percent.

Monopsony buying power — where a single buyer controls the bulk of the market, like that used in the Australian Pharmaceutical Benefits Scheme — helps keep costs for individual drugs 9 percent lower than those in Canada.[107] Other measures, like tendering for generic products available from multiple companies and cross-price subsidization (requiring lower prices for already listed drugs in return for accepting new listings), that have cut the New Zealand drug budget by almost 50 percent stand little chance of success in a world of multiple payers.[108]

Finally, pharmacare has the potential to help improve the way that doctors prescribe. Pre-marketing trials test drugs on selected groups of patients, but when the products are released on the market they are the object of intense promotional pressure and as such often end up being prescribed to large numbers of patients who were excluded from the clinical trials. This heavy prescribing takes place long before the full safety profile of new drugs is known and therefore exposes patients to potentially serious problems. In the United States, it's estimated that Vioxx caused an additional 88,000 to 140,000 excess cases of serious coronary artery disease in the five years it was on the market.[109] New drugs not only pose safety problems, but for the most part they also fail to offer any major new therapeutic benefits. Figures from the

2005 annual report of the federal Patented Medicine Prices Review Board show that only slightly more than 10 percent of all new drugs are significantly better than existing medications that are generally much less expensive.

Economic incentives and disincentives can be used to limit prescribing of new drugs, but once again these disincentives are only going to be successful when they apply to the majority of prescribing decisions. Furthermore, if government was paying the bulk of the drug costs, it would probably have much more of an incentive to ensure appropriate use, if for no other reason than to keep costs down. In Australia, the federal government provides about $25 million annually to the independent National Prescribing Service, whose mission is to improve drug prescribing by doctors and drug use by consumers.

The usual argument mounted against a first-dollar pharmacare system, similar to what already exists for doctor visits and hospitalizations, is that it is unaffordable. To begin with, this line of reasoning simply ignores the reality that we are already paying for prescription drugs to the tune of almost $18 billion per year. The question is not whether the country can afford the cost, but rather how will the cost be met?

Currently, government accounts for a little under half of all costs, private insurance covers 34 percent, and the rest is paid out of pocket. If government were to pick up the entire tab, then it is inevitable that public spending would increase, probably by about $7.7 billion annually. However, even allowing for increased use of prescription drugs by groups now not covered at all or under-covered, total spending on medications would actually *drop* by between 9 to 10 percent because of lower administrative costs and the lower prices that could be achieved through national bargaining power.

Right now we are funding prescription drugs the way that Americans fund their entire health care system. We have rejected the American approach for doctors and hospitals because we have recognized that it is inefficient and inequitable. It's time to reject that approach to paying for prescription drugs. Pharmacare makes sense on all three grounds: equity, economic efficiency, and effective prescribing. It's time to stop waiting for it.

CHAPTER 24

Federal Pharmacare: Prescription for an Ailing Federation? [110]

Greg Marchildon

Health care has been at the top of the federalism music chart for almost a decade. During this time, first ministers' meetings have become a set piece. Before the meeting is called, the premiers demand more money for health care from Ottawa — knowing that they will not get what they are asking for. The prime minister brushes off these initial demands in public, but meanwhile the federal government enters into private negotiations with the provinces to reach an agreement. Once the dollar figure is in the federal ballpark, the prime minister schedules a formal meeting.

The exception to this pattern was the September 2004 first ministers' meeting that produced the so-called "Ten Year Plan to Strengthen Health Care." In contrast to earlier meetings, Prime Minister Paul Martin made no real attempt to get even a rough agreement in advance. The premiers went into the meeting with their largest ever demand: that the prime minister put enough money into the Canada Health Transfer to close what they called "the Romanow gap" and, at the very same time, that the federal government also take over provincial drug plans. While no precise dollar figure was produced for the drug proposal, the provinces were in effect asking Ottawa to pony up close to $8 billion annually, the amount they were collectively spending on prescription drugs for their respective residents.

At the time, Premier Ralph Klein of Alberta congratulated himself and the other premiers for their "stroke of brilliance." Indeed it might have been, but only if the premiers had walked in with a workable blueprint of how such a major innovation would improve prescription drug coverage at a reasonable cost and simultaneously facilitate health reform. Instead, they came to the first ministers' meeting without even a sketch of what a federal pharmacare program would look like, much less accomplish. They thereby confirmed the skeptics' conclusion that the premiers' offer was about cost-shifting, not about improving health care for Canadians.

Given the ephemeral nature of the provincial pharmacare proposal, it was relatively easy for Martin to brush it aside and focus on the reduction of wait lists. This was the item at the top of his agenda, even though it fell entirely within provincial control and jurisdiction. On the pharmacare proposal, the prime minister stuck to the short-term recommendations in the Romanow and Senate reports of 2002, and asked that some of the federal money be used to improve catastrophic drug coverage while shunting consideration of the pharmacare proposal to a federal–provincial ministerial committee. Here, it has become dead easy — and publicly justifiable — for Ottawa to veto any ambitious proposal on federal pharmacare given the already huge amount that it is transferring to the provinces as part of the Ten Year Plan deal.

It is also unfortunate. Only by transforming public drug policy will we be able to tackle the real sustainability problem in health

care. Going one step further, by initiating major reform to the way
in which drugs are currently prescribed and used, we can dramatically improve primary care, home care, and long-term chronic
care. Without major changes to our federal–provincial arrangements for the administration, delivery, and funding of public
prescription drug programs, we are unlikely to ensure "that the
right patients are getting the right drugs ... at the right price," at
a reasonable and sustainable cost to governments and taxpayers.[111]
As can be seen in figure 1, drugs — including over-the-counter
and prescription drugs — already constitute the second biggest
piece of the health care pie, less than hospital care but more than
physicians' care.

Figure 1: Total health expenditure by use of funds, Canada, 2006

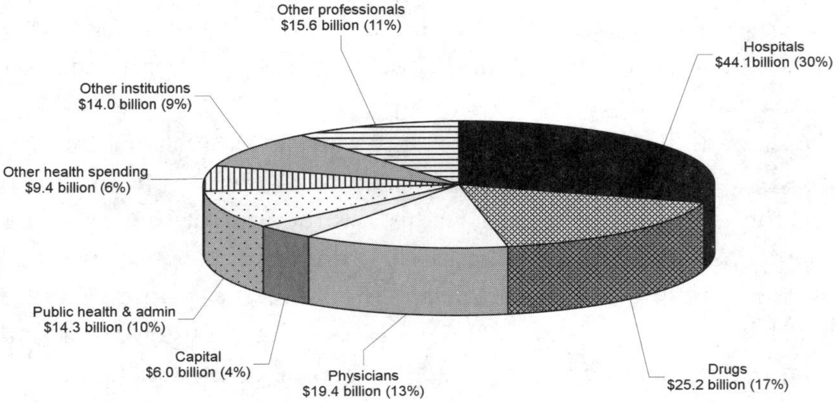

Other professionals
$15.6 billion (11%)

Hospitals
$44.1 billion (30%)

Other institutions
$14.0 billion (9%)

Other health spending
$9.4 billion (6%)

Public health & admin
$14.3 billion (10%)

Capital
$6.0 billion (4%)

Physicians
$19.4 billion (13%)

Drugs
$25.2 billion (17%)

Source: CIHI, *National Health Expenditure Trends 1975-2006* (Ottawa: CIHI, 2006), 96.

The Romanow Commission laid out an incremental strategy
to achieve significant change in how we organize the use of pharmaceuticals in the provision of health care. The catastrophic drug
transfer program it recommended was to be only the first step
toward creation of a National Drug Agency, establishment of a

national drug formulary, introduction of more effective management and monitoring of drug utilization, and regulatory changes aimed at lowering the price of generic drugs and limiting the inflationary impact of new patented drugs.[112]

There has been little to no movement on this transformative agenda in part because of the current division of responsibilities for prescription drug care. The federal government has virtually all the regulatory tools, while the provinces are responsible for designing, administering, and funding their respective prescription drug subsidy plans. Alone, neither order of government is capable of addressing the financial sustainability problem or initiating thoroughgoing change in drug utilization patterns. Given the current stalemate, the time may have come to consider a more radical proposal in which one order of government assumes responsibility for prescription drug policy in Canada.

Prescription Drugs: The Real Sustainability Problem

The debate concerning sustainability of a primarily publicly funded universal health care system has been raging in Canada since the late 1990s. In the early to mid-1990s, all provincial governments restrained spending in their efforts to end deficits. As the largest spending envelope in each province, health care was not spared. In constant inflation-adjusted dollars, per capita public health spending declined over these years. After 1997, with their accounts balanced, governments began to loosen the fiscal purse strings and spend on health care again.

On the basis of the growth in overall public health spending since 1997, some commentators and governments have argued that medicare — defined as medically necessary hospital, diagnostic, and physician services covered under the general principles of the Canada Health Act — is no longer fiscally sustainable. These arguments ignore the fact that private health care spending has been growing even faster than public spending. Indeed, as can be

Figure 2: Average annual per capita growth of health
expenditures in 1997 dollars, 1992–2006

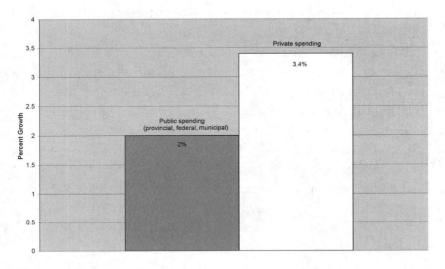

Source: CIHI, *National Health Expenditure Trends, 1975-2006* (Ottawa: CIHI, 2006), 95.

seen in figure 2, private per capita spending grew 1.7 times faster
than public spending.

Table 1 documents rates of growth of expenditure in various
health sectors. From 1998 to 2004, spending on provincial and
territorial public drug plans and private drug insurance plans has
grown, on average, by almost 12 percent annually. This is virtually
double the rates of growth in core medicare hospital and physician services.[113] Despite this enormous difference, governments
tend to focus on medicare spending because they feel they have
some ability to control expenditures of their publicly administered
and financed single-payer systems. In contrast, prescription drugs
inhabit a multi-payer world of mixed public/private funding and
administration.

The federal government runs its own public drug plan for Inuit
and registered First Nations individuals. This is the fastest growing

Table 1: Annual growth rates (in current prices) of prescription
drug plans v. medicare, 1998-2006

	1998	1999	2000	2001	2002	2003	2004	2005	2006	1998-2006 average
Public Drug Plans	11.6	13.7	16.5	14.6	12.8	11.2	9.4	9.5	7.7	11.6
Private Drug Plans	15.6	5.2	14.2	16.1	11.6	12.9	10.6	10.0	9.9	11.8
Hospital Expenditures	5.2	3.9	8.3	6.3	7.5	6.5	7.3	5.6	4.8	6.2
Physician Expenditures	4.2	4.0	6.2	7.7	7.7	7.1	6.5	5.6	7.1	6.2

Source: CIHI, *Drug Expenditure in Canada, 1985-2006* (Ottawa: CIHI, 2007), 60; and CIHI, *National Health Expenditure Trends, 1975-2006* (Ottawa: CIHI, 2006), 96.

component of the Non-Insured Health Benefits (NIHB) programs administered by the First Nations and Inuit Health branch
of Health Canada. Currently, that growth rate matches the growth
rate of the provincial and territorial drug plans.

What does all this mean? The growth in public and private
drug plan expenditures greatly exceeds the rate of growth in
medicare expenditures — despite significant remuneration gains
by health providers in recent years. Meanwhile, prescription drug
plan costs continue to soar. Growing at an annual average of over
20 percent between 1997 and 2004, the Quebec drug plan has
been in a league of its own in terms of both budget growth and
program design. Implemented in 1997, the Quebec plan is in fact
a public–private social insurance scheme rather than the tax funded plans found in Quebec before that date, and in the other
provinces today.[114]

Extrapolation of these trends leads to the conclusion that
provincial and territorial governments are caught on the horns of
a dilemma. They can continue to earmark an ever-growing share
of their health budgets for their drug plans and try to improve
their existing single-payer medicare systems with less money. Or
they can increase co-payments and reduce drug plan benefits (and
beneficiaries) so that they can earmark more money for core
medicare services.

The decision by the Supreme Court of Canada in *Chaoulli v*

Quebec (Attorney General) has raised the possibility that provinces will have to permit parallel private insurance for core medicare services unless they significantly shorten waiting lists for medically necessary elective surgeries. *Chaoulli* may have loaded the dice against any significant pharmacare initiative and in favour of judge-decreed priorities. Investing more public money in medicare at the expense of public investment in prescription drugs may be the path of least resistance, but it will mean offloading costs to private individuals and private insurance plans — and may actually end up raising total health care costs. Managers of private plans can be expected to pass on cost increases by use of larger co-payments and higher premiums. For sure, the Supreme Court has hampered the ability of the provinces to make strategic health care decisions. In these circumstances, it is probably wise for the provinces and territories to transfer their public drug plan responsibilities to the federal government and for Ottawa to accept that, for the first time, it must assume administrative responsibility for delivering a major "slice" of public health care in Canada.

Federal Pharmacare: Putting the Pieces Together

Before describing a federal pharmacare program, it is worth reviewing the existing pieces of the $21 billion prescription drug expenditure pie in Canada shown in figure 3. The size and nature of each piece could change depending on the design of any new pharmacare program — with the devil in the details.

The largest slice is the almost $9 billion spent (in 2006) by the provinces and territories (including Quebec) on their public drug plans. Between 1970 and 1986, every province introduced a prescription drug plan. Most were drug subsidy programs aimed at seniors and individuals receiving social assistance, two high-risk groups generally without access to private health insurance (which most often comes in the form of employment-based

group plans). In the 1990s, provincial governments limited benefits and hiked co-payments and other user fees associated with
their drug plans, often hurting the poorest and most vulnerable.
Almost all provinces shifted costs from the public purse to private
pockets. Their experience with these short-term cost-saving
measures followed a consistent pattern: drug plan costs originally
declined only to surge upwards again within a year of the changes.

In contrast to single-payer medicare programs, there is considerable variation in the administration, delivery, and benefits of
provincial and territorial drug plans. In addition, each jurisdiction
has its own drug formulary, and makes its own final decision concerning what pharmaceutical products it will list on the basis of
clinical efficacy and, to a more limited extent, cost effectiveness.
Recently, in another cost-saving effort, all provinces except Quebec have agreed to a Common Drug Approval assessment

Figure 3: Canadian prescription drug expenditures, 2006

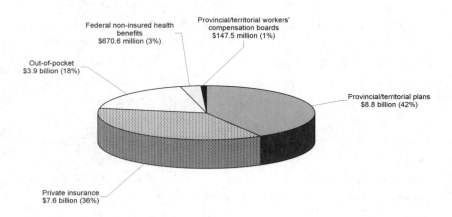

Source: CIHI, *Drug Expenditure in Canada, 1985-2006* (Ottawa: CIHI, 2007), 60.

conducted by an intergovernmental body, the Canadian Agency for Drugs and Technologies in Health. While the Common Drug Approval provides assessments on the clinical and cost effectiveness of new drugs, the actual decision whether to include any new drug in its formulary, and the extent to which the assessment shapes the final decision, remains in the hands of individual provinces and territories.

A further provincial expenditure of $1.7 billion takes place on medicare-covered prescription drugs. Since these drugs are dispensed within hospitals and are considered medically necessary, there is no "patient participation" in paying for them. Individuals who are Inuit or registered First Nations receive over $600 million in drug benefits not covered under the provincial and territorial plans. Finally, provincial and territorial workers' compensation plans cover $148 million worth of drug benefits. All of these public plans supplement or complement $7.6 billion of private health insurance, most of which is in the form of employment-based benefit plans.

There is also the critical regulatory role played by the federal government. On the basis of clinical evidence of a given drug's safety, efficacy, and quality, Health Canada's Therapeutic Products Directorate decides whether any new prescription drug can be marketed in the country. A quasi-judicial, arm's-length federal tribunal, the Patented Medicine Prices Review Board, regulates the retail prices of new patented prescription drugs. Currently, generic drug prices are not regulated because neither level of government has clear constitutional jurisdiction. Ottawa's authority to regulate the prices of patented prescription drugs comes from the explicit mention of patents as being under federal jurisdiction in the Constitution, but this authority does not extend to generic drugs. Nor do the provinces have any obvious constitutional foothold that would allow them to regulate generic drug prices.

Federal pharmacare would ensure that one level of government would be responsible for the regulatory functions as well as administering, delivering, and funding a single national drug plan. With the simple administrative agreement of the provinces (if this is even necessary), price regulation could be extended beyond patented drugs to generic drugs, something desperately needed for a country whose generic prices are among the highest in the world.

Regulatory power over prescription drug prices may be necessary but is not the ideal means to control the cost of a major pharmacare program. Many OECD countries with national drug plans negotiate discount prices from pharmaceutical companies on large-scale orders. The bargaining leverage exercised by national drug plans arises from the size of the market at stake and the power to include or exclude drugs from the national formulary. Discount prices negotiated between drug manufacturers and government are common practice in Australia, New Zealand, and many Western European countries. They are also common practice among the larger Health Maintenance Organizations (HMOs) in the United States. But not in Canada: with few exceptions, governments in Canada do not purchase prescription drugs in bulk. Instead, they rely on user fees and formularies to control costs. With a national pharmacare plan, Ottawa could undertake such bulk purchasing at discounted prices.

The Advantages of Federal Pharmacare

From the perspective of improving the workings of Canadian federalism, a pharmacare scheme operated by Ottawa presents several clear advantages over the status quo. First, this realignment would clarify roles and responsibilities in an area of health care where they have been ambiguous. While the provinces currently pay for almost all public drug coverage in Canada, they lack the regulatory powers of the federal government. Federal pharmacare would ensure that the order of government with the constitutional powers of regulation would also administer and pay for public prescription drug coverage.

Second, federal pharmacare would address the provincial claim of a vertical fiscal imbalance — the claim that while Ottawa enjoys rapidly increasing tax revenues, the provinces face increasing spending responsibilities that are endangering the fiscal health of all but the most prosperous jurisdictions. A federal pharmacare program would be of particular benefit to "have not" provinces that can least afford such a rapidly growing program.

Since the late 1990s, the provincial governments have argued that there is a structural fiscal imbalance between the revenue-generating capacity of the provinces and their expenditure responsibilities relative to the federal government. Although Conservative Prime Minister Harper seems to have more sympathy for the provincial case than past Liberal prime ministers, he would do well to keep in mind the last time the federal government made a major tax transfer to the provinces in the Established Programs Financing (EPF) deal of 1976/1977. At the time, Ottawa lowered its taxes to give tax room so the provinces could raise theirs. Ever since, Ottawa has reminded Canadians of this major re-jigging of the tax system by calculating transfers to the provinces as the sum of cash plus so-called "tax transfers." Thirty years on, the provinces offer no recognition of the fiscal benefits they received from this deal.

Federal pharmacare would be a proactive and constructive way of addressing the fiscal imbalance argument without repeating the EPF. Potentially, this is a win-win solution. The provinces would obtain significant ongoing fiscal relief while Ottawa would deliver a service that directly touches most Canadians and would be able to influence, very directly, the sustainability of public health care.

The advantages of federal pharmacare to Canadians should be obvious. The current patchwork of provincial, territorial, and federal drug programs has created, in the words of one researcher, a "dog's breakfast" of benefits and exclusions that vary across the country.[115] In particular, there exists a major east–west cleavage: drug coverage programs are considerably thinner in the four Atlantic provinces than programs offered in all the jurisdictions west of those provinces. To the extent that federal pharmacare can both eliminate the disparities of public drug coverage across the country and level up to one of the more generous provincial programs, it will act as a national unifier.

Costs and Other Downsides

The single largest impediment to federal pharmacare is the program cost. In fact, the potential cost of a pharmacare program has perennially deterred the federal government from proceeding with a cost-shared provincial–territorial program for prescription drugs in the traditional medicare mould.

The annual operating cost of a federal-only pharmacare program could range from a low of $9 billion to a high of $21 billion, depending on the public program's relationship to private prescription drug insurance, the level of co-payments and other user fees, and changes in prescription and utilization patterns in response to the new system of public coverage. The lower figure of $9 billion is the current cost of all provincial and territorial drug programs and assumes that the federal program would not disturb any of the other pieces in the prescription drug pie and would be about midway or less in its program benefits. The higher figure of $21 billion is the total prescription drug pie and presumes that federal prescription drug insurance replaces all other public and private plans in the country as well as all out-of-pocket costs in the form of the insurance co-payments and deductibles paid by individual Canadians. Using 2001 data, a consultant's study arrived at a figure of $13.6 billion for universal, first-dollar-coverage (no co-payments, deductibles, or other user fees) federal pharmacare. After inclusion of drug price inflation since 2001, this amount is very close to the higher figure of $21 billion.[116]

Unless federal pharmacare "levels up" coverage and accessibility to the most generous provincial program today, some groups will see no advantage in the reform. To take an obvious example: if Ontario residents, who already have one of the more generous programs in the country, end up receiving fewer benefits while paying the same taxes, they will be understandably dissatisfied. By the same token, if federal pharmacare means levelling up to a more generous national drug plan, it should be possible to eliminate current federal NIHB drug benefits and the differential benefits and expenditures associated with it, and the questionable distinctions it makes among Canadians — including the distinction between registered and non-registered Indians.

One scenario is a universal program with co-payments in line with one of the more generous provincial plans but one nonetheless designed to minimize the displacement of current private insurance arrangements. From the beginning, it would make sense to include hospital-based prescription drugs in federal pharmacare. If that were not done, provincial and territorial governments would have a built-in incentive to cost-shift from inpatient to outpatient prescription drug therapy. A very rough back-of-the-envelope calculation would put the cost of this type of federal pharmacare at $14 billion.

What would we get for this money? A truly universal program in which Canadians receive medically necessary drug therapies on the same terms and conditions wherever they live in the country, whatever their history and risk profile, and whether they are inside or outside a hospital. These conditions of access could be spelled out in a new Federal Pharmacare Act that would parallel the Canada Health Act.

Beyond money, we would need to avoid a federal pharmacare program operated in isolation from provincial health reforms. As it is, provincial drug plans, administered in a silo separate from other health services, are generally disconnected from the provincial health reform agenda. Moving pharmacare to a different level of government could exacerbate this problem by creating even more separation between prescription drug policy and health reform. To counteract this tendency, it will be essential for the two orders of government to have a meeting of minds as to how prescription drug therapy fits in the larger health reform agenda.

Those interested in primary care reform, in particular, need to address prescription and drug utilization patterns and behaviours as part of a larger effort to improve diagnosis and monitor ongoing treatment. With federal pharmacare, Ottawa would still depend on the provinces and regional health authorities to influence drug prescribing and utilization. While costs would be the federal government's primary concern, the provinces' primary focus should be on the overall health impact of prescription drug therapies. To avoid strategies that focus on cost-shifting, the two orders of government would benefit from a common reform strategy that simultaneously aimed at improving health outcomes and containing health costs.

Taking the broad view, federal pharmacare should be one element in a larger strategy of transforming and sustaining public health care in Canada. After hospitals, prescription drug therapies now constitute the largest sector of health care expenditures. Indeed, we now spend over $2 billion more on prescription drugs than we do on all physician care. We now have a prescription drug therapy for virtually every illness or injury. Paradoxically, there is little evidence that this huge expenditure is leading to better health.[118] This raises the question of whether Canadian-style medicare systematically over-weights the value of prescription drug therapy relative to alternatives.

Pharmacare would give the federal government a powerful incentive to fund an independent research institute capable of systematically and regularly testing prescription drug therapies against promising non-drug therapies. Public research that is not funded or compromised by the pharmaceutical companies is essential to determining whether there are superior alternatives to prescription drug therapies to treat certain conditions. If it were responsible for administering and funding pharmacare, the federal government would have a strong incentive to examine more effective and lower cost alternatives to prescription drug therapies. For example, there is clinical evidence indicating that non-drug cognitive behaviour therapy (CBT) administered by psychologists can be at least as effective as antidepressant medication in treating severely depressed outpatients.

Quebec: A Separate but Equal Solution

In September 2004, one province stood outside the premiers' consensus in asking the federal government to take over responsibility for prescription drug care. Quebec Premier Jean Charest gave few reasons for his objections, but they can easily be inferred. On one level, his opposition simply reflected his province's historic opposition to federal involvement in all areas of social policy. On another level, Charest was protecting a provincial policy environment that has been supportive of the research-and-development-based pharmaceutical industry, almost half of which is located in Quebec.

The simple solution would be to proceed without Quebec's collaboration. This could take two forms. The first would be to impose a federal pharmacare program on Quebec. It is difficult to see how this could be done. Although the federal government has a strong constitutional foothold in this particular policy domain, it does not have sole jurisdiction. Moreover, any Quebec government would resist — strenuously — any unilateral initiative as an invasion by Ottawa of Quebec's jurisdiction over social policy.

The second, more plausible approach is simply to build a federal pharmacare program around the existing Quebec drug plan. While some might trumpet — or decry — this as asymmetrical federalism, the more important criticism is that such an approach could undermine the objectives of federal pharmacare. It would create an enormous policy doughnut in which program benefits varied enormously inside and outside Quebec. It would reduce Ottawa's negotiating leverage with a pharmaceutical industry either based in Quebec or threatening to move its manufacturing capacity from other parts of Canada to Quebec — or offshore. Finally, given two disparate health and industrial policy regimes, it would put Quebec and Ottawa on a major collision course, and generate new intergovernmental conflicts over prescription drug regulation, health policy, and industrial development.

The best approach is neither of the above. Instead, we need to negotiate a compromise between Quebec and the rest of Canada. A precedent is the Canada Pension Plan/Quebec Pension Plan (CPP/QPP) in which two programs, with very similar (but not identical) objectives and administrative design, are implemented simultaneously. This solution would require the Quebec government to deal with the potential wrath of some pharmaceutical companies for replacing its industry-friendly policies with a more health-oriented prescription drug program and policy environment. It would also require a resolute federal government, willing to pick up the tab only on the explicit agreement that Quebec fundamentally redesign its current drug program and that the other provinces, in turn, accept the CPP/QPP-style arrangement. The *quid pro quo* would be clear. For replacing its current program — likely unsustainable in any event — Quebec would retain control and receive an annual federal transfer for a Quebec drug plan that would be portable (and interchangeable) with the federal plan.

A Constructive Response

During the past decades, we have seen continual intergovernmental squabbling over public health care, federal transfers, fiscal imbalance, and equalization. These disagreements have produced very little in the way of improved programs and policies for Canadians. Federal pharmacare offers not only a constructive response to evidence of a growing fiscal imbalance between the provinces and the federal government but also a project whereby Ottawa could enhance national unity by "touching Canadians directly." More than this, given its existing regulatory powers, the federal government is the only level of government able to contain, effectively, the cost of a public prescription drug plan in the long term. Whether it would have the political will to use its power to exact concessions from the pharmaceutical industry remains an open question, but federal pharmacare would provide the capacity and the opportunity.

Federal pharmacare would, overnight, give each of the provinces the fiscal breathing room within its health budget to increase its investment in medicare, home care, long-term care, mental health, and public health, where necessary, as well to focus more heavily on the "upstream" determinants of health. With prescription drug plans removed from the equation, the annual growth of public health care costs in the provinces would diminish significantly, reducing or eliminating the crowding-out effect that health care budgets have had on other public budgets during the last few years. As for Quebec, federal pharmacare could help the provincial government curtail an unsustainable program that is already seen as providing limited coverage for seniors and the poor because of its high user fees.

Federal pharmacare is not only good health policy, it may be the right prescription for an ailing federation.

CHAPTER 25

A Strategy for Mental Health [119]

Patricia J. Martens

The SOS Medicare 2 conference devoted a great deal of attention to a variety of issues, but rarely did it include issues of mental health. It reminded me of a sign that was formerly at the airport in Thompson, Manitoba, just beside the front entrance, which stated: "Don't even think of parking here." We need to make sure that mental illness is truly brought out of the shadows and into any national discussion about health.

First, let's have a look at the size of the issue (see figure 1). In Manitoba, we have the ability to look at patterns of health and the use of the health care system for the entire population (i.e., population-based) through the use of the Population Health Research Data Repository housed at the Manitoba Centre for Health Policy in the University of Manitoba's Faculty of Medicine. This repository houses many different databases (made anonymous) originally collected for purposes of running various government

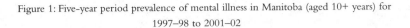

Figure 1: Five-year period prevalence of mental illness in Manitoba (aged 10+ years) for
1997–98 to 2001–02

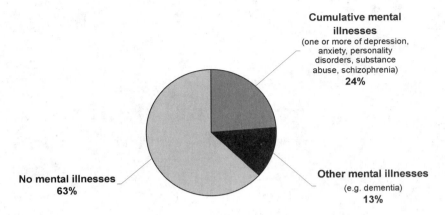

**Cumulative mental
illnesses**
(one or more of depression,
anxiety, personality
disorders, substance
abuse, schizophrenia)
24%

**No mental illnesses
63%**

Other mental illnesses
(e.g. dementia)
13%

programs, but now used by researchers. The mental illness study
used Manitoba records for hospitals, physicians, pharmaceuticals,
and registry records over the five-year period from 1997/1998 to
2001/2002.[120]

We grouped the population of Manitoba into three groups —
those who had cumulative mental illnesses, other mental illnesses,
and no mental illnesses. People in the cumulative mental illness
group are those who have one or more of depression, anxiety, personality disorders, substance abuse, and schizophrenia. Basically,
one in four (24 percent) of Manitobans over a five-year period
had one or more of those diagnoses. Another 13 percent had other
mental illness diagnoses, like dementia. So about one in three
Manitobans over a five-year period had some sort of mental illness diagnosis. Hence, message one is: "Houston (or is it Ottawa?),
we have a problem."

And what is the impact on health care? In our Manitoba study,
those not having mental illness go to see a physician about four
times a year if female, and three times a year if male, for a variety
of reasons. Those in the cumulative mental illness group go more

than twice as often — about nine times a year for females, and seven times a year for males. But only around one or two of those visits are actually coded as visits for reasons of mental illness. Visits for most other illnesses occur at twice the rate — twice the visits for respiratory problems, twice the musculoskeletal, and so on. There appears to be strong comorbidity (that is, intertwining) of mental and physical illness (see figure 2). Hence, message two is: "We need to look at primary health care models for mental illness treatment."

Our Manitoba study also looked at access to physician specialist care. Who accesses the physician specialists of mental illness, for

Figure 2 Physician Visit Rates by Sex and Cause for Manitobans in the Cumulative Disorders Group Versus No Disorders Group, 1997-98 to 2001-02

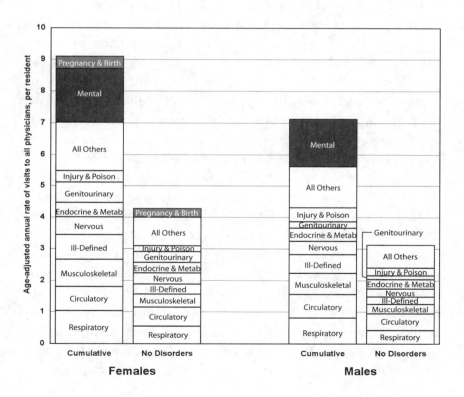

example, psychiatrists? If you take 100 people with mental illness, they would make 100 visits to psychiatrists if they live in the richest urban areas, 70 in the poorest urban areas, 30 in the richest rural areas, and only 10 in the poorest rural areas. By age, they would make 80 visits if they're middle-aged, and only 15 if they are elderly. So who sees psychiatrists? Probably the group that needs them the least uses them the most — urban people living in the highest socioeconomic areas, middle-agers — while the group that needs them just as much, if not more (rural, lower socioeconomic area residents, elderly, and youth), has the lowest rates of use. Especially for rural residents, we should be looking at increasing the use of tele-health. So, message three is: "If we are serious about universal and accessible mental health care, figure out how to make this happen and make it needs-based."

Now let's turn briefly to community and long-term care. Manitoba has one of the most long-standing home care programs through universal, public health insurance. That's the really good news. But those with mental illness experience a huge risk of using such services — three to five times the normal rate. If we look at another community-based program, nursing (personal care) homes also show the impact of mental illness, especially on the elderly. For Manitoba's nursing homes, 75 percent of the people walking in the door of a nursing home for the first time in 2002/2003 had a mental illness diagnosis five years prior to that.[121] Moreover, 87 percent of the residents of nursing homes in 2002/2003 had some sort of mental illness diagnosis.

Looking at staffing for home care and personal care homes, very few home care workers are trained or allowed to deal with mental health needs, and very few nursing homes have psychiatric nurses on staff. According to table 1, the current rate of RPNs per capita (per 10,000 population) varies tremendously, from a low of 0 in Churchill, and around 2 in South Eastman and Burntwood, to a high of 41 in Brandon. Hence, message four is:

Table 1: Per Capita Allocation of Registered Psychiatric Nurses (RPNs)
by Regional Health Authority (RHA) Manitoba

RHA	RPNs*	Population of RHA in 2000	RPN per ten thousand population
South Eastman	10	54427	1.8
Brandon	195	47337	41.2
Central	146	97865	14.9
Assiniboine	34	71544	4.8
Parkland	41	42909	9.6
Interlake	167	74944	22.3
North Eastman	18	39369	4.6
Burntwood	10	45051	2.2
Churchill	0	1008	0.0
Nor-Man	9	25233	3.6
Winnipeg	329	649012	5.1

* Count of RPNs provided by Laura Panteluk, 2007

"Community-based services are essential, and staffing must reflect mental health needs, not just physical needs."

So what's the good news? Senator Kirby's 2006 national report brought the issue of mental illness to the fore.[122] There's also been a lot done to look at the idea of primary care models for mental health. The Canadian Collaborative Mental Health Initiative group (which includes consumers and providers) has put a huge amount of thought into how to go about this in its Canadian Collaborative Mental Health Care Charter (www.ccmhi.ca). Its commitments include informing, advising, and supporting primary health care reform initiatives, as well as advocating for mental health provider education and evidence-based practice.

And, of course, there's the recent budget announcement in March 2007 that takes Senator Kirby's work to the next stage of a Canadian Mental Health Commission. The upside is that $10 million has been promised over the next two years, and $15 million a year thereafter, to establish the Commission (to be headed by Senator Kirby). The potential downsides: it will probably be grossly underfunded, non-uniform, have no national framework, and reinforce volunteerism.

The Manitoba Provincial Mental Health Advisory Council's key message to all of us is message five: "Quit assessing and start helping!"

Up until now, we have talked too much about the problem, and not enough about the solution. We have siloed mental illness into bits and pieces of programs and funding. We have let other interests, like acute care, crowd it out. What we need to do is herd those cats, and actually start singing from the same songbook, with an integrated approach.

We have the tools. We have some funding through recent Canadian initiatives. Now let's look for models to integrate mental health issues into a seamless, universal, comprehensive, public, accessible, and portable mental health program.

CHAPTER 26

Home and Community Care in Canada: The Unfinished Policy [123]

Judith Shamian

Tommy Douglas envisioned the implementation of medicare as occurring in two phases. The first phase dealt with implementing the public financing of the medical system and the second phase was to deal with revamping and reorganizing the delivery system beyond acute care.[124] While the first part of this vision has been implemented, decades later the second part remains to be completed.

Home and community care has become an increasingly essential part of a comprehensive integrated health care system. As noted by Monique Bégin, leaving home and community care out of the discussion, and the Canada Health Act, was unintentional. That home and community care was not deemed medically necessary is reflective of the context within which the medical system operated at the time of its creation.[125] Decades later, as the balance of care increasingly shifts from an institutional setting to a community setting, it is essential to examine whether the current policy framework is optimal to keep Canadians healthy and to also appropriately fund that needed care.

If Tommy Douglas's agenda had been fully implemented, it would be safe to assume that we would have a policy safety net that would include all aspects of a comprehensive and integrated health care system, including home and community care. If we do not deliberately discuss home and community care within the context of revamping the system, we run the risk of continuing to ignore what is a very integral and medically necessary part of the health care system. There needs to be a full discussion and exploration of what appropriately funded and supported home care can do to improve access and reduce cost. There is a need for a complete national policy protecting access to publicly funded home and community care.

The home and community care sector is one of the fastest growing parts of the health care system. Since 1995, home care use has increased 60 percent in Canada and this is expected to grow as it adapts and responds to a number of demographic, social, and environmental changes.[126] In spite of this growth, home care and community-based care are underdeveloped in this country because they have historically been starved of adequate funding in order to fuel expensive, institutional-based care.[127] While some steps have already been taken across Canada to enhance and strengthen funding for home care, much more work needs to be done in this area to ensure that home care is truly comprehensive and that it permits providers to deliver the broad continuum of services that people require in order to be able to stay at home and retain maximum independence.

In September 2000, the First Ministers Meeting Communiqué on Health described home care as a critical component of a fully integrated health system and commitments were made by the provincial and territorial governments to strengthen investment in this area. However, little progress has been made in establishing national standards or a national definition of the range of home care services to be funded. After meeting in February 2003, the first ministers signed an Accord on Health Care Renewal that developed into their 2004 Ten Year Plan to strengthen health care, which included a shared agreement that home care at the national level should constitute:

- short-term acute home care for two-week provision of case management, intravenous medications related to the discharge diagnosis, nursing, and personal care;
- short-term acute community mental health home care for two-week provision of case management and crisis response services; and
- end-of-life care for case management, nursing, palliative-specific pharmaceuticals, and personal care at the end of life.

These three areas of home and community care do not comprehensively meet the needs of Canadians requiring home and community care, and do not deal with the integration into the health care system that the first ministers have repeatedly committed to.

There are three categories of Canadian home care that provide three different functions — prevention and maintenance care for people with low-level care needs who would otherwise deteriorate, acute care substitution for hospital care, and long term/chronic care substitution for residential facility care.[128] The first ministers have agreed to provide only limited acute home and community care, including end-of-life care. This limited approach to home care gives priority to those with post-acute medical needs and ignores those who require more personal care and practical support such as, bathing, dressing, food preparation, and housekeeping in order to be able to remain at home and out of institutions.

The original Royal Commission lead by Mr. Justice Emmett
Hall from 1961 to 1964 that issued the report forming the basis
of our modern medicare system did not seek to limit the types or
nature of services to be covered by a national system of health
insurance. As stated by the Commission at page ten of its report:

> And the device must be used ultimately to finance the
> whole spectrum of health services, not merely hospital
> and physicians' services. To make certain that all our cit-
> izens have access to the necessary health services is now
> clearly a matter for the public interest.[129]

Despite this, home care has historically been largely ignored by
the Canadian public health sector and programs, outside of post-
acute and end-of-life, have not received the attention and funds
they need. Further, because home care services are not deemed
medically necessary under the Canada Health Act (CHA), there is
no federal restriction against cancelling public funding for these
programs, making them vulnerable to cuts and restrictions.

As a result of the current policies in place, access to home and
community services is limited. Most individuals and families who
require ongoing home and community services find themselves
purchasing services in a market that is mostly unregulated and
thus, these services can be not only costly, but the quality of care
can vary greatly. According to the Romanow Report, Canadians
pay out of pocket for about 30 percent of total yearly health care
costs in Canada and about 70 percent of total costs are covered by
public funds. While according to CIHI only 50 percent of home
care patients in Canada receive publicly funded care.[130] If we add
to it the hours of caregiving provided by unpaid family caregivers
annually, saving the Canadian health care system about $5 billion
each year,[131] it can be argued that at least 70 percent of the care
provided in the home and community is financed privately, or

provided by family members, while only 30 percent of the burden is borne by public funding. Home care is medically necessary, and prior to the restructuring of the system in the 1990s, many of these services were provided in the hospital, and protected under the Canada Health Act. With the increasing trend toward providing more health care in the home and community, individuals requiring care, and their families, are forced to shoulder the majority of the cost both financially and physically.

Although not recognized as a formal part of the health care system, today there are at least 2.1 million unpaid family caregivers in Canada.[132] Without the unpaid labour provided by family caregivers, the Canadian health care system would long since have been unable to cope with the increasing demands for care. With an aging population, fewer beds and facilities, a crisis situation in supply of health human resources, and more people wanting to be cared for in their own homes, the number of family and friend caregivers is expected to continue to increase. Despite the obvious value of the contributions being made by caregivers, there are few services aimed at helping them maintain their health and balance. Some studies suggest that as many as one in five adult Canadians, mostly women who also work outside the home, provide unpaid care.[133] These caregivers provide the vast majority of home care.[134] Fifty percent of unpaid family caregivers report health problems due to caregiving, 79 percent report some emotional difficulty such as increased stress, sleep disturbances, and other problems, 25 percent report that their employment situation has been affected by their caregiving responsibilities, and more than two-thirds of caregivers spend more than $100 per month on caregiving.[135]

Recent national and provincial reviews including the final report of the Romanow Commission, Senator Michael J. Kirby's 2002 Report on the Health of Canadians, the 2001 report of the Quebec Health Review (the Clair Commission), and others have touched on the need for an expansion of home and community services. Health Canada estimates that public home care expenditures grew by 11 percent per year between 1990 and 1998 as federal, provincial, and territorial governments began to see home care as a more efficacious and cost-effective alternative to institutional care.[136]

As we work to reform the system in the spirit and vision of Tommy Douglas, it is paramount to reduce the burden on families while we make sure that they are integrated into the care we provide and empowered to partner with the established health care system. While both Canadian data and various national and provincial reports point to the urgent need to deal with the policy issues and policy gaps related to home and community care and services, there seems to be a limited appetite to deal with the unfinished policy challenges. The lack of political will to close the policy gap will further complicate issues and will lead to further system breakdown, resulting in unnecessary pressures on the expensive acute care system.

Home and community care policy in Canada remains unfinished. If policymakers are serious about ensuring the sustainability and quality of our health care system they must turn their attention to the role that home and community care plays. Failing to do so will result in a fragmented, weakened health care system.

CHAPTER 27

Completing the Vision: Prevention and Community Health Centres

France Gélinas

Once upon a time, there was a great man, a visionary, who wanted to make sure that no one was denied health care because of their inability to pay; a visionary who believed that governments had a role to play in keeping people healthy. This great man, of course, was Tommy Douglas, the founder of medicare in Canada.

According to Tommy, medicare was to be implemented in two stages. The first stage was to remove the financial barriers between the provider of health care and the recipient. During the implementation of the first stage, we saw provincial and territorial governments assume payments for hospitals' and physicians' services. Those services became universally available to all Canadians based on their needs, not on their income or ability to pay.

It did not come easy. The first phase of his vision was fiercely opposed by physicians and other groups, but Tommy's vision prevailed and medicare was implemented. Medicare is now considered one of our country's finest achievements and a program that defines us as Canadians.

But the vision is not completed. The second stage is still waiting.

> Let's not forget that the ultimate goal of medicare must be to keep people well.
>
> —Tommy Douglas

That Was Then. Now ...

Canada has a network of over 300 Community Health Centres (CHC), which are committed to completing medicare's original vision and want to move as swiftly as possible to the second stage of medicare — the stage where we implement reforms to keep people well.

Community Health Centres are primary health care organizations. They are community-governed, non-profit organizations that group a team of health care professionals, including physicians, nurses, social workers, dietitians, physiotherapists, health promoters, community development workers, early childhood educators, and others — all under one roof. The different professionals work in an interdisciplinary team to offer primary health care services, health promotion programs, and community development initiatives.

A Community Health Centre's programs and services are developed according to community needs. Community Health Centres (CHCs) work in partnerships with social services agencies, hospitals, and other health care providers in order to deliver integrated and coordinated care. They are focused on prevention. Their work is grounded in the determinants of health, the root causes of illness and poor health.

The Second Stage of Medicare will Focus on Prevention
The goal of the second stage is to prevent needless illness and
needless suffering.

> Only through the practice of preventive medicine will
> we keep the costs from becoming so excessive that the
> public will decide that medicare is not in the best inter-
> est of the people of the country ... We need to
> reorganize the health delivery system.
>
> –Tommy Douglas

Community Health Centres can report on many positive
impacts of the second stage of medicare in action, on the positive
impact of keeping people well.

Pathways to Education is a program in Toronto's Regent Park
CHC. The program supports kids in their studies in order to make
sure they do not drop out of school. Their work is based on the
importance of education as a determinant of health. The program
encompasses the following principles:

- it is focused on population health;
- it is centred on the kids;
- it is equitable, effective, and accessible to all;
- it is safe; and
- it is empowering to the kids, their families, and
  their community.

Another large area of work in the second stage of medicare
focuses on the reorganization of the system. One example of this
is the prevention of chronic diseases and their multiple complications.

Chronic diseases are the most frequent, most expensive, and
the most avoidable health problems. Their causes are uncertain
and are linked to multiple risk factors. Chronic diseases have long
latency periods and are long-term afflictions. They bring physical

deteriorations and functional incapacities. Most people afflicted
with a chronic disease live in the community.

By working at all three (primary, secondary, and tertiary) levels
of prevention, the London Community Health Centre has been
able to decrease the rate of diabetes (a common chronic disease in
Canada) and its complications in the local Latino population. This
population is facing a disproportionate rate of diabetes. Their
health promoters have been working on issues like housing,
schooling, and immigration. These interventions in the social
environment of the people are part of the primary prevention
efforts. They have had a huge impact on the development of diabetes in the Latino community.

Other members of the primary health care team hold clinics
and education sessions on diabetes management for people who
have been diagnosed with the disease. Those programs are based
on established best practice for the management and care of diabetes. The goal is to prevent complications linked to poorly
managed diabetes and support people in their efforts to stay
healthy. This is an example of secondary prevention in action. In
other words, working with the individual risk factors of people
who have been diagnosed with the disease in order to prevent
complications.

Lastly, an interdisciplinary team of physicians, nurses, nutrition-
ists, chiropodists, and others, continues to support and follow
closely people living with diabetes who are developing complications, in order to avoid further illness and suffering. The program,
in aiming at averting further complications, is an example of the
third level of prevention.

In the second stage of medicare, we will do a better job at keeping seniors healthy by reorganizing the health delivery methods
and system.

The Centre de santé communautaire de Sudbury, a Community Health Centre targeting the Francophone population of that

city, has adopted the Hand-in-Hand program. It is a non-medical Adult Day Centre model designed to keep seniors healthy and living in the community. It is based on the determinants of health that most affect francophone seniors, such as isolation and a sense of belonging. Hand-in-Hand incorporates activities and programs that touch all levels of prevention. Programs focusing on physical activity, nutrition, and security are designed for seniors by seniors.

These are only three examples of what is happening in CHCs. There are second stage examples happening in all kinds of community-based agencies. Unfortunately, those examples continue to be the exception, not the rule.

How Do We Move Forward?

We want all Canadians to benefit from the second stage of medicare, but it is not happening and will not happen without appropriate action.

There are many reasons why the second stage of medicare is not yet in place. There are those who have ferociously resisted the kind of change envisioned in the second stage of medicare. There are those who see two-tiered health care and for-profit delivery as the solution.

There are other reasons of a completely different nature that explain why the second stage of medicare is not happening. Community Health Centres and other parts of the health care system where the second stage of medicare is already happening have to work harder at telling the story.

We have to work harder at inspiring Canadians with our vision. We have to start talking more like Tommy Douglas.

What Does It Mean?

It means talking about the solutions our non-profit, public health sector can provide — solutions that cannot and will not be provided in a private system.

It means talking more about the original vision, keeping people well, and the two stages of medicare.

It means showing Canadians how the benefits of the second
stage of medicare are achievable and in some cases already happening.

It means working together to develop an advocacy campaign
that will excite and engage Canadians about the second stage of
medicare and strengthen the values that unite us all.

PART V

Inequality and Social Determinants of Health

CHAPTER 28

It's About Equity and
Going Upstream:
Health for All

Monique Bégin

We now spend some $148 billion in total (public and private expenditures) for health care in Canada, representing 10.3 percent of our GDP (2006). Outside of the United States, we are regularly among the top spenders, usually with (in no particular order) France, Germany, Switzerland, and Sweden. Through first ministers' accords on health care in 2000, 2003, and 2004, even in the last federal budget, billions of additional dollars — cash, not tax points — have been added to federal transfers to the provinces, re-establishing Ottawa as a committed and responsible funding partner. And we still complain.

Granted, incremental reforms to medicare and local innovative approaches do not give us the sense that we are overcoming our bad micromanagement — replacing solo medical practice by team practices, developing primary care access, introducing IT — moving ahead with medicare. It's also true that, since the passage of the

Canada Health Act in 1984, many political leaders have forgotten not just the spirit, but the letter of the law. And, to my chagrin, many Canadians mistakenly consider American health care's costly disaster the norm, thinking Canada is unique in having a universal, "free" health care system.

What really counts is that, despite the billions we put into our medical care system, we still witness thousands of people in Canada who die before their time, who don't enjoy the good health they could have, who suffer from diseases that are avoidable, and who are prevented from enjoying a much better health status.

So we have to ask: Where does good health come from? As Bob Evans so aptly put it: *Why Are Some People Healthy and Others Not?*[1] If genetics and individual risk factors are not the best predictors of staying healthy or becoming ill, what are the predictors society should know about? I want to refocus the question with population health at the centre, and doctors and hospitals as only one determinant of good health among several others, each as important, if not more so. Not that I don't recognize the critical role of free (collectively prepaid) universal medical care as a must in any society, but we know that there is much more to health than health care, however good its quality.

We need to think more clearly about equity in the health status of people in Canada. We need to start "going upstream" to achieve the best standard of overall health — "downstream" being the medical care provided by doctors and hospitals. No matter how good their care may be, they cannot do much more than treat and try to cure people after they become sick. Other than giving advice on lifestyle changes — such as, lose weight, stop smoking — they can't do much to address the causes of ill-health. That is not their role in our system, as Dr. Robert McMurtry, a former Dean of Medicine at the University of Western Ontario, noted in the 1st Annual Amyot Lecture, *Medicare and Wellness: The Odd Couple.*

The Scientific Evidence

I'll always remember my astonishment at discovering something fundamental and new to me, when in 1981 I visited the Montreal Diet Dispensary (MDD), a volunteer organization. Agnes C. Higgins was still its executive director at the time (she passed away in 1985). Before joining the Dispensary in 1948 as a dietician, she worked in prenatal clinics where she observed that disadvantaged mothers very often gave birth to babies who were underweight and sickly. In 1948, she began questioning why so many poor women in the Greater Montreal Area were two to three times more likely to have low birth-weight (LBW) babies than women in the general population. The answer, of course, was that without sufficient income women couldn't afford adequate diets and were unable to meet pregnancy's high nutritional demands.

There were additional risks of malnutrition associated with teen pregnancies — for both mother and child — because teenage mothers are themselves still growing. LBW babies were a greater burden on the health care system than healthy weight babies because they:

- had longer hospital stays at birth;
- more frequently required costly neonatal intensive care;
- were hospitalized more often, and for longer periods, during their first year of life;
- experienced greater developmental disabilities; and
- were more likely to develop chronic health problems as adults (for example, diabetes, hypertension, cardiovascular disease).

To attack this problem, Agnes Higgins persuaded the Dispensary to give priority to disadvantaged expectant mothers. (The MDD, founded in 1879, and its volunteers, used to prepare and distribute meals to the sick and to convalescents free of charge or at a very low price.) She developed a model which combined nutritional assistance with counselling: expectant mothers were given basic foods such as milk and eggs, as well as nutritional supplements and advice on nutrition and budgeting. She established that key barriers to improved nutritional status among pregnant mothers included:

- a lack of income;
- feelings of guilt associated with eating scarce family food;
- a lack of role models for — or lack of knowledge about — preparing nutritious meals;
- lack of proper cooking facilities;
- addiction to cigarettes, alcohol, and/or drugs;
- social isolation and depression;
- emotional stress due to abusive or unstable relationships;
- ambivalence towards/denial of pregnancy;
- lack of time (such as raising a family with no support); and
- a mistaken belief that weight gain should be limited during pregnancy.

Ten years ago, MDD was assisting over 2,600 clients — an estimated two-thirds of all low-income pregnant women in Montreal who required support. Clients included teenagers, newly arrived immigrants, single heads of families, and women living alone without any family or social support. To me, such an initiative was about health promotion, a desirable goal in health policy, but one totally outside of our departmental main considerations and budgets — that of doctors and hospitals and the medicare system itself.

Little did I know that a new science demonstrating the links between socioeconomic factors and health status was already developing, in particular in the UK with the Black Report and later the Whitehall studies. Sir Michael Marmot, chair of the

World Health Organization's Commission on Social Determinants of Health, of which I am a member, has been at the forefront of research into health inequalities for the past twenty-five years. He started his research on the Whitehall data trying to identify, in a rather conventional way, individual risk factors — cardiovascular function, smoking, car ownership, angina, leisure/hobbies, ECG measurements, diabetes — for cardiovascular and respiratory disease in British civil servants. The research team had grouped the (male) respondents by their grade in the hierarchy of the civil service, from the highest administrative ranks (deputy ministers, permanent secretaries) to professional and executive (such as senior executive officers), clerical, and others (unskilled manual workers, porters, messengers). His observations proved the opposite of his starting hypothesis.

Let me quote him from an interview he gave in 2002:

> So I spent quite a lot of time looking at ... the first Whitehall study, and the remarkable finding — which ran counter both to my expectations at the time, and I think most other people's — was firstly, just looking at heart disease, it was not the case that people in high-stress jobs had a higher risk of heart attack. Rather, it went exactly the other way: people at the bottom of the hierarchy had a higher risk of heart attacks. Secondly, it was a social gradient. The lower you were in the hierarchy, the higher the risk. So it wasn't top versus bottom, but it was graded. And, thirdly, the social gradient applied to all the major causes of death ... to cardiovascular disease, to gastrointestinal disease, to renal disease, to stroke, to accidental and violent deaths, to cancers that were not related to smoking as well as cancers that were related to smoking — all the major causes of death ... This finding of a gradient not only ran counter to

thinking at the time about heart attacks — that high-
status people were supposed to get more heart disease
— but also ran counter then, and still does, to the way
most people think about inequalities in health.

Yes, we all tend to have a very polarized view of life in society: it's "we" and "they." "They" are the poor, and of course they
have all sorts of problems. "We," the better off, have better health
(except for our preconceived notion that people with jobs at the
top are more prone to heart attacks). We have no idea whatsoev-
er that we are all involved in a health status graded according to
where we stand in the social pecking order. To borrow again from
Bob Evans, we Canadians like to think that ours is a classless, very
egalitarian society, but it is not. [2]

Social Determinants at Work in Canada

Let's turn to Canada, starting with a few images from the international scene of the role played by socioeconomic classes when
it comes to health status. A classic example used by our Commission goes like this: if you catch the metro train in downtown
Washington, DC, to your suburb in Maryland, life expectancy is
fifty-seven years at the beginning of the journey. At the end of the
journey, it is seventy-seven years. That means a twenty-year difference in life expectancy between the poor, predominantly African
Americans of downtown Washington, and the richer and predominantly white people of the suburbs. By the same token, if
you are a fifteen-year-old boy in Lesotho, your chance of reaching the age of sixty is about 10 percent. If you are a
fifteen-year-old boy in Sweden, your chance of reaching the age
of sixty is 91 percent. Although poverty is not the same in Lesotho
and in Washington, DC, and poor people's living conditions are
different, they both suffer from a lack of opportunity in their
respective lives and a lack of control over their respective futures,

because of the social conditions that shape the physical environment they live in.

These health gradients apply between countries — rich and poor, as well as within countries — between social classes.

So what about us in Canada? Like everywhere else, "life expectancy is shorter and most diseases are more common the further down the social ladder in each society."[3] Reconnecting with the Whitehall studies, Louise Lemyre and her team at the University of Ottawa confirmed the gradient theory when they recently studied levels of psychological stress in federal civil servants. The research sample was divided in five classes of bureaucrats, all at the executive level; there was a clear graduation of the degree of stress — the highest ranking officials showing the least stress.[4]

We know that 40 percent of chronic illness can be prevented and that 25 percent of direct medical costs are attributable to a small number of risk factors such as smoking, obesity, physical inactivity, and poor nutrition. From the Canadian Population Health Initiative, I have drawn some vignettes of domestic bad health status due to bad social conditions:

- Compared to those in subsidized housing, children still on waiting lists for subsidized housing are six times more likely to have stunted growth and 50 percent more likely to be iron-deficient.
- Canadians from lower-income families have an increased risk of asthma and more asthma exacerbations necessitating an emergency department visit or admission to hospital.
- In Montreal, if you live in the well-to-do west end, your life expectancy is close to eighty years. If your home is in the centre-south (CLSC Des Faubourgs), it is only sixty-six years.
- Immigrant women report very good to excellent

health upon arrival to Canada. Ten years later, those with high income report their health has diminished by 8 percent, while those with low income say theirs has deteriorated by 20 percent.

- In BC First Nations communities where there are no identified Cultural Continuity Factors, the youth suicide rate is 140 per 100,000. In communities listing at least five Cultural Continuity Factors, such as cultural practices and community control over resources, the rate drops to some 40 per 100,000.[5]

- In Nunavut, the average lifespan for women is twelve years less than the average for Canadian women; for males, the gap is eight years.

- Inuit have infant mortality rates that are triple the all-Canadian rate.

- The largest cause of Potential Years of Life Lost (PYLL) for First Nations on-reserve is injuries. This group has 4,909 years of life lost per 100,000 population, compared with 1,271 years of life lost in the Canadian population as a whole — leading causes being motor vehicle accidents, suicide, drowning, and fire.[6]

We could go on depicting situations quite shocking for a country as rich as ours. Food insecurity exists among 10.2 percent of Canadian households representing 3 million people. According to the Canadian Association of Food Banks' (CAFB) 2006 Hunger-Count survey, more than half of the food banks participating in the survey are located in rural communities, serving a total of 65,387 people. In the month of March 2006, over 753,000 different people accessed food banks, 41 percent being children. Monthly food bank use serves 2.4 percent of the total Canadian population, double the 1989 figure.[7]

I certainly don't like to see the UN criticize us in front of the whole world, but we must face some unpleasant facts. Here is what the UN Committee on Economic, Social and Cultural Rights' 2006 report printed about Canada:

- Over the last ten years, welfare benefits have dropped in most provinces below half of basic living costs.
- In 2001, just 39 percent of unemployed Canadians were eligible for unemployment insurance benefits. The program must be made more accessible.
- Minimum wages are inadequate to achieve a decent standard of living.
- Homelessness and housing constitute a national emergency.

In other words, the First Nations, Inuit, and Metis pockets of urban poverty, the rural poor in some regions, and immigrants after ten years in Canada — these are the principal groups of our society who are cheated of optimum health. Translated into academic concepts, as we explained to the Senate Committee, the strongest predictors of health disparities are socioeconomic status (SES), gender, Aboriginal status, and geographic location.[8]

I put a lot of stress on poverty, although there are some ten other social determinants — education, housing, environment, gender, early childhood development, social inclusion, to name only a few — because the Whitehall studies show that income, and income distribution in a society, is more important than total income earned. Large gaps in distribution or steep gradients lead to increased social problems and poorer health. In the ten years of 1990 to 2000, the wealthiest 10 percent of Canadians increased their income by $23,000 per person per year while the poorest 10 percent of Canadians increased theirs by $81 per person per year.

In the last 20 years, the income gap has been growing. This is very troubling. What is more troubling is that the 46.3 percent of families that are raising children under the age of eighteen — almost half of all Canadian families — "are putting in more work time, yet most — 80 percent of them — are getting a smaller share of Canada's growing economy," says a recent study by the Canadian Centre for Policy Alternatives (CCPA). In this economic study, Armine Yalnizyan demonstrates that: "Over the past two decades a social experiment has unfolded in Canada: governments have actively pursued policies that support market dynamics and willingly decreased their role as a buffer against markets, particularly for the economically vulnerable."

At the best of economic times — ten consecutive years of budget surpluses — and throughout the income spectrum, it becomes clear that these Canadian families are prisoners of "an economic system that is failing the majority while disproportionately benefiting a select few."[9] The neutral, objective, and scientific term to qualify this state of affairs is inequality. There is greater inequality in Canadian society at the very time we have solid evidence that the healthiest and happiest societies are those with the most equitable distribution of income.

Going Upstream: From Inequality to (In)Equity

Inequality in society, as well as health inequality, refers to an observable, often measurable, difference in (health) status between individuals or between groups, whatever its cause. On the other hand, inequity (of health or otherwise) is a moral category rooted in values, social stratification, and embedded in political reality and the negotiations of social power relations. Consequently, health equity can be defined as the absence of unfair or unavoidable or remediable differences in health among populations or groups defined socially, economically, demographically, or geographically.

Moving from the observation of inequality to a philosophy or an ethic of equity implies making a choice. And choices cannot be made that do not rest on a set of values. Canadian elites — whoever and wherever — rarely discuss values these days, and this since a good twenty-five years ago. Or rather, what is being implicitly if not explicitly praised is taking risks and becoming competitive, not collectively but as individuals. There is nothing inherently wrong with that, but it certainly does not reinforce solidarity, sharing, fairness, inclusion, caring, or compassion. It refers to "me," not "them," not "us." It speaks to individualism. Roy Romanow is one of the few leaders who speak out for a more broadly based and collective approach. In an essay in *Walrus* magazine, "A House Half Built," he appealed to Canadians to rebalance their values "between the individual and society," and denounced "unbridled competition (as) the new orthodoxy."

Other challenges, much easier to tackle than reviving the collective values on which Canadian society has developed, await us on the road of going upstream to tackle the causes of avoidable bad health outcomes. But they take innovation and political will. One such challenge is how do we tackle the "silos" approach to public policy when most determinants of health are outside the purview of health ministries?

Many of our policymakers envy the Québec Public Health Act (2001) for its famous article 54 as a way of making social determinants of health a whole-of-government affair. The article reads as follows:

> The Minister (of Health and Social Services) is by virtue of his or her office the advisor of the Government on any public health issue. The Minister shall give the other ministers any advice he or she considers advisable for health promotion and the adoption of policies capable of fostering the enhancement of the health and welfare of the population. In the Minister's capacity as government advisor, the Minister shall be

consulted in relation to the development of the measures provided for in an Act or regulation that could have
significant impact on the health of the population.

An operational impact assessment tool kit has been developed
and adopted, but only time will tell what article 54 actually
accomplished to promote the social determinants of health.

We can also learn from the Manitoba "Healthy Child Committee of Cabinet" established in 2000 by Premier Gary Doer and
composed of eight "social determinants" ministers.[10] To my
knowledge, it is the only such cabinet committee in Canada dedicated to the well-being of children and youth. They have bridged
government and communities and appear to be an effective inter-
sectoral tool of policy implementation and program development.

Putting equity and a sense of the common good back into politics and policymaking, along these lines, appears to me the
ultimate challenge for today's Canadian society.

Conclusion

The question of shared collective values brings yet another observation which I am offering as a conclusion.

Most of us know that Canada is a big spender when it comes
to medicare and other health expenditures. But how many Canadians know that we have a shameful record when it comes to our
total social expenditures? Comparative national statistics, such as
those of the OECD, rank us near the bottom of the list of industrialized countries, just above the United States. We do not invest
much in what is now called human capital. Roughly speaking, we
spend less than half of what each of Denmark, Sweden, Norway,
Finland, even Iceland, as well as France, Germany, and Belgium,
spend yearly for public social expenditures measured as a percentage of GDP.

The Nordic countries, in particular, stand out in terms of both public health and welfare state institutions. Sweden, for example, epitomizes the welfare state. The monetarist policies that took over North American, as well as most European countries, some twenty-five years ago and which are now either well entrenched or regularly revived by private interests, have inflicted more or less damaging blows to most welfare states. Unfortunately, Canada's safety net did not escape this fate. Still, the Nordic countries, despite cuts, kept and developed their welfare states.

Today, their successes in generalized good health outcomes, as well as their economic prosperity and the stability of their societies, have made researchers pause and think. Maybe these countries have something to teach us. Although there are indeed some clear differences between these nations, the similarities still warrant a consideration of the Nordic model. But what are the links between Nordic welfare state arrangements on the one hand and public health and health inequalities on the other?

The project NEWS (The Nordic Experience: Welfare States and Public Health) is intended to shed more light on that question. The project will draw on existing knowledge and new analyses from leading researchers in social policy and welfare state research, as well as from public health, social epidemiology, and health inequalities research.[11]

More and more policymakers in the European Union and in international organizations, as well as some individuals in Canada, regard "social policy as a productive factor." This new discourse frames the economic argument in favour of going the route guided by the social determinants of health. "In short, poverty and inequality are regarded as evidence of an inefficient society," as David Hay concluded in his review of the literature for the Public Health Agency of Canada and the Canadian Policy Research Network.[12] So the development of an economic argument also helps the cause of more social equity.

I don't want to finish on overly negative feelings about us in

Canada. Have we done something right in matters of social policies these past decades? Yes we have. Without government income
programs such as Old Age Security, the Guaranteed Income Supplement and its provincial variants, and the Canada and Quebec
Pension Plans, 58 percent of Canadians sixty-five and older would
be poor. Because of public pensions, only 6 percent of seniors live
on low incomes. This places Canada fourth in an international
comparison of the percentage of seniors with low incomes after
government assistance. This example of enlightened social policy
demonstrates that, when there is a will, there is a way!

CHAPTER 29

Poverty and Health: Implications for Health and Quality of Life [13]

Dennis Raphael

Introduction

Canadians have traditionally considered their nation to be among the most humane and caring on the planet. Compared to the public policies of their American neighbour to the south, Canadians view their public policies concerning the provision of health care and social services and other supports to citizens to be responsive, fair, and equitable. These supports to citizens constitute what has come to be known as the modern welfare state. Yet Canada has one of the highest poverty rates for individuals and families among wealthy industrialized nations[14]. In reality, Canada's approach to public policy in a wide range of spheres — including public policy concerning the prevention of poverty — is quite undeveloped as compared to most European nations.[15] And poverty is the strongest determinant of health.[16] Poverty is also the strongest determinant of a variety of other indicators of societal well-being,

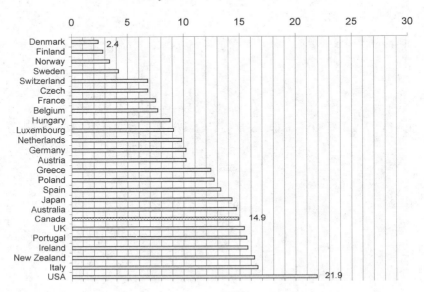

Figure 1: Child Poverty in Wealthy Nations, Late 1990s

Percentage of Children Living in Relative Poverty Defined as Households with

<50% of the National Median Household Income

such as literacy levels, crime and safety, social cohesion, and community solidarity, as well as general well-being;[17] these latter indicators are often described as measuring the quality of life.

The degree and depth of poverty within Canada, the provinces and territories, and local municipalities are strongly influenced by these public policies.[18] An increasing body of scholarship reveals that governmental decisions concerning how to allocate and distribute resources within the population of a jurisdiction are the primary determinants of poverty rates within a jurisdiction.[19] Why is it that a wealthy industrialized nation such as Canada has 15 percent of its children living in poverty while far-less-wealthy nations such as Denmark and Finland have less that 3 percent of their children living in such conditions (See figure 1)?[20] These differences are a result of public policy decisions that directly influence the lived experience of those living in situations associated with poverty.

These public policy decisions affect the availability of supports to children and families, benefits for those experiencing disability and unemployment, the amount of taxation and revenue available for programs, wages and employment security and benefits, and the distribution of economic and social resources within the population. The incidence and experience of poverty have direct effects on the health of individuals, communities, and societies, and on a variety of other indicators of quality of life.

Poverty and Health

Studies show that the living conditions experienced by those living in poverty are associated with a very wide range of health indicators. Poverty is a strong predictor of life expectancy and of individuals' perceptions of their health. Poverty predicts the incidence of, and death from, a staggeringly wide range of diseases. Poverty also predicts incidence of and death from injuries, levels of health literacy, and use of health services. And experiencing

Figure 2: Life Expectancy of Males and Females by Income Quintile of Neighbourhood, Urban Canada, 1996

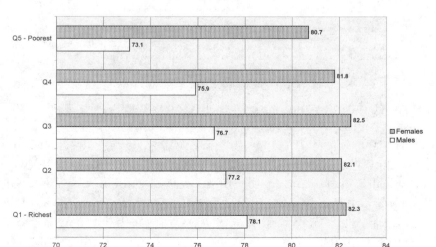

Table 1: Age-Standardized Mortality Rates per 100,000 Population, for both Sexes, or for Males and Females when Rates Differ by Gender, for Selected Causes of Death by Neighbourhood Income Quintile, Urban Canada, 1996

Both Sexes

Cause of Death	Q1	Q2	Q3	Q4	Q5	RR[1]	RD[2]	Excess[3]	% excess[4]
All causes	450.0	472.8	474.6	505.1	593.1	1.32	143.1	51.9	10.3
Injuries (excluding MVAs and Suicides)	12.7	14.7	13.3	15.4	23.5	1.85	10.8	3.3	20.8
Perinatal conditions	2.4	3.7	3.8	3.3	4.7	1.94	2.3	1.2	33.6
Pedestrians in MVAs	0.9	1.1	0.8	1.4	1.8	2.13	1.0	0.4	31.5
MVA Occupants	6.6	7.1	5.0	4.8	3.5	0.53	-3.1	-1.2	-22.3
Infectious diseases	6.0	7.5	7.6	11.0	20.5	3.41	14.5	4.5	42.7
Ill-defined conditions	6.7	7.3	8.2	10.6	17.0	2.52	10.2	3.3	32.8
Mental disorders	7.7	7.5	7.1	8.8	10.1	1.30	2.3	0.5	6.2

Males

Cause of Death	Q1	Q2	Q3	Q4	Q5	RR	RD	Excess	% excess
All causes	567.9	608.5	630.6	672.8	813.5	1.43	245.6	96.0	14.5
Ischemic heart disease	126.8	137.0	140.6	149.7	165.7	1.31	38.8	18.5	12.7
Cirrhosis of liver	6.7	7.3	8.9	11.2	16.7	2.50	10.0	3.5	34.2
Lung cancer	51.5	56.6	60.7	67.2	80.1	1.56	28.6	12.1	19.1
Suicide	15.6	13.8	17.3	18.4	27.5	1.76	11.9	3.2	16.9
Diabetes	13.5	13.5	14.5	16.8	21.2	1.56	7.6	2.6	16.1
Prostate cancer	24.4	21.6	21.0	20.0	18.0	.74	-6.4	-3.5	-16.5

Females

Cause of Death	Q1	Q2	Q3	Q4	Q5	RR	RD	Excess	% excess
All causes	367.2	376.6	363.0	383.7	427.7	1.16	60.5	18.0	4.7
Ischemic heart disease	61.7	64.4	61.8	68.3	77.0	1.25	15.3	5.6	8.3
Cirrhosis of liver	3.6	3.3	3.4	3.5	3.4	.95	-0.2	-0.2	-5.6
Lung cancer	27.0	30.0	30.4	30.5	34.8	1.29	7.8	3.7	12.0
Suicide	3.5	4.3	4.1	6.6	8.6	2.53	5.2	2.1	38.4
Diabetes	9.1	7.8	9.5	8.9	13.4	1.47	4.3	0.7	7.7
Breast cancer	30.4	25.5	26.2	25.8	26.6	.88	-3.7	-3.7	-13.8
Uterine cancer	4.3	5.1	5.6	5.1	6.4	1.50	2.1	1.1	20.2

[1] Inter-quintile rate ratio (Q5/Q1). This is the ratio of years lost between the poorest to richest neighbourhoods.
[2] Inter-quintile rate difference (Q5 - Q1). This is the difference of years lost between the poorest and richest neighbourhoods.
[3] Population-attributable risk (Total-Q1). This is the amount of years lost associated with income differences between the richest neighbourhoods and all others.
[4] Population-attributable risk percentage [100 x (Total-Q1)/Total]. This is the percentage of years lost associated with income differences between the richest neighbourhoods and all others.

Source: Wilkins, R., Berthelot, J.-M., & Ng, E. (2002). Trends in mortality by neighbourhood income in urban Canada from 1971 to 1996. Health Reports (Stats Can), 13(Supplement), 1-28.

poverty during childhood is a good predictor of poor health not just in childhood, but also during adulthood.

In 1996, life expectancy differed widely among urban neighbourhoods of varying incomes.[21] Lower life expectancy was especially likely among the fifth or lowest-income quintile of neighbourhoods. Among males in this lowest income quintile, life expectancy of 73.1 years was 2.8 years shorter than the next quintile group, and a full five years shorter than males in the wealthiest quintile group (figure 2). Females living in the lowest income quintile had a life expectancy 1.1 years less that those in the next group, and 1.7 years shorter than the wealthiest income quintile.

A particularly interesting finding was that the gap in life expectancy between men and women is 7.6 years in the poorest, fifth income quintile group. It is less so in the fourth and third income quintile (6 years), even less in the second income quintile (4.5 years) and the least in the wealthiest income quintile (4.1 years). Income interacts with gender to predict life expectancy. Poverty seems to be a much stronger threat to life expectancy for men than for women.

These differences in life expectancy reflect findings that Canadians living within the poorest 20 percent of urban neighbourhoods die earlier from a wide range of diseases that include cardiovascular disease, cancer, diabetes, and respiratory diseases — among other diseases — than other Canadians.[22] Table 1 provides specific findings of income-related differences in mortality.

As shown in table 1, the burden of ill health is concentrated in the lowest income quintile of neighbourhoods in urban Canada. For just about every cause of death, the poorest neighbourhoods fare much worse than the others. Q1 is the richest quintile, Q5, the poorest. RR shows the ratio of premature years lost between the Q1 and Q5 quintiles. RD shows how many years are lost between the Q1 and Q5 quintiles. Excess figures show how many years are lost between the richest quintile and all others, and the final column shows the percentage of all premature years of life lost that can be attributed to differences between the richest and the other quintiles.

The overall effect of income differences on years of life lost in urban Canada was also calculated.[23] In 1986, 21 percent of years of life lost for all causes prior to age seventy-five in Canada could be attributed to income differences and this estimate increased to 23 percent by 1996. This figure is obtained by using the mortality rates in the wealthiest or first quintile of neighbourhoods as a baseline

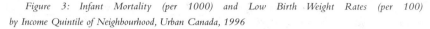

Figure 3: Infant Mortality (per 1000) and Low Birth Weight Rates (per 100) by Income Quintile of Neighbourhood, Urban Canada, 1996

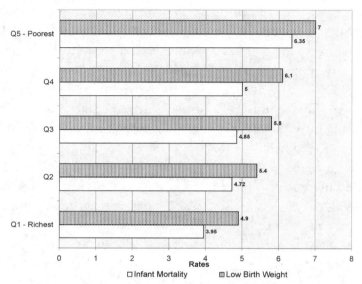

and considering all deaths above that rate to be excess related to income differences. The magnitude of income effects (23 percent) approaches or exceeds that associated with the major killers such as cancers (30.9 percent) and heart disease (17.6 percent).

Excess in mortality associated with income manifests itself in a wide range of diseases. Wilkins and colleagues took the excess lost years of life associated with income and examined which diseases these were associated with. They found that 21.6 percent of this income-related excess manifests itself in circulatory disorders; 16.9 percent, in deaths from injuries; 13.4 percent, in cancers; and 12.2 percent, in infectious diseases.

The data for infant mortality and low birth-weight rates showed similar trends (figure 3). The gap between the lowest-income quintile and the next quintile was the largest for infant mortality and low birth-weight rates. The infant mortality rate is 60 percent higher in the poorest income quintile than in the richest quintile areas. The low birth-weight rate is 43 percent higher

Figure 4: Odds Ratios for Risk Factors Associated with Self-Rated Fair or Poor Health and Poor Scores (50 Percentile) on the Health Utilities Index

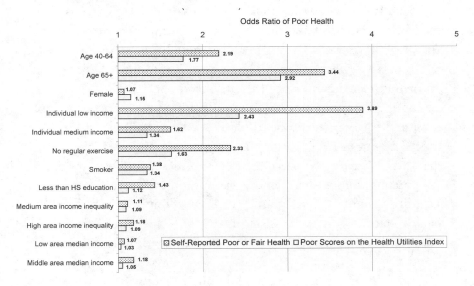

in the poorest income quintile than in the richest quintile areas.

A recent study reinforces the finding of the strong effect of income upon health status. In this Ontario study, self-reported health status as well as an objective measure of functional health (for example, vision, sight, mobility, pain) was examined in relation to both personal and area variables.[24] Findings indicated that individual level of income was a primary determinant of both self-reported and functional health (figure 4). Self-reported health is exactly that: a person rates their health as excellent, very good, good, fair, or poor. Functional health is an objective measure of motor, sensory, and pain-related health.

The analysis showed that having a low income gave an individual almost a four-times greater risk of reporting fair or poor health than high-income individuals. An individual of low income also had a two-and-a-half-times greater risk of having poor scores on the health utilities index. These low-income effects were much stronger than the effects of no regular exercise, smoking, and having less education. Income-related health inequalities such as these in Canada are generally higher than would be expected from income-distribution and health data derived from other nations.[25] This may have to do with Canada's generally less developed social safety net and weaker approach to economic and social provision, compared to other wealthy industrialized nations.

Living in poverty has important health consequences for children and for their health as adults.[26, 27] As noted earlier, the infant mortality rates of those living in the poorest 20 percent of Canadian urban areas is 60 percent higher and low birth-weight rate is 43 percent higher than in the richest urban areas.[28] Low birth weight (weight <2500 grams) is a very important measure of health status, as it is consistently related to the experience of chronic disease such as heart disease and type 2 diabetes in adulthood.[29]

And Wilkins reports that the low birth-weight rates range from 4.9 percent in the wealthiest urban areas to 7.0 percent in the poorest quintile of urban neighbourhoods in Canada.[30] Data from the National Longitudinal Study of Children and Youth paints a similar picture. Children from the lowest income families had a 13 percent chance of having poor functional health as measured by a composite measure of eight basic health attributes: vision, hearing, speech, mobility, dexterity, cognition, emotion, and pain and discomfort.[31] The rate for the wealthiest group of children was only 5 percent.

Indeed, the Canadian Institute for Child Health reports that children living in poverty are the most likely to have asthma or other chronic diseases, visit emergency rooms, and die from injuries.[32] Quebecois researchers, using data from the 1998 Longitudinal Study of Child Development in Québec, found that both overall and perceived health varied with income in five-month olds, even after taking into account health at birth and other socio-demographics.[33]

Longitudinal studies carried out in Europe have found that children living in poverty are more likely to develop cardiovascular disease, type 2 diabetes, respiratory problems, and some forms of cancer as adults.[34] These poverty and health relationships are robust and persist regardless of income status as adults. These same findings indicate that early childhood experiences of living in poverty are of more importance to later health than the presence of behavioural risk factors in adulthood.[35] In essence, experiencing poverty as a child provides a health risk that is carried into adulthood.

Addressing the Poverty and Health Relationship

Despite Canada's reputation as a leader in health promotion and population health, elected officials, health care and public health officials, and the media do not usually see poverty as a health issue. Instead, the health problems of people living in poverty are usually seen as reflecting their risk behaviours. This is the case even though evidence indicates that poverty is a much stronger determinant of health than these risk behaviours.

As one example, a report from Statistics Canada devotes most of its content to documenting how health behaviours (for example, smoking, exercise, weight) and psychosocial variables (for example, stress and depression) helped explain differences in health status among health regions.[36] This was done even though data from the same study showed that self-reported income — with the health of people of lower income especially poor — was far and away the best explanation for these regional differences in health outcomes.[37]

This emphasis is also puzzling given that poverty has been identified as a key determinant of health in many federal and provincial statements.[38] Similarly, Canadian Public Health Association (CPHA) policy statements stress the importance of the societal determinants of health, including poverty.[39]

Yet, despite the best continuing efforts of Health Canada and CPHA document writers to promote the importance of poverty as a health issue, the country's focus remains on behavioural change. There are some very important issues raised by this focus. First, evidence indicates that these behavioural risk factors play a rather small role in understanding the poor health of people living in poverty.[40] Second, focusing on behaviours rather than life situations leads to "victim blaming" whereby disadvantaged people are blamed for their own health problems, a concern raised in Canada over twenty years ago.[41] Third, emphasis on risk behaviours fails to address underlying issues of why disadvantaged people adopt these behaviours.[42] Fourth, these approaches are generally unsuccessful in developing effective interventions for behaviour change in disadvantaged groups.[43] Fifth and perhaps most important, an emphasis on behavioural risks diverts attention from poverty including its causes, its health effects, and the need for societal action to reduce and eliminate it.[44] Labonte states:

> The argument was simple. The health of oppressed people (poor, women, persons from minority cultures, workers, and others) was determined at least as much, if not more, by structural conditions (poverty hazards, powerlessness, pollution, and so on) than by personal lifestyles. Moreover personal lifestyles were not freely determined by individual choice, but existed within social and cultural structures that conditioned and constrained behaviour. Behavioural health education, social marketing, or wellness approaches to health promotion fostered victim blaming by assuming that individuals were entirely responsible for their choices and behaviour. They also blamed the victim indirectly by ignoring the structural determinants of health, those causes that

are embedded within economic, class- and gender-based patterns of social relationships.[45]

Why is there this blind spot? Health care and public health officials downplay poverty because raising its profile may be seen as threatening their relationship with governments who provide their status and funding. The denial of poverty as an important health issue is consistent with the ascendance of governmental commitments to neoliberal and neoconservative ideologies that position societal issues, including health and health promotion, as individual issues beyond the concern of governments and their institutions.[46] While centre-left governments may be more prone to lifestyle approaches (NDP-led provinces Manitoba and Saskatchewan have healthy lifestyles initiatives), conservative governments also promote similar approaches even though they may have other social policies and programs that end up undermining population health in the long run.[47]

There are instances in Canada where poverty has been raised as a health issue by health authorities. The Public Health Agency of Canada has established a National Coordinating Centre for the Determinants of Health in the Maritime Region which will be hosted by St. Francis Xavier University in Antigonish, Nova Scotia. Public health units in Alberta (for example, Chinook, Edmonton, and Calgary); Ontario (for example, Peterborough, Waterloo, Sudbury, and Perth); British Columbia (Interior Health); and Quebec (for example, Montreal) have raised poverty as being a key health issue. At a recent meeting of the Ontario Public Health Association, delegates voted to urge the provincial Medical Officer of Health to incorporate poverty and other determinants of health as issues to be included in the mandatory guidelines for public health practice. This view was endorsed by the association that represents provincial health officers. There may be other examples of such activity.[48]

Conclusion

Poverty is associated with a wide range of health issues. These relationships are so strong as to suggest that poverty is the primary
determinant of health, however defined. Poverty is an especially
important issue for children, as it not only threatens their health
and well-being as children but passes on health risks that can be
manifested during adulthood. Despite these findings, and numerous governmental and health-association documents and reports
acknowledging these findings, there is little if any action being
directed towards raising poverty as an important health issue.

In contrast to other nations where research and policy concern
with poverty and health has a long standing history such as the
UK, few Canadian researchers explicitly focus on the health of
people living in poverty.[49] And when these researchers do, many
are likely to attribute such differences to behavioural risk factors
such as tobacco use, physical activity, and diet. Nevertheless, there
is Canadian work that looks to understand the health of people
living in poverty as reflecting societal structures and processes.
There is research that focuses on the political economy of health
inequalities and how changes in economic structures and processes associated with increasing economic globalization and the
adoption of neoliberal public policies create and maintain high
poverty levels in Canada.[50] There is increasing interest in poverty
as a health issue in various non-health sectors.

Considering the increasing concern with the sustainability of
the health care system, it would be expected that the incidence of
poverty, and its profound effects upon health, would be taken
more seriously.[51] To date, this has not generally been the case.
However, the importance of the poverty and health issue, and the
increasing evidence of the effects of poverty upon health and
quality of life, suggest some hope for the future.

CHAPTER 30

Growing Inequality, Basic Needs and Health

Armine Yalnizyan

In March 2007, the Canadian Centre for Policy Alternatives released a reprise of the work I did, in 1998 and 2000, looking at what has happened to the incomes of families raising children in Canada.

In 2004, the richest 10 percent of families raising children in Canada earned incomes 81 times that of the poorest 10 percent. In 1976, a time of a strong economy that was arguably not as robust as today's, the richest families made 31 times the earnings of the poorest families.

In after-tax terms, income inequality has grown faster in the last decade than it has at any time in the past thirty years for which we have kept data. It is now at record high levels at a time when it should be declining and at record lows.

This is a period of unparalleled economic prosperity. Our economy is performing better than it has in forty years. This generation of parents raising children are better educated than the past generation, and they are spending more time in the labour market — and less time with their families — than the past generation. These are precisely the conditions under which the income gap between rich and poor should be shrinking.

The story is not limited to those at the extremes of the income spectrum. The bottom 40 percent of families raising children saw their household earnings fall behind their counterparts a generation ago. Even after taking into account the redistributive role of governments, after-tax incomes of the bottom 40 percent of Canadian families are either worse, or just barely better, than the incomes of families in the bottom half of the distribution a generation ago. Overall, the bottom half of families raising children saw little or no improvements to household incomes — though they worked more and were better educated. The benefits of economic growth accrued primarily to the richer half of the distribution. Those in the richest 10 percent of the income spectrum saw the biggest gains.

These findings suggest there are real limits to economic growth as the only mechanism for benefiting a population, even a well-educated, hard-working population. Markets may be powerful mechanisms for growth and expansion, but they are not in the business of delivering social or economic justice. That is not their role. It is up to people, through the institutions we create and the representatives we elect to send to legislatures, to articulate and enforce social and economic objectives. It is up to us to make sure the benefits of economic growth — to which we all contribute — are distributed more widely.

For the moment, however, we are sleepwalking through the converging effects of market forces and institutional change. We risk accepting these trends as the "new normal," deepening poverty even as affluence soars to unprecedented heights.

That acceptance may change, because the story of the growing gap is not only about greater poverty in a time of plenty. It is also a tale of increased economic insecurity and financial worry for a growing number of Canadians. And when more people are involved, more possibilities for change exist.

Those who receive social assistance are, without doubt, most harmed by these trends I have described, but the working poor are not far behind; and close behind them are those who consider themselves middle class. More people are feeling the pinch. As incomes become more polarized, income inequality triggers inequalities in access to a range of determinants of health, leading to greater disparities in health outcomes along the whole spectrum of incomes. More decision makers are starting to take notice.

The growing concentration of economic power among those already most advantaged is echoed in household incomes, in family wealth, as well as in corporate incomes and assets. Rising inequality has become a fact of life, between nations, within nations, among households. More people are starting to connect the dots. Polls show they don't like where we're headed, and they want something to be done.

The solutions to the growing gap are not just income related. They centre on the affordability of the basics in life. The short list of these basics includes shelter, education, child care, clean water, and health care. For the individual, we know that secure access to the basics assures better health. We also know that better access to basics across a population means better population health.

The Determinants of Health

Tommy Douglas knew better than most that the determinants of health are not just social. They are also genetic, environmental, and economic. Saskatchewan built this into their approach to health care.

Tommy often said his greatest legacy was to bring electricity to Saskatchewan. Long before medicare was in place, he knocked down outhouses and put up power lines all over the province. In so doing, Tommy Douglas electrified the nation, with a vision both straightforward and radical, offering a "can-do" platform that was grounded in both fairness and pragmatism.

A couple of years ago, CIDA (Canadian International Development Agency) commissioned me to write a handbook for development workers who are seeking to improve the health of citizens in developing nations. It's called *Getting Better Health Care*, and is co-published by CIDA and the Canadian Centre for Policy Alternatives. Writing something relevant and actionable was challenging, since there is such a range of experience among developing nations. The provision of health services for citizens can vary from nothing to quite elaborate public systems. So I decided to trace our history over the past one hundred years, looking at the lessons learned on our path to what we have today.

Like all nations, we started from nothing. In fact, our response to health care was in response to poverty, not plenty. We created what we have now in incremental steps, every few years undertaking something different, building on what we already had. We are still experimenting — though sometimes it seems that the current experiment is testing how much we can undo before the wheels fall off the little red wagon. But if we heed the lessons learned from our own history, the path to better health, and better health care, is not hard to see.

Tommy Douglas tore down the outhouses and set up systems of clean water and waste management. Since the turn of the last century, that has *always* been the first step to better health — better access to clean water and better disposal of waste assures better health. It is appalling that in 2007, right here in Canada — a country blessed with an abundance of water beyond most countries' wildest dreams — we cannot assure access to clean water for all Canadians, most particularly those who live on reserves. It is an incomprehensible situation; yet still people all around the world turn to us and say: "What can we do to get a 'Canadian-style' system of health care?" And they ask that question because we have a reputation for making things better for *everyone* ... when we *want* to do it better for everyone. That takes us right back to that can-do attitude that has existed in the past and can exist again — an attitude that knows the score, knows what it takes to change the scorecard, and does it. And that takes me to my final point.

The New Jerusalem

Tommy Douglas understood that, if the people of Saskatchewan were to enjoy better health, he had to invest in the determinants of health. These are the very areas in which, as Madame Bégin has reminded us, we have actually reduced investments over the last twenty years. We have forgotten the importance of reflecting on where we've been, in order to better see where we are heading.

Saskatchewan was where commitment to the social gospel first flourished in Canada. While it might not have been called the social gospel elsewhere, that same ethos echoed across the country in those early post-war years. In 1948, Canada signed on to the Universal Declaration of Human Rights — a document that most people don't know was written by a Montreal lawyer, originally from New Brunswick, named John Humphrey.

In the wake of the Second World War, the whole of Canada seemed taken by a particular view of what needed to be done. The province of Saskatchewan, under the inspiring leadership of its premier, Tommy Douglas, saw the task as nothing less than building the road to what Tommy called the "New Jerusalem."

If we improved people's access to the determinants of health throughout this nation, we would simply be doing today what we committed to do in 1948, when we signed on to the Universal Declaration of Human Rights. Every human being needs adequate shelter, access to clean water, enough food, access to health and education, freedom from violence, freedom to associate. That is as true today as it was in 1948.

I would contend that there are more Canadians who do not have access to these basics in 2007 than there were in 1948. And it is not because we can't afford it.

Tommy's government had no money when he did what he did, but he and his electorate knew where they had to head. Many decades later, we are wallowing in affluence, both economically and fiscally; everyone knows what is needed, but there is little progress.

But there are enough people in Canada to help gun the engines that have been idling too long. The road map is not about going back to a sentimental past, or settling for the best of what we have today. It's about moving forward, building the road to the New Jerusalem.

We know where we're headed, and we know how to get there. Let's get going.

CHAPTER 31

People Are Dying
for a Home

Cathy Crowe

A Toronto media outlet recently asked me what I thought of a new hospital mobile outreach program that would bring health care to homeless people. I replied, "Well, as long as we have homelessness, we will have two-tiered health care. As long as we have mobile vans and health workers with knapsacks providing curbside care, we should face the fact that we really have two-tiered health care in this country."

In 1909, J.S. Woodsworth, the first leader of the CCF, wrote a letter to the *Manitoba Free Press* about a "little foreign girl [*sic*]" whom he had seen living in filth in a North Winnipeg tenement. His letter asked if anyone could help her. This little girl was living in deplorable conditions with her family, sharing one bed which doubled as table and chairs, and she was languishing with horrible open sores on her body.

In subsequent decades, Canadians participated in social justice campaigns that led to the birth of many of our national social programs, including medicare. The development of our social programs has always been based on the belief that Canadians should not have to rely on luck or the benevolence of others for life's very basics, like food, water, shelter, and health care. Most Canadians know about the medicare story — how it was achieved and how it is now under threat.

One of our great social justice campaigns gave birth to our national housing program, yet most Canadians don't know the story of how it came to be. It is a riveting story, a story just waiting for a film to be made about it.

Returning World War II veterans, facing a housing shortage, fought for their right to housing across Canada. In Ottawa, Montreal, and Vancouver, women's groups joined in. They demonstrated, and they actually took over empty buildings like the Hotel Vancouver and the Kildare barracks in Ottawa.

The campaign led to empty military buildings being freed up for housing; it led to a federal agency, Wartime Housing Ltd., that built 19,000 temporary rental homes over four years. It led to the creation of the Central Mortgage and Housing Corporation, now the Canada Mortgage and Housing Corporation, which came to be our national housing program. CMHC helped to build affordable housing for close to 2 million Canadians until that program was quietly destroyed.

Our housing program was taken from us in 1993, and we have to get it back, because people are dying for a home, literally.

Canada remains one of the few countries in the world without a national housing program. Canadian NGOs pointed this out in their 2005 submission to the United Nations Committee on Economic, Social and Cultural Rights Working Group. Canada has:

> no coherent policy of national standards to ensure that
> the right to adequate housing is enjoyed by all, and

particularly by poor and disadvantaged groups, such as low-income women.

The 2007 federal budget was entirely silent on homelessness. The hundreds of pages of budget documents barely even mention housing, except to repeat some previously announced spending. Perhaps more frightening is that no one seems to have noticed: there were no headlines in the papers saying *"Harper ignores 4 million Canadians in core housing need!"* or *"300,000 homeless people left with no hope for housing!"*

What this means, with no national housing program and no political will to recreate one, is that the following hotspots will continue to erupt unchecked throughout Canada.

1. Shelter conditions

Each year over 300,000 men, women, and children are homeless and are forced to live, sometimes months but more often years, in crowded and inadequately funded emergency shelters. Across this country, bunk beds, dormitory rooms, tuberculosis outbreaks, bedbug infestations, noise, violence, and mental trauma are all too common in our shelter system.

2. Outside sleeping/squats/tent cities

An overflow of perhaps several thousand people are forced to sleep outside, in squats, tent cities, or sporadically in hotel rooms or church basements, facing the additional risk of violence, isolation, and exposure to the elements. To make matters worse, this visible group, often labelled as street people, face new and harsh municipal and provincial laws on where they can sleep and how they must behave. More hate crimes against homeless people are being reported, which seems to parallel these new punitive laws.

3. Charity

My mother was a nurse, so I know about the days before medicare. I know that we could not rely on donations, volunteers, or the private sector to provide life-saving services to Canadians needing health care. I also know that we cannot rely on donations, volunteers, or the private sector to provide Canadians with housing or emergency shelter. Most major cities in this country rely on huge charitable endeavours to provide life-saving services for our people. The most obvious, the Out of the Cold or In(n) from the Cold faith-based programs, provide single-night shelter on the floor of their place of worship.

That little girl in the North Winnipeg tenement is now a little girl or boy staying with her parents on a church basement floor in Calgary, being bused to school, only to be bused after school to a different church basement floor, and so on, and so on.

4. Pandemic flu and emerging viruses

Social disasters like overcrowding, hunger and homelessness are usually paired with plagues, scourges, and emerging viruses. We have already witnessed clusters of tuberculosis and TB deaths among the homeless population; we have seen lockdowns in Canadian shelters during a Norwalk virus outbreak, and during SARS we saw an attempt to "home quarantine" the homeless.

Those relying on day and night shelters or food banks might wonder how our stretched infrastructure will hold up should another SARS-like event occur, or how their health unit's Pandemic Plan is relevant when there already exists a shortage of soap, toilet paper, and paper towels in the daytime drop-in that serves 300 people.

5. Heat/global warming

Heat deaths are one more consequence of homelessness, poverty, and social isolation and the withdrawal of social programs.

Temperatures in Toronto rooming houses last summer were recorded at thirty-four to thirty-five degrees Celsius.

6. Deaths

Anecdotal reports suggest that homeless deaths are rising all across the country. The victims are disproportionately young and Aboriginal compared to the housed population in Canada. These deaths are widely ignored and under-reported. Coroners routinely dismiss a homeless person's death as due to "natural causes," seemingly unaware that a pattern of social neglect is taking place.

For those ill and dying who are fortunate enough to live in Toronto or Ottawa, there are shelters with palliative care components and hospice — but still no housing.

Some front-line workers are beginning to face the realization that their current work includes a palliative component, despite the lack of a terminal medical diagnosis for the people they care for.

A National Program

Given these horrific circumstances and outcomes that I have only touched on, I want to send out an SOS, and emphasize that the fight we face now for adequate housing is like the fight for medicare. *The fight for housing must be included in our continuing fight for basic health care in Canada.*

CHAPTER 32

Miyo-Mâhcihowin: Self-determination, Social Determinants, and Indigenous Health

Willie Ermine and Eber Hampton

Thus far, indigenous conceptions of health have had little influence in the construction of the Canadian model of medicare. In determining the content and direction of the second phase of medicare, the time has come to incorporate an indigenous understanding of health. Based upon the Cree language, we provide a living example of an indigenous approach to health and the implications this holds for all of us, as we look forward to the second phase of medicare, in which the social determinants of health take centre stage and self-determination is recognized as one of those key social determinants.

The late Lionel Kinunwa taught that indigenous language is our philosophy book, our political science text, our self-help pamphlet, and policy manual. He taught that speaking is an exercise of power and as such should be done with responsible intent. To know that power can reside in speech is also to understand the nature and influence of the words that are uttered. In some measure, the wellspring of speaking meaningfully, of exercising responsible power, resides in our capacity to link our outward expression with our philosophical and cultural foundations. Paulo Freire also discussed the notion that words have capacity to transform. He stated that, "within the word we find two dimensions, reflection and action, in such radical interaction that if one is sacrificed–even in part the other immediately suffers."[52]

In other words, we need to act and perform the health philosophies that are inextricably linked and grounded to our basic humanness. We cannot ground words and actions about human health to institutional or colonial underpinnings that have no passion or spirit for human well-being in the way that humans can relate. Here we present one way of gaining insight into the thought worlds of Indigenous Peoples that addresses health from the human perspective. Through this exercise we attempt to examine the philosophical undercurrents of language that gives us insight and reflection on notions about human health. The languages of Indigenous Peoples such as the Cree can offer a glimpse into the value of words in helping us in our desire to be human and to understand the frameworks that uphold our beings.

The undercurrent of word meanings, words that say more than the uttering, are a storehouse of perceptions about our humanity and about our healthiness and well-being. Indeed, the strategic actions that communities will take concerning their health can be largely based on these philosophical foundations. These cultural precepts are embedded in words and can be revealed through an examination and the unfolding of embedded concepts found within indigenous languages. Words that evoke thoughts, feelings, and reveal historical and philosophical pictures are dissected and discussed to "unpack" their meaning. These meanings not only explicate Indigenous/Cree thought but also describe the processes and the codes governing the Indigenous reality and all of its relationships.

To provide a specific example, we can examine the Cree word *Miyo-Mâhcihowin,* sometimes translated as *good health,* or as *living well*. This word has at least four embedded concepts that contribute insights to the notion of healthiness. We take the notion of healthiness and feed the concept to the Cree language to see what comes out from that thought world. It asks the question: "What is good health?" Beyond the literal translation and describing the term, the word also provides us with the process that must be undertaken in order to actualize well-being and good health.

The Cree word *Miyo-Mâhcihowin* contains the following concepts: *Miyo-* is a root form that refers to the unfolding of something in a good way; that things are the way they should be as arranged by whole flow of universal energy. It also means being good or competent at something, or being good at unfolding in a good way. It is a verb that describes an active process, and its usage always signifies a positive outcome. Miyo is always good.

Mâci — is the root verb that describes motion, or movement. It is the constant stirring and movement of the human form in a certain direction or with purposeful action, usually in concert with the flowing movement of all that is. This root word, taken to higher philosophical levels, can also be broken into two separate roots. *Mâ* — is the root that speaks about a repeating pattern. *Ci* — is the root that talks about "parts of," or particles, if we want to think in that way. Thus, *mâci* — is the repeating movement, or continuous shifting of particles (such as our selves). It is the dance with the universe.

Ho — is the root that unifies these concepts and declares that unity as a model of being, a way of being human, or a state of being. It is the state of achieving this movement (*mâci*) in the good way. At the philosophical level, the good way (*miyo*) of unfolding, and movement (*mâci*) is tied to the notion of a universal order. This universal order is the implicate order as discussed by Bohm.[53] The implicate order is the natural (univer-

sal) unseen process, the stirring of all energy, or the whole flowing movement of the universe, which moves all things and with
which all things must flow in unison. This movement with the
universal flow is consistent with synchronizing the human with
flowing universal energy. The result is a well-tuned human or
"healthy" human being because of the universal order. Therefore,
the way of "being"'and the way of healthiness is understood as
"moving well with the natural processes of the universe."

Finally, *win* — is the root that accounts for the procedure or
process to achieve the way of being — being healthy in this case.
This root describes the system, or the human endeavour, that creates or enables the way of being healthy to unfold. It is to
recognize and acknowledge specific determinants of this universal
impulse for healthiness. It is a system or blueprint to achieve a certain state of being that we categorize as healthiness. However, this
root word only provides us with the pointer, or the direction, to
go and does not actually give us the process or the actions
required to achieve the state. It should be understood that, in the
Cree world, as in many others, this system or process is to be
found in the ethos of the community, or the collective agreement
we call the tradition, within the whole spectrum of its knowledge
system. The process of achieving healthiness is to be found in the
tradition of the people. To understand and achieve Cree/Indige-
nous health requires Cree ethos, to know the contours of Cree
culture and tradition and its philosophical contributions to human
well being, and to follow these precepts. Unfolding this kind of
health knowledge and knowing its determinants can be enhanced
through the self-determination of the people that hold that spark
of insight.

We may continue the example by imagining a Cree speaker
who understands the intent of *miyo-mâhcihowin* and a speaker of
English for whom *good health* means "free from disease." Let's
imagine our speakers as individuals that are neither unusually

typical nor unusually atypical in their language communities. Since we are writing in English, it may help to suggest simple contrasting analogies that these particular imaginary speakers might use to explain their intent.

CREE SPEAKER	SPEAKER OF ENGLISH
Miyo-mâhcihowin	Good health
Is like being a good dancer in that one moves pleasingly and in sync with the rhythm of the drum	Is like being a well oiled bio-chemical system in that all subsystems are operating within normal specifications
Speaking of miyo-mâhcihowin in the present context our intent is to hear, speak and act on what works for the well being of all our relations	Speaking of good health in the context of second phase medicare we naturally speak of primary care and the prevention of disease
By asserting self-determination we reject imposition of control and welcome mutual assistance and learning	By knowing and manipulating the social determinants of health we can prevent disease

This, or any, difference of intent immediately calls forth ethical space.[54] Settler colonialism made a futile attempt to forestall ethical space, the space of dialogue between human communities, by imagining the other with nothing to say. Difference entails ethical consequences of choices in word, action, and intent, and human ethics remind us that it is these choices we make that invariably infringe on the sacred spaces of other humans and communities. We make choices within an ethical space inevitably created by our differences. However, we must also be reminded that ethical space concerns the capacity to know what harms or enhances the well-being of sentient creatures. Consciously acknowledging ethical space gives us the opportunity of negotiating higher quality problems and achieving solutions that have mutual benefit. The imaginary speakers of table 1 might negotiate an inclusion of self-determination in the list of health determinants.

From our perspective, an even more propitious outcome would be a mutually enhanced understanding of community. Community is a structure of the support mechanisms that include the personal responsibility for the collective and reciprocally, the collective concern for individual existence. Cajete suggests that, "the community is the place where the forming of the heart and face of the individual as one of the people is most fully expressed."[55] Community is a primary expression of natural context and an environment where exists the fundamental right of personhood to be what one is meant to be. Movement within this community context allows individuals to discover all there is to discover about oneself. It is crucial to understand that human communities hold their own models of humanity.

Our imaginary English speaker may more acutely feel tension between the individual and the group. Citing Kawachi and Kennedy, Dennis Raphael describes a social comparison approach to understanding social determinants of health: "The perception and experience of hierarchy in unequal societies lead to stress and poor health."[56] It is unfortunate that many of our communities have been altered by past experiences, but many are now at the stage of "memory work" to recover the philosophies and practices that gave strength to our people. Revitalizing our knowledge systems requires the support for self-determination so that diverse human communities can have resources to actively engage with their own social determinants of health.

Perhaps David Bohm could mediate the discussion.[57] He refers to the idea of community as a process of participatory thought. He recognizes participatory thought as a people's participation in some of the things they saw, and that one cannot be part of something unless that thing in some sense accepts one's participation. In this sense, community is participatory thought in action. *Miyo-mâhcihowin* calls for a collective effort and requests unity of human communities in the dance with the universe.

The ethical space urges us to dialogue from the position of our humanity. This is to recognize that the institutionalization of our health systems has appropriated our freedom to speak to each other from our humanness. Hierarchy in unequal societies is a problem spawned by institutionalization. The ethical space offers the opportunity for us to detach from these mental traps to be able to dialogue across cultures as way of finding solutions to mutual existence.

In summary, the Cree language, known for its precise idiom, has an array of embedded concepts within its word structures that speak about the nature of our human existence. For this reason, Indigenous words (and language) become rich resources for providing direction to processes that would enable Indigenous Peoples to engage meaningfully in health practice. Words, in this case, become texts, or blueprints, by which we study and analyze concepts that can provide us with perspectives relating to our human condition. There is a need to understand that these cultural precepts are always in the background, haunting the systems and processes that obstruct the self-determination necessary to good health. Through the concept of the ethical space, dialogue can occur between worldviews to find the relevant course to good health or Miyo-mâhcihowin — the universal movement.

Miyo-mâhcihowin is both a promise and a challenge. The promise is that, at their best, our communities offer values and knowledge to creatively unfold the next phase of medicare in a good way. The challenge is fundamentally ethical. We must speak, listen, choose, and act in ways that work for the health of ourselves, our communities, and our society. As we work to unfold the next phase of medicare it is natural to think of public policy as a contested arena. It may be useful to think not always of arena, but also of ethical space that calls to us in the words of the elder, "to put our minds together and see what kind of world we shall make for our children."

PART VI

Getting There
from Here

CHAPTER 33

Canada's Shared Destiny and the Future of Medicare

Roy Romanow

To place the debate over medicare in its full context — to underline the importance of the task ahead of us in reinvigorating our shared commitment to medicare — I would like to also put Canada's values on the table. I see the choice that we as Canadians make about medicare as one that is fundamentally intertwined with our nation's values and its future.

Every day, Canada faces new challenges that ask questions about what kind of people we are, and what kind of future we wish to shape. Today we are wrestling with the renewal of medicare. But we could just as easily be discussing the integrity of our ecological environment, our role in Afghanistan and the world at large, or our domestic choices with respect to other social and economic policies.

Because what all these debates have in common is that they all return to a basic and fundamental question: What are the values of

Canada and how do we build a more progressive and united
nation?

In seeking to answer these important questions, we should
never act as if we are starting from scratch. Every nation has a narrative. Canada's narrative offers us a strong and rich legacy of
success that has forged our nation. It is a legacy that I describe as
a "shared destiny" — a legacy that is key to understanding the
future of our yet young country. It is this same legacy of "shared
destiny" that remains the roadmap to our future, at home and
abroad.[1]

For those of you who, like me, came of age in our Prairie communities, I don't have to tell you about the importance of the
notion of "shared destiny." The harsh, often snow-blown conditions, droughts, distance and isolation, and small population,
forced us together, like poplar trees huddled on a windswept plain.
We all learned to see survival and progress as a test of our ongoing ability to organize collectively and to remain united around
shared values.

Although Canada has other regions with their own challenges,
I suspect the same is also true for them.

And so, through the years, as we lived together, worked together, and built together, this notion of "shared destiny" was
transformed into the foundation of a nation. Generation after
generation of Canadians have seized on the cornerstone idea that
our future and our society is frequently best shaped through community action — that the sum of Canada is often greater than its
remarkably diverse parts.

John Whyte, in making the Saskatchewan government's argument to the Supreme Court of Canada in the post-1995 Quebec
Secession reference case, summed up this notion of "shared destiny" when he said:

A nation is built when the communities that comprise

it make commitments to it, when they forgo choices and opportunities on behalf of a nation ... when the communities that comprise it make compromises, when they offer each other guarantees, when they make transfers, and perhaps most pointedly, when they receive from others the benefits of national solidarity. The threads of a thousand acts of accommodation are the fabric of a nation.[2]

This, then, is our nation's narrative and it resides in our collective DNA. In recent years, however, the soil has been tilled for the sprouting of views at odds with shared destiny. Today, we witness a palpable momentum toward individualism, decentralization, and privatization.

All of these are described as the new ways to deal with today's world, but, in truth, they represent an abandonment of our accomplishments and a parting of the ways with the belief in our collective capacity to meet our future challenges and to forge a stronger and more unified nation.

Medicare, which is the product of this narrative, is also now caught up in this so-called new thinking. And, just like with today's other major issues, it is the manner in which we choose to inform our way forward, the set of values that we draw on to shape our progress, that ultimately will become an expression of who we are as a nation.

That is why the debate over medicare is not just about effectiveness and efficiency. It is not simply about the irrefutable evidence showing that our single-payer public system delivers excellent outcomes, which it does. The medicare debate is not even just about basic Canadian values like equity and fairness for all citizens.

Yes, it is about all these things. But it is also about much more. For medicare holds such a central role in our narrative of shared destiny that how we deal with our social programs will determine the future progress of our nation.

Canada's Medicare System: Separating Fact from Fiction

So, keeping this history in mind, what is the road to progress on medicare? Well, let's begin by making sure that we separate truths from myths.

First, there is a myth that we have one big, monolithic public health care system. Some even believe it to be an overly expensive and unwieldy behemoth unable to keep up with the demands of today, and utterly unfit for tomorrow. But we don't have one system. We have thirteen health care systems: one for each province and territory. And if you add in the federal government as a deliverer, we actually have fourteen systems.

All, however, are bound together by the shared principles enunciated in a federal law called the Canada Health Act (CHA)[3], thanks to the leadership of Monique Bégin, which outlines the five pillars of Canada's medicare: universality, comprehensiveness, portability, accessibility, and public administration.

The CHA also states that all patients are entitled to "medically necessary services," delivered by doctors and hospitals, and paid for from the public purse. And, while the federal government can enforce the CHA by withholding from the provinces the cash transfer payments it makes for health service delivery, in recent times it has rarely done so. Thus, each province and territory exercised its new grants of autonomy to shape its health care system in whatever way it saw fit.

In fact, outside of the core basket of CHA services that covers doctors and hospitals, provinces can and do — in varying degrees — fund, subsidize, and deliver a range of other programs. Lately, some provinces have become increasingly more bold in implementing important changes to medicare, with impunity. As a result, we don't have a single public health care monopoly. And it's certainly not "socialized medicine" or "state-run medicine" in the common understanding of those terms.

It is not state-run because many hospitals and other health care institutions are community-based non-profit bodies. Moreover, the vast majority of doctors are effectively independent contractors paid according to fee schedules.

And there is another myth: that the whole thing is publicly funded. In fact, it's a complex structure of three main categories of financing. At the first level — or core CHA — are those services to which all Canadians are entitled as a right of citizenship, rooted in the fundamental Canadian value that health care is a social good. These core CHA services, as Greg Marchildon has documented, add up to 43 cents on every health care dollar spent in Canada. Essentially, this is the single-payer system, publicly financed through progressive taxation, which is at the heart of medicare.[4]

The second level, worth about a quarter of our total health care bill — or 28 cents out of every health care dollar — represents a mixture of public and private spending and delivery. Drug costs are a prime example of expenditures in this segment. They are covered by the provinces in the case of seniors or low-income people, employment-based group plans, or private insurance. But the coverage is highly variable from region to region.

Home care, rehabilitation, and long-term care offer similar examples of mixed, or blended, public and private funding. The provisions of the CHA cover none of the services in this second tier, except as they relate directly to doctors and hospitals.

Yet another level of health care services, the third, is paid for almost entirely by private funds. Most dental and vision care, as well as a range of other services from chiropractic to psychological, are not covered by Canada's public plans even though Mr. Justice Emmett Hall, in his seminal report, urged this extended coverage over forty years ago.

About 50 to 60 percent of Canadians are fortunate to have work-based insurance programs to cover some of these costs. Others pay directly out of their own pockets, or don't receive them at all.[5]

So, to recap, only 43 percent of total health care expenditures in Canada are publicly funded through the single-payer system, approximately 27 percent involve a mixed public/private model, and 30 percent are paid for completely by private schemes, or directly out of our own pockets. As we can see, it is a myth to argue that our medicare system is entirely financed by public funds.

Canada's Medicare System: Towards Sustainability

There is yet another myth that needs to be addressed. It tries to speak to the very real rise in total health spending in Canada, which must be acknowledged, and says that public health care costs are spiraling out of control. That, the myth says, is "unsustainable" — that the spending is crowding out other areas of public programming. So, it says, we must look to even greater private financing and private delivery of care to ensure medicare's sustainability.

This mantra has been repeated so frequently that we should not be surprised if many Canadians believe it to be true. Once again, however, the facts prove otherwise. The federal finance department, in projecting health care costs into the year 2040, discounted "theories that rising health-care costs will bankrupt federal and provincial governments ... Governments' share of total health care spending for the country will likely remain less than 10% of the size of the Canadian economy."[6] That's Ottawa's Department of Finance.

A recent study in *Canadian Public Policy* examined this issue from a retrospective view, namely, what the actual expenditures were over a given period, as opposed to a prospective analysis as Ottawa's was. This study looked at public spending from

1988/1989 to 2003/2004 and concluded that "there is no evidence that increased provincial government health expenditures resulted in lower levels of spending on other categories of government-provided goods and services."[7]

So the evidence demonstrates, both prospectively and retrospectively, that public financing does not cause limitations on other essential government services. Then what does?

To answer this question, we must clearly understand this extremely important, but little reported, fact: that, among the three tiers of service that I described earlier — publicly funded, privately funded, and mixed groups of services — it is in the publicly funded system that the costs have actually risen the *least*.[8]

Over the past five years, the Canada Health Care Association says that it is in the privately funded sector that growth rates have been climbing much higher and faster, averaging a 6 percent annual rise in the private sector as compared to 4.5 percent on the public side.[9] So why have public-service costs not grown as fast as expenditures in other sectors?

One explanation is that a lot of care has shifted out of hospitals, because of technical advances, and is being moved to home-based and ambulatory care. Many interventions are now being handled by prescription drugs, which means, as I have explained, that more costs are being passed directly on to individual Canadians.

The second reason — and perhaps the most important one — has to do with the administrative efficiency of the single-payer public insurance model. While private insurance and multi-payer systems, as in the United States, spend a lot of money on the extensive infrastructure required to deal with multiple insurance companies, by contrast, a single insurer for the core services in Canada is spared most of these administrative outlays. And the paperwork costs are considerable. Writing in the *New England Journal of Medicine*, Harvard University researchers estimated that, in 1999, total administrative costs per capita in the United States were well over three times the costs in Canada: US$1,059 per capita in the United States compared to US$307 per capita in Canada.[10]

Until the introduction of medicare in Canada, health spending as a percentage of GDP in the two countries grew in lock-step throughout the 1950s and 1960s.[11] But after medicare was introduced in Canada, our health spending began to grow at a very different pace. Today, health spending in Canada amounts to under 10 percent of our GDP, while in the United States it amounts to over 15 percent of GDP, and rising.[12] And on top of all of this, the latest 2006 US census shows that nearly one in six Americans, or 15.9 percent of the population, were uninsured for some or part of the census year.[13] Also revealed was that half of the 1.5 million of American families who filed for bankruptcy in 2001 — many of whom, by the way, had private insurance that just ran out or was inadequate — cited medical causes as the reason for filing bankruptcy.[14]

In contrast, according to a study of the OECD last year, the Canadian system contributes to health outcomes that are, on the whole, more often than not, better than those produced by the United States, and in fact better than much of the rest of the world.[15] And let's not forget that Canada's publicly funded health system also provides significant economic advantages thanks to reduced health costs to Canadian employers. For example, the auto industry, a sector that generates billions of dollars for the Canadian economy, holds an advantage that amounts to about $4 per hour per worker compared to the United States.[16]

So, instead of viewing public spending in health innovation and reform as unsustainable and as a burden, let's acknowledge that it is both sustainable and crucial to our nation's social and economic well-being. It is a reinforcement of our values, and an investment in the future of a stronger Canada.

The Royal Commission's Solutions for Reform

There is much at stake in this debate. The good news is that the solutions are at hand, ready to be seized by our policymakers, just as soon as they can muster the political will to act.

The Royal Commission on the Future of Health Care that I headed made forty-seven recommendations for reform, but, rather than detailing them all, let me simply outline the five enduring lessons that I believe remain central to the Canadian debate about health care reform.

1. The universal single-payer advantage

My first point is to reinforce the advantages of a universal single-payer system for all the reasons that I advanced. Our task is clear, if not without difficulties: we must bring aspects of home care, access to advanced diagnostic services, and catastrophic drug coverage — the areas of fastest rising costs — within the single-payer system.

Let me illustrate, using pharmaceuticals. Since 1990, the cost of prescription drugs as a percentage of total health expenditures has increased to 14.6 percent from 8 percent. Canada's private spending on prescription drugs now outpaces that of most other OECD countries.[17]

So we must lay the groundwork now for including these and other elements under the umbrella of public funding, or their costs will continue to escalate without restraint and relentlessly abandon those in need.

2. Keeping the focus on total costs

We still have to control total health care costs and avoid shuffling expenditures between the public and private sectors of the health care system. Until the mid-1990s, some provincial governments, including my own in Saskatchewan, were successful in restraining the growth of public health care costs. We rationalized our services and improved efficiencies, while trying to preserve access to quality services. Our fiscal position obligated us to do this.

It turned out, however, that we pushed some of these costs out of our own provincial budgets and onto the personal budgets of the residents. It was, in other words, a *false economy*. Because, in the end, the total bill for health care is paid by all citizens, whether through their taxes, their premiums on insurance policies, or out of their own pockets, through direct payment.

3. Tackling wait times

My third point is that we must do everything possible to improve timely access to quality services within the public system. Although we have focused too much on this, to the detriment of other areas of concern, wait times still represent one of the significant proxies of public trust in medicare. And, while the vast majority of Canadians are happy with the service they receive, a sizeable number of them feel they have wait too long.[18]

Improving timely access to care will require, above all, a more integrated approach to health care delivery, as opposed to attempts to target only selected categories.

4. Addressing the determinants of health

Fourth, we have to pay more attention to prevention. There are several important pathways to achieving a healthier nation. A quality health care system is certainly part of the answer. But equally important in achieving this goal is attention to prevention and to the "determinants for a healthier population" — from income status, to education, early learning and child care, to housing, to the state of the environment, and, yes, to the quality and accessibility of our health care system.

I've been working with a group of exceptionally dedicated and talented national and international experts on the important task of creating a Canadian Index of Well-being, the CIW. It's our hope that the CIW will be accepted as a credible barometer on the social, health, and environmental conditions that shape our communities.

What we need to measure is what counts, because that determines what makes it onto the front pages of newspapers and the front desks of decision makers. Right now, we tend to measure our well-being primarily through a narrow set of economic indicators, particularly the gross domestic product, or GDP. Imagine, however, if every time we heard about the GDP, we also heard the results of the Canadian Index of Well-being. Perhaps it would help us integrate this information into the economic decisions.

My hope is that the CIW will raise our overall understanding of the importance of a holistic response to health. It is a bold vision, and a first step will be the launch of the CIW in October of 2007 — look out for it.

5. Transformative change

My final point is that governments must show the will and leadership to achieve what I call transformative change. They must do so based on our values, and they must respond to the public will.

Since the Commission: How Are We Doing?

Some of you may be asking yourselves: What has transpired since the release of the final report of the Royal Commission? The short answer is that, while we are making slow progress in some areas, Canada still has a long way to go.

There are some positive developments that we should acknowledge and build on. For instance, we now have a Health Council of Canada to monitor and publicly report upon our successes and failures, even though Alberta and Quebec have not agreed to participate.

Primary health care reform is slowly taking shape and some positive work can be highlighted. Information technology and tele-health are being developed. Wait times are being addressed, as difficult as this is proving to be. Hospital and other health services are being reorganized, in order to become more responsive to patients' needs.

We are slowly — perhaps too slowly — breaking down the silos within our health care system. And the so-called "Health Care Deal for a Generation" infused $41.3 billion over ten years for action in areas of shared priority. This was a major recommendation of the Royal Commission. It restores financial cutbacks to the provinces by Ottawa. Sufficiency of public funds should no longer be an obstacle for our provinces to implement the reforms — especially if they are encouraged by Ottawa.

Privatization: Debate Reignited?

Yet we know that there continues to be a hard-hitting debate about the appropriate balance between public and private funding and delivery. The most recent development of note was the Supreme Court's decision in the *Chaoulli* case, in which four of the seven presiding justices ruled in favour of Dr. Chaoulli and his client/patient, Mr. Zeolitis. They ruled that the Quebec government's ban on private health insurance was in violation of the Quebec Charter of Rights and Freedoms and, by direct implication, the constitutionally entrenched Canadian Charter of Rights and Freedoms.[19]

I won't delve here into the complex legal issues raised by this controversial decision, except to say that many observers argue that the Supreme Court has made a major and unfortunate intrusion into the development of Canada's social policy.[20] The majority seemingly relied on the evidence and arguments provided by some members of the Senate of Canada, the Canadian Medical Association, and individual physicians who long ago chose to practise private for-profit care outside the medicare system.

It is notable, however, that all these interveners steered clear of the American experience in their arguments and pointed instead to Europe and a so-called blended system of public and private care.

But what of the European model? Testifying at the trial level of this particular case, noted Yale health economist Ted Marmor described the European model as follows:

> the experience of private supplementary insurance in Europe is that parallel financing persistently raises questions of fairness. They are never ending sources of complaint as illustrated by the controversies over pay beds in British NHS hospitals, private insurance coverage of co-payments in France, and the exiting from the public insurance "pool" of those in Germany's top ten percent of income earners.[21]

This description confirms the overwhelming findings of many other studies, and supports the evidence and conclusions contained in my Royal Commission Report.[22] In fact, while Canada's total health care bill remains higher than the OECD average, at 9.9 percent of GDP, our health care costs are well in line with those of other wealthy nations. Total health spending as a percentage of GDP remains above 9 percent in Australia, France, Sweden, and the Netherlands, among others.[23]

Furthermore, if we accept the argument that the best road to sustainability is to contain the spiraling costs of pharmacare and home care by bringing them into the public system, then Canada still has plenty of room to manoeuver. Canada, at 70 percent public funding, falls below the OECD average when it comes to health spending financed by public dollars as a share of the total pie.[24] This share is more than three-quarters of total costs in France and Germany, and well above 80 percent in the UK and Sweden.

This evidence was ignored by the majority of the Supreme Court, which appears to have given undue weight to those who clamour for privatization, for the markets to rule, for more private delivery, for more private payment, for more private choice. Thus the case of *Chaoulli v Quebec* has re-energized a powerful group of pro-two-tier-care Canadians.

Citing the *Chaoulli* decision and other authorities, they cite this market-based vision for health care as something new, as "out-of-the-box," innovative thinking. But just how "new" is this particular approach? Let me give you a quote, and then pose a question. The quote reads:

> What is meant by 'universal' is that the plan arbitrarily includes everybody, whether they need the benefits and whether they wish to be included or not. It is a compulsory program in which participation is compelled by the state and not left to the voluntary choice of the citizen himself ... This violates a fundamental principle of free society, namely, the right of each citizen to exercise freedom of choice.

Do you know who said that and when? It was former Alberta Premier Ernest Manning in 1965! Suddenly, the old has once again become the new. Suddenly, we witness decisions driven by ideology masquerading as evidence. Well, just ask the parents or guardians of the millions of American children who are not covered by health insurance if they are enjoying their exercise of freedom of choice!

Returning to "Shared Destiny"
Monique Bégin, author of the Canada Health Act, reminds us that the true guardians of medicare — this most cherished expression of what it means to be Canadian — are the people of Canada. She

is right. Today, the overwhelming majority of Canadians continue to support the universal, single-payer approach to public health care.[25] Few buy the argument that things will improve if we move to a categorical, multi-payer system. Deep down, Canadians know that choice in such a system would be based on ability to pay.

There are two competing visions and guiding values about health care. Each would take our nation down a fundamentally different path. One view, high on rhetoric but low on evidence and masquerading as something new, is based on the premise that health care is a commodity — that medical needs ebb and flow with markets, and they determine who gets care, when, and how.

The other vision, rooted in our narrative as a nation, backed by evidence and public opinion, strongly believes that health care is a public good. It believes that democratically elected governments, as representatives of the public, not corporate bottom lines, should define common needs, provide equitable services, and a reasonable allocation of resources. Fairness, equity, compassion, and solidarity: these are the values that were adopted and nurtured throughout Canada's history of shared destiny.

These values gain their expression in our core belief that everyone should have access to our health care system on the same terms and conditions, and that this access is ultimately a right of Canadian citizenship. These values are manifested through our view that medicare is a truly national program — a nation-defining and nation-building enterprise.

Ultimately, the success of medicare reforms will be determined by whether we recognize the central importance of values in this debate. I was a premier once. I know the pressures that militate against taking the longer view of things and of reaching beyond one's particular place at a particular point in time. It's not easy and, among other things, it does indeed require leadership that is committed and responsive to a progressive society.

But now, more than ever, is the time to recapture the moral and political strength to see ourselves in our own place, in our own time, informed by our own values, and within our own actual narrative, as an independent nation, worthy of the respect of a world that needs an even better Canada. In doing so, we shall once again put our nation's policies on track and resume the task of building an even greater Canada.

CHAPTER 34

Medicare as Mainstream Agenda: The Second Stage and the Role of Physicians

Danielle Martin

Implementing the second stage of medicare is clearly vital to health policy experts, to the labour movement, to nurses, to governments, and of course to ordinary Canadians who so deeply support the principles of the Canada Health Act, but who also know our system is not yet providing the level of health and health care they want and deserve.

We must be careful not to assume that all of the groups who should be with us *are* with us. To move forward, we need to ask some uncomfortable questions: *Who has not yet joined us in our efforts to preserve and improve medicare? Why not? Who else must we invite to the table if we are going to move this discussion forward?*

At the historic SOS Medicare 2 conference in Regina, there were many people who described themselves as front-line health care workers, yet there were virtually no physicians participating in the discussion — indeed, there was no *formal* representation from the world of organized medicine.

Why is it that one of the most important groups in health policy and health care delivery did not participate in this important conference to revitalize and extend medicare? And, what should we do about it?

To be sure, organized medicine has a not-very-proud history of resistance to the establishment of medicare, particularly to phase one of medicare, where the introduction of single-payer insurance and the banning of extra-billing led to organized physician strikes, as well as less public forms of protest.

Even today, when the research shows our publicly funded single-payer system is equal to or better than the alternatives, the leadership of the organized medical community appears reluctant to embrace what most Canadians believe to be their most important national asset. Indeed, the election of Dr. Brian Day to the presidency of the Canadian Medical Association last year again opened up a debate at the CMA as to whether private insurance for medically necessary physician and hospital services should be permitted. This, despite the evidence that such a move would benefit very few Canadians, at the expense of the vast majority.

At a time when just about all Canadian health care organizations are trying to move medicare forward into phase two, we should not take for granted that the compelling evidence for medicare has penetrated the consciousness of organized medicine or front-line physicians. To be sure, it is the role of groups like Canadian Doctors for Medicare to help with the physician education and the advocacy necessary in this regard. But it is also the role of every group represented here today. Because, without doctors, it will be very hard to move medicare into phase two.

This is not to say that the vast majority of Canadian physicians don't support medicare. It is my belief that they believe wholeheartedly in the principle that health care should be delivered based on need, not ability to pay. On this there has always been a disconnect between the beliefs of the average doctor and the leadership of organized medicine. But it's also true that physicians — like so many health care workers — are frustrated with the health care system and want something better for their patients and for themselves. If medicare is not made better, they may be willing to consider something else.

It's important to understand this context to figure out how to approach physicians to gain their support for phase two of medicare — the phase that will involve moving more care out of institutions into the community, moving beyond doctors and hospitals, implementing better management of chronic illness, focusing on disease prevention, and perhaps even establishing a national pharmacare program.

While phase one of medicare was implemented despite the strenuous objections of a vocal minority of physicians, it will be *very* difficult to accomplish phase two without the support and participation of this powerful group of health care providers. Fortunately, we can expect widespread support for phase two from physicians at the *front lines*, who, like all of you, know our system must be reformed if we are going to meet the future challenges of health care.

You don't need to work hard to convince a front-line physician of the need for the electronic health record, for inter-professional teams, for primary care for every Canadian, for a strategic approach to home care programs. So it seems to me that we can use phase two as a means of igniting doctors' optimism about what a publicly funded health care system is capable of when it is funded properly and managed well.

It's also true that, while physicians may be advocates for health system reform, they are unlikely as a group to become radical advocates of social justice — though there are many physicians who work for social justice in Canada and throughout the world. Fortunately, there are others who can take on that part of the advocacy work that needs to be done.

An inclusive phase two would broaden its language to include the kinds of terms that doctors would feel comfortable embracing, terms like *evidence-based policy, improved health outcomes, respect in the way the system treats patients and workers*. In other words, the movement for medicare must make space for multiple approaches, including those that *non-activist* supporters of medicare would feel comfortable with — and whose support we must gain.

Finally, we must acknowledge that this broadening of the medicare agenda should not stop at physicians. We also need Lawyers for Medicare, Big Business for Medicare, and the participation of all the other groups who have access to levers of power that can help move our agenda forward.

The second phase of medicare demands these partnerships, and we must have the courage to build them together.

CHAPTER 35

The Wrong Kind of Rights: The Charter Threat to Medicare

Andrew Petter

If we hope to preserve and advance medicare, we must face the fact that Canada is a very different place today than it was forty-five years ago when medicare was introduced in Saskatchewan. In the early 1960s, Canadians were imbued with a strong sense of national purpose, collective responsibility, and faith in public institutions born out of the experience of the Second World War. Memories of the Great Depression lingered, and with them suspicions of unbridled market capitalism and acceptance of the need for a vibrant state presence to preserve the public good.

The rise of neoconservatism in the 1980s, which paved the way for economic globalization in the 1990s, eroded the fiscal and regulatory capacities of government, shifted powers back to the market, and ate away at Canadians' sense of national purpose and collective responsibility. In the new reality of the 1990s, the main role of government became to reduce its involvement in the economy, and to convince Canadians that the best hope for improving their well-being was through increased participation in the global marketplace.

These developments were aided and reinforced by the adoption in 1982 of the Canadian Charter of Rights and Freedoms, an instrument that constitutionally entrenched generalized rights such as liberty, security, and equality within the ideological architecture of liberal legalism. According to liberal legalism's blueprint, the main threat to Canadians' freedom is presumed to be the state, rather than disparities in wealth or concentrations of private power.

Not surprisingly, therefore, Charter rights are predominantly negative in nature, with little in the way of positive economic or social entitlements. Moreover, these rights are animated by a belief that existing distributions of property are a natural product of private initiative. Such property distributions are therefore regarded as the pre-political foundation upon which Charter rights are bestowed and against which the constitutionality of state action is judged.

The ideological assumptions of liberal legalism remove from Charter scrutiny the major source of inequality in our society — the unequal distribution of property entitlements among private parties — and direct the constraining force of the Charter against the institutions of the state best equipped to redress such inequality: governments and legislatures. In doing so, they also give political meaning to the Charter's open-ended provisions.

Shaped by these assumptions, the right to "equality" in section 15 of the Charter does not give citizens the right to be made equal in condition, but rather the right to be treated equally by government. Thus section 15 places no positive duties on the state; it is satisfied by equal inaction as much as it is by equal action. Similarly, according to these assumptions, the right to "security of the person" in section 7 of the Charter does not require government to implement measures to *make* people secure. Courts are to disregard threats to personal security emanating from the market. It is only when the "normalcy" of the market is disrupted by state action that section 7 rights are engaged.

The Charter's impact was to entrench a framework of rights that was hospitable to government cutbacks, privatization, and deregulation, and to provide constitutional "cover" to governments that pursued these polices. In addition, the Charter opened up opportunities to challenge all manner of state action in the name of protecting rights. Thus, corporations (which the courts unthinkingly accepted as rights-bearing "persons") have made effective use of the Charter to resist state regulation by, for example, invoking privacy rights to strike down search-and-seizure powers in anti-combines legislation,[26] using free speech rights to strike down legislative restrictions on tobacco advertising,[27] and relying upon rights to freedom of religion to strike down laws limiting Sunday shopping.[28]

While the Charter has provided comfort to governments pursuing neoconservative policies and has been used by corporations and others to chisel away at certain aspects of state regulation, even Charter skeptics did not, until recently, believe that it posed a serious threat to core social programs such as medicare. This was due less to legal limitations (which are only as constraining as the courts say they are[29]) than to assumptions that judges would recognize that they lacked the capacity and expertise to evaluate complex social policies, and that they would not want to risk incurring the political costs associated with challenging such policies.

These assumptions were shattered with last year's decision of the Supreme Court of Canada in *Chaoulli v. Quebec (A.G.)*, [30] in which a majority struck down provisions of Quebec health care legislation prohibiting persons from purchasing private health insurance and gaining access to private health care services. Four of seven sitting judges held that these provisions violated rights to "life" and to "security of the person" in the Quebec Charter of Human Rights and Freedoms, and that they could not be justified where patients were not guaranteed timely access to medicare services.

Three of these four judges held that these provisions also violated corresponding rights in section 7 of the Charter (with the fourth majority judge declining to address this point). In doing so, they dismissed as mere "assertions of belief" and "socio-political discourse that is disconnected from reality" evidence suggesting that a single-payer model of health insurance was necessary to preserve the integrity and viability of Canada's universal public health insurance system.

In addition to threatening a central tenet of medicare, *Chaoulli* provides disturbing evidence of just how far we have come as a country in our embrace of market capitalism, and how far our courts are prepared to go in tipping the scales of justice against state intervention of any kind. As Justices Binnie and LeBel pointed out in their vigorous dissenting judgment, nothing in the Charter prevents Canada from adopting a US-style market model of medicine in which millions of citizens would be denied access to required health care services because they could not afford them. Yet once government replaces this market model with a single-payer public health insurance system, that system becomes vulnerable to constitutional challenge if it denies timely access to required health care services to even one citizen who could afford to purchase those services in the marketplace. In the legal culture of the Charter, the ability of one person with money to purchase health care services in the marketplace commands greater constitutional attention than the ability of millions of people who lack financial resources to gain access to such services through a public health insurance system.[31]

How are we to preserve and advance medicare in the face of a political and legal culture that glorifies the market, demonizes the state, and demands perfection of government programs that limit the ability of those with money to vindicate their constitutionally protected rights through commercial means? I will leave it to others to discuss how best to address the broad policy challenges posed by the current political environment, and will focus instead on the particular legal threat represented by the Charter. Here I believe the best strategy is more obvious. If we wish to preserve a single-payer system of health care in this country, governments and interveners must in future litigation make every effort to challenge the reasoning of the majority in *Chaoulli*, and to get medicare as far away from the courts and the Charter as possible.

Fortunately, there is some cause for hope in this regard. The Supreme Court of Canada's judgment in *Chaoulli* involved only seven judges (as opposed to a full bench of nine) and is not conclusive in relation to the Charter. Only six judges based their decisions on the Charter, with these judges splitting three-three on whether single-payer health insurance violates the Charter. Moreover, one of the judges who found a Charter violation has since retired and been replaced. Even if one assumes that the seventh judge, who found a breach solely on the Quebec legislation, would in a future case arrive at the same conclusion with respect to the Charter, the votes of the *Chaoulli* judges would again be tied, leaving the outcome in the hands of the three judges who did not take part in that case.

This does not mean that it will be easy to persuade a majority of the Court in a future case to oppose the decision of the three judges in *Chaoulli* who found a Charter violation. It will not, particularly given that the Chief Justice, who co-authored that decision, recently referred to "accountability" in health services as one of the ways in which the Charter had made Canada a more just society.[32] On the other hand, the vociferous reactions to

Chaoulli on all sides of the health care debate have highlighted the politically contentious nature of the issues at stake. These reactions, plus two new cases being launched against medicare legislation in Alberta and Ontario, should cause judges to worry about how much deeper they will be drawn into the political minefield of health care policy if they do not take advantage of the opportunity to extricate themselves now.

Citizens can play an important role in influencing this decision. Those judges who found a Charter violation in *Chaoulli* relied upon the appellants' claim that single-payer health insurance "precludes the vast majority of Canadians (middle-income and low-income earners) from accessing additional care." Not only is this reliance unjustified, but it also exposes the lack of a rights-based foundation for the majority's decision. Whatever purpose an entrenched charter serves in a liberal democracy, by no established theory of rights does it authorize judges to shield majorities from universal policies that have been established — and can be disestablished — through democratic processes.

This is a point that citizens can reinforce through their advocacy. By speaking out forcefully and effectively in defence of a single-payer health insurance system, citizens can both challenge the claim that such a system is contrary to their interests and stand up for a value that seems to have been overlooked by the majority in *Chaoulli:* the right of citizens to govern themselves by democratic means.[33]

CHAPTER 36

It's All About People

Elizabeth Ballerman

To finish Tommy Douglas's vision of medicare, we will have to demonstrate similar vision, determination, and tenacity. Not only do we need to clearly define what we are fighting against, but, as importantly, what we are fighting for.

And what we are fighting for is all about people:

- the public who depend on the system (all of us),
- the providers of care,
- the decision makers, and
- the funders, who also are us.

In Alberta, we've fought privatization for decades. The determination of a broad spectrum of grassroots Albertans, with the support of strong coalition partners, beat back the worst aspects of the infamous Bill 11, its predecessor Bill 37, and more recently the "Third Way."

There have actually been several reversals of privatization

within our province:

- for ten years, Calgary Laboratory Services was a public–private partnership, which has been brought to total public ownership. This represents a real gain, because community labs were private before the privatization, and are now public;
- Capital Health has also repatriated laboratory services that it contracted out ten years ago;
- in two of the nine regions, emergency medical services, which included a mix of public and private operators, were regionalized and the quality of those services is excellent;
- the College of Physicians and Surgeons reacted surprisingly quickly and decisively to kibosh a Copeman style "Club Med" clinic, where an annual fee would have provided preferred access;
- and finally, in Calgary, where we blew up a hospital, a new construction that was originally slated as a P3 will be built as a public asset.

These successes, however, don't mean the forces of privatization have gone away.

It's all about people. Without health care workers of every description, whether direct caregivers or the multitude of support personnel — without them, a bed is just a piece of furniture, a new MRI unit just a photo-op, and the dream of comprehensive primary care and prevention are just that: a dream.

If one could fix the system in five minutes, someone would have done it, but here are six key concepts from the perspective of my union's members.

1. *The Canada Health Act must be updated*
Or, a companion piece of legislation is needed to reflect current and changing methods of health care delivery. As supporters of

the Act, we have been reluctant to advocate that it be "opened," due to a "be careful what you wish for" concern that this would be used as an opportunity to let in privatization. Expansion of the system to include pharmacare, primary, continuing, and home care, as well as pre-hospital, for example, ambulance, dental, and vision care are self-evident needs. And, as unions, if these were part of the public system, we wouldn't have to fight for them at the bargaining table. But make no mistake: whatever is de-listed, whatever is privatized, and whatever is still missing — these will be on the table.

2. Allied health workers are essential, but commonly omitted in conversations about the health care system

Consider what would be missing if they were not there. They have tremendous contributions to make, some as self-directed and primary access professions, others in diagnostic, therapeutic, and rehabilitation roles. Appropriately utilized, they can relieve some of the pressure from physicians, both in institutional and primary care settings, in mental health, and in health promotion and prevention initiatives.

3. There are very significant shortages

Which, among allied health professions, often outstrip, on a percentage basis, those of doctors and nurses. The Alberta government predicts (optimistically in the opinion of some) a 10,000-person shortage among all health workers by 2016. Vancouver Coastal Health Region predicts a shortage of up to 85 percent among laboratory technologists by 2015. Across the country, some vacancies have continued not only for months, but for years. At one point last year, within our professional technical bargaining unit in the Northern Lights Region, over 25 percent of the positions were vacant.

4. We need a comprehensive, national health workforce strategy that will cross federal and provincial jurisdiction, and several ministries, including, Advanced Education, Labour, and Health

Poaching from each other's provinces or from other jurisdictions is not a comprehensive strategy. We need to "grow our own" and therefore we need to develop careful predictive models to determine our needs and to train enough health professionals for those needs. Retention must be seen to be as important as recruitment. A number of studies, including a comprehensive study by my organization last year, demonstrate the toll that working in health care takes, in terms of both physical and mental health. We must ensure that those already in the system are, and feel, valued, and that they are safe, so that they will stay with their career as long as possible, and that they will be ambassadors for young Canadians facing career choices.

5. We must keep the system public

This is more than just a philosophical statement, particularly in light of the major staffing shortages that we see. I absolutely believe that ownership does matter. In practical terms, we have seen technologists and professionals go to the private sector, sometimes for dramatically higher pay, sometimes simply because the private system does what all of us know it does — cream-skimming. The private system can sometimes offer little or no shift work, and patients who are mobile and relatively healthy, making life a whole lot easier, and causing an ever increasing load on the public sector's already stressed workforce. It's not just we "left wing nuts" who know this. Even the CEO of the Calgary Health Region, who was once Ralph Klein's chief of staff, has stated unequivocally, that as long as there are staffing shortages privatization will simply pull more workers out of the public system.

6. And finally, politicians have to be honest with Canadians, and Canadians with ourselves
We cannot continue to provide topnotch public services at the same time as we clamour to reduce our personal tax burden and cave in to industry demands for tax breaks. We need to acknowledge our taxes for what they are: a pooling of resources so that collectively we can do what none of us could do individually.

It's all about people, and if the people who make the decisions don't get it and act on it, if the people who deliver the services are not there, then we — the people who depend on the system — have just bought ourselves some very expensive furniture.

CHAPTER 37

The Continental Deep
Integration Threat

Maude Barlow

The historic gathering at the SOS Medicare 2 conference, represents a revitalizing of our collective will to stand on guard for medicare, the jewel in the crown of our social legacy. Never has the danger to public health care been greater. Not only are several major provinces openly courting private service delivery, but we also have a prime minister in Ottawa who was once head of the National Citizens' Coalition, an organization founded to fight public health care, and which predicted that thousands of Canadians would die if we adopted a public system.

Not unconnected to the health care crisis is another development that is of great concern: the increasing pressure to create a Fortress North America, led by the big business community on both sides of the border, against the perceived threats that George Bush and Stephen Harper see to our current "way of life." In a reaction to American security concerns post 9/11, the big business lobby in Canada, led by Tom d'Aquino and the Canadian Council of Chief Executives (CCCE), convinced the Paul Martin government to undertake an extensive project of deep continental integration with the United States in order to keep the border open for Canadian exports.

The Security and Prosperity Partnership (SPP)

What both the CCCE and the Task Force on the Future of North America recommended was the eventual creation of a North American common market; common immigration and refugee policies; a North American security perimeter; one common passport for the bloc; harmonized defence operations and policy; a harmonized regulatory framework for food, health and safety rules, and environmental standards; a North American resource pact, which is to include energy, hydroelectricity, and water; and to negotiate within the WTO as one trade bloc. (The latter would mean negotiating the General Agreement on Trade in Services (GATS) with the very country that wants to use the WTO to force open Canada's health care services to American corporations.)

The Security and Prosperity Partnership (SPP) signed in Waco, Texas, by the governments of Canada, the United States, and Mexico in March 2005 did not go as far as this corporate blueprint for the continent, but it did set out to begin the process on many of these fronts, co-governed by the North American Competitiveness Council (NACC), which was set up at the second "Three Amigos" summit held in Cancun, Mexico the next year, this time attended by Stephen Harper. The NACC is represented by the CEOs of thirty major North American corporations, including Wal-Mart and Lockheed Martin, and is the only sector of society consulted by the three governments in the whole process.

Already dozens of cross-border government working groups

have laid out a far-reaching program for continental harmonization and integration, and the US government has hired the
right-wing Center for Strategic and International Studies, to prepare a policy blueprint for the bloc called *North American Future
2025.* The Fraser Institute recently called for a shared border security and defence pact between Canada and the United States, and
David Dodge, governor of the Bank of Canada, has speculated
favourably on a common North American currency.

The Security and Prosperity Partnership has potentially more
far-reaching ramifications for Canada than NAFTA, yet it has not
come back to the legislatures of the three countries. When I asked
senior officials from the American Embassy (who had requested a
meeting with us after seeing media criticism of the SPP from our
March 2007 teach-in on deep integration called *Integrate This!*)
why the SPP was not being ratified in each country, they said that
the three governments and the business community didn't want
"another bruising NAFTA battle." This attitude speaks volumes to
this profoundly undemocratic process. No doubt the political and
business elites in the three countries know that the SPP would not
gain popular support if it were to be put to the people and their
elected representatives; instead, a small cadre of mostly unelected
insiders is designing a new competitive global bloc based on the
worst values and policies of the Bush administration.

Internally, Canada is being prepared for this continental bloc by
a series of initiatives that have had very little public debate.

SMART Regulations

Every federal government department has gone through an exercise called SMART Regulation, which stands for Specific,
Measurable, Attainable, Realistic, and Timely, and is a WTO trade
tool favoured by big corporations to harmonize (almost always
downward) global regulatory standards. In 2006, the federal government went through a massive review of all current regulatory

practices and policies in order to set the stage for North American regulatory harmonization to eliminate different (that is, higher) domestic regulations — what the business community calls the "tyranny of small differences." Every area of public policy has gone through this review, which is now with cross-border committees for further harmonization. As one example, Canada has recently moved to lower its standards on pesticide residues on food to reduce the "tyranny" of our former higher standards under this process.

Trade, Investment, and Labour Mobility Agreement (TILMA)

Other provinces are lining up to join a new trade and investment treaty that Alberta and British Columbia have signed, which gives private companies operating in one province the right to challenge higher regulations in the other as an unfair barrier to trade. The Trade, Investment, and Labour Mobility Agreement is a mini-MAI (Multilateral Agreement on Investment), which civil society groups around the world defeated a decade ago as the most anti-democratic global tool ever devised. TILMA places the responsibility on provincial governments to ensure that "all government measures, laws, acts, regulations, standards, requirements, guidelines, programs and policies" are not a restriction on trade and investment, and gives governments, companies, and individuals the right to sue for up to $5 million for existing or future regulations that "restrict or impair" trade. Unlike NAFTA, public health care is not exempt from TILMA.

Atlantica, Cascadia, the Pacific Gateway, and NAFTA Corridors

The stage is being set to create North American regional free trade zones, as well as super-conductor NAFTA highways from Canada's far North to the southern tip of Mexico. Led by the

North American Super-Corridor Coalition, plans are afoot to build several massive multi-functional corridors to move goods, services, temporary workers, and resources along North-South lines. At their heaviest, the corridors will house six passenger-vehicle lanes, four truck lanes, six rail lines, as well as utility and pipeline capacities. Already talks are underway to harmonize labour, health, and safety rules throughout the continental system.

The Atlantic Institute for Market Studies has joined business groups in the northeastern states to promote Atlantica, a free trade zone that would harmonize labour, health, and safety standards of the Atlantic provinces and the northeastern states to the lowest common denominator (including minimum wage). It calls for the economic and political integration of the whole northeastern region. Halifax will be an expanded port of entry for goods and resources bound for the United States, and the Canadian section of this free trade zone will house LNGs — Liquefied Natural Gas Terminals — all likely to have very serious environmental consequences for the region. Atlantica proponents want to adopt a TILMA deal among the Atlantic provinces and the northeastern states.

British Columbia's Gordon Campbell is promoting a similar Western zone dubbed Cascadia, with joint entry policies, harmonized trade practices, and a common ports authority. Working with the Harper government, the BC Liberals and the big business community are behind the $1 billion Pacific Gateway Project that will see a massive expansion of the Port of Vancouver to move Asia's goods — not through Canada, but through a super-corridor into the United States.

Public Health Threatened

While none of this may seem to threaten public health care at first glance, collectively these undertakings pose a very serious threat to any universal Canadian program. The free trade zones and

SMART regulation pose a direct threat to higher health and safe-ty standards in Canada, and TILMA poses a threat to higher standards in any given provinces. The SPP, if successful, would eliminate the ability of Canada to withstand the invasion of US health care corporations. The merging of all other economic, reg-ulatory, tax, and environmental policy will render a separate social infrastructure very hard to maintain over the long haul. To protect Canada's public health care system requires an all-out fight against the Security and Prosperity Partnership and all of its manifesta-tions in Canada.

CHAPTER 38

Talking Solutions

Marcy Cohen

We can't stand still. We can either go back or we can go forward. The choice we make today will decide the future of medicare in Canada.

–Tommy Douglas, 1984

We are at a key turning point in medicare's history. Talking about how to reform rather than privatize our public health services is critical to ensuring the long-term sustainability of our public system. This is a key message to emerge, not only from the SOS Medicare 2 conference, but also from the Health Council of Canada's 2007 report that synthesizes four years of public opinion polling (2002 to 2006) on the Canadian health system.[34]

The overall results from the report suggest that, while there has been an increased focus on private provision, "Canadians remain firmly committed to universal health care," but believe that substantive changes are urgently needed, as a priority, to reduce wait times and improve quality.[35] There is also "strong" agreement that additional home care services are needed, and "moderate support" for a national pharmacare program.[36]

Backing up this need for reform of public health services is the "overwhelming" consensus that increased spending on health care, from both levels of government, is necessary.[37] This includes support for higher transfer payments from the federal to provincial governments, conditional on the development of national standards.

We are clearly in a teachable moment. As progressive organizations representing health care providers, consumers, and academia from across the country, we need to be at the forefront in defining the substantive changes needed to sustain our public system and in developing the concrete strategies for achieving these changes. In moving this agenda forward, I have three points and two concrete suggestions to make.

First, I think it is critical to begin by talking about progressive innovations already in place in Canada and elsewhere that link to the priority concerns of Canadians — access to timely care and quality — and to include strategies for how these innovations could be scaled-up and broadly implemented across the health system.

One example is evident in the innovations in elective surgeries in both the Calgary and Vancouver Coastal Health Authorities.[38] Successful programs have been implemented that have proved to be very effective in reducing wait lists and improving efficiencies at each stage of the surgical process (for example, before, during, and after surgery). They depend on establishing multidisciplinary team-based care and shifting wait-list management from the individual surgeon's office to the multidisciplinary team and health authority. What is needed now, and still missing, is leadership from the provincial and federal governments to scale-up and replicate these innovations throughout the system.

Similarly, in building support for the second stage of medicare, it is important to be clear how the development of a comprehensive integrated Community health system will take the pressure off emergency and in-patient beds, thereby reducing wait times and improving quality. In residential care, for example, there is considerable international evidence showing that transfer rates to hospital can be dramatically reduced with appropriate staffing levels and the introduction of a multidisciplinary team of primary care professionals into residential care.[39] Similarly, admission and readmission to hospital for people living with a mental illness can be avoided when access to social, as well as medical, support is readily available in the community, particularly for people in the early stages of a psychosis.[40] In Denmark, where they have successfully implemented a comprehensive system of community services to care for the frail elderly, they passed a law in 1998 requiring local governments to offer every senior seventy-five years and over services twice a year, because they found that people usually wait too long to seek help and then require more expensive acute interventions.[41]

Each of these innovations is inspiring, doable, and cost effective. What is needed, to ensure that innovations like these can be adopted and then disseminated throughout the system, is leadership and infrastructure support from both the federal and provincial governments. This is the key message that we need to communicate to the public, and it brings me to my second point.

Over the last thirty years, because of reduced federal funding, the transfer of tax points to the provinces, the expansion of community (in other words, non-medicare) health services, and the signing of the social union agreement, there has been a reduced role for the federal government and an expanded role for provinces and regional authorities in establishing health policy. As a result, it often seems that we have not one, but ten or more different health systems in this country. As a result it is more difficult for progressive groups working in different provinces to agree on priorities at the national level, despite the steadfast commitment to medicare among mainstream Canadians.

This is where I would like to place my first suggestion: a project that highlights the best of public health systems from across the country, such as the Community Health Centres in Ontario, home support in Manitoba, reference-based pricing in BC, the Alberta Bone and Joint Institute in Calgary, and the Quality Council in Saskatchewan. This project could be a very effective vehicle for communicating what our public health system could look like if we just took the best of what already exists in different parts of the country and implemented these initiatives more broadly. Although this would likely begin as a research and policy project, the goal would be to link with the mainstream media and educational institutions to bring this message to ordinary Canadians and begin a dialogue (within the public and between the public and health care providers) about the barriers and facilitators to broader implementation of "positive public" solutions.

This focus on public dialogue leads to the third point I want to raise as essential in moving forward a progressive agenda of health care reform: the need for more democratic forms of governance to support greater public involvement in evidence-based decision making. While there is very broad lip service paid within health care to the importance of evidence-based decision making, in many cases the evidence does not guide practice on the ground. This may be because the evidence challenges the established interests within health care such as the pharmaceutical industry, physicians' organizations, hospital administrators, or comes up against the inertia of large bureaucratic systems.[42] Whatever the reason, evidence does not, very often, carry the day in the current environment, where key decisions are made behind closed doors with little opportunity for public input or scrutiny.

To ensure greater public accountability and involvement, a

number of changes in health care governance are required. This brings me to my second suggestion: the need for progressive organizations across the country to develop a policy document outlining the basic tenets of a more democratic, evidence-based process of health care governance. This document would likely call for broader public involvement in establishing a reporting requirement (such as, the evidence-based indicators) to improve quality and comparable, publicly available information on issues such as hospital re-admission rates for specific populations, hospital-acquired infection rates, transfer rates from long-term and community care to hospital, and the link between staffing and resident/patient outcomes.

It might also include a template of provincial legislation needed to guarantee ongoing public input into health authority service plans, language for ensuring that these service plans are evidence-based, and that health board appointees are representative of the population demographics in the communities where they are located. This document would be an important common starting point for health care providers, unions, community coalitions, and progressive policy institutes advocating for more democratic and effective forms of health care governance.

Quite clearly, what is needed, and still missing, is provincial and federal leadership to ensure that evidence-based reforms are broadly implemented and more democratic forms of governance are put in place. To echo the words of Bob McMurtry: "what we have is not a crisis in medicare, but a crisis in leadership and democracy."

CHAPTER 39

A Political Agenda for Building Medicare's Next Stage [43]

Doris Grinspun

In 1979, twenty-two years after the introduction of hospital insurance in Saskatchewan, Tommy Douglas urged us to "work to get medicare as it was intended to be, a program that would provide, in Canada, a society in which we would have freedom from fear and freedom from want." [44] The key message conveyed in this quote is that we need to transcend the silos of medicare (our publicly funded and administered health care system) on the one side, and social and environmental factors that have a decisive impact on our health (the social determinants of health, or SDOH), on the other. In particular, we must broaden the intellectual and institutional spaces for joint social activism — the kind of activism that will advance both medicare and SDOH — because, as Tommy Douglas insisted, when people's health is at stake, both are indivisible and indispensable.

The union of medicare and SDOH will require:

- an understanding that both spheres of social intervention are crucial and interrelated;
- urgently engaging diverse communities and creating the political will for action in both areas; and
- moving from a narrow sectoral and disciplinary
  approach to a broad inter-sectoral and interdisciplinary one.

These are the essential tools to build the next stage of medicare
and a healthier society. Only when we have engaged with these
tools will Tommy Douglas's legacy be fulfilled: "Let's not forget
that the ultimate goal of medicare must be to keep people well
rather than just patching them up when they get sick."[45]

The elements of a political agenda that must be present to further the second stage of medicare, at both the provincial and
national levels,[46] include:

- addressing growing social inequalities;
- responding to a growing and aging population;
- resolving health human resource shortages;
- protecting medicare from the forces of privatization;
- building a national pharmacare program;
- addressing environmental threats to human health;
  and
- securing the financial capacity to address SDOH
  and medicare.

Addressing Growing Social Inequalities

The gap between Canada's rich and poor is at a thirty-year high
and growing. In Ontario alone, 1.7 million people live in poverty,
including the working poor, those living on social assistance, and
the homeless. Large disparities in infant mortality, the burden of
disease, and life expectancy between groups of people or populations are not random, but are socially determined. For example, the

infant mortality rate in Canada's poorest neighbourhoods in 1996 was two-thirds higher than that of the richest neighbourhoods.

Medicare's next stage must tackle SDOH. Governments need to implement a comprehensive poverty strategy that includes meaningful increases in minimum wages, liveable social assistance rates, affordable housing, as well as health and social policies that support children. There can be no health for children who go hungry, for mothers who must choose between feeding their children and paying their rent, or for homeless people who suffer the indignities of social exclusion and violence.

Responding to a Growing and Aging Population
As the population ages, the incidence of chronic illness increases. By age sixty-five, 77 percent of Canadian men and 85 percent of women have at least one chronic condition. Moreover, people with chronic diseases, such as diabetes, heart disease, or emphysema, use the majority of health care resources. Chronic disease is currently managed within an illness model often characterized by frequent emergency department visits and hospital readmissions with long lengths of stay. This "illness model" is focused on diagnosis, treatment, and cure. It's an approach that is appropriate for acute illnesses, such as heart attack or stroke, but it is costly and ineffective for the management of chronic disease. As we build the next stage of medicare upon Tommy Douglas's vision to increase the health care system's focus on wellness, prevention will become the new priority at all points along the continuum of care.

Numerous studies show the benefits of a preventive model in managing chronic illness. This includes: improved quality of life for patients; decreased health care utilization (fewer emergency department visits, fewer hospital readmissions, and decreased length of stay), improved quality of care, improved patient satisfaction, and improved health care provider satisfaction. Nurses are well equipped to manage and deliver care to patients with chronic ailments, from diagnosis and management to caregiver and family support and end-of-life decision making. Community-based programs focused on prevention will enable persons with chronic conditions to remain vibrant members of our communities while reducing hospital utilization.

These programs include current models such as Community Health Centres, Home Health Care, and new models such as Nurse-Led Clinics (NLCs). Research shows the effectiveness of NLCs when compared with out-patient and in-patient care for the management of chronic disease. They have been found to be more cost-effective, and to result in higher patient satisfaction, fewer deaths, improvements in care and patient lifestyle, increased access to care, and reduced wait times.

Regressive groups claim that we can no longer afford medicare because we have a growing and aging population, and that we must build a parallel system to "free up space for those who cannot afford to pay." Progressive groups, nurses included, say that we must and we can create the necessary programs to serve those who built this nation. Moreover, we say that these programs are the only way to sustain and strengthen access for all.

Resolving Health Human Resource Shortages

Canada's RN workforce is aging. The average age for RNs in 2006 was 45.6 years. Efforts are required to retain the current workforce, absorb and retain new graduates, attract more individuals to nursing, and reduce workloads. However, it is imperative that Canada not engage in strategies to address the shortage in health human resources, improve access to care, and maintain sustainability that involve foreign recruitment by "poaching" nurses from abroad. Our organization — the Registered Nurses' Association of Ontario — is mindful of our responsibility not to contribute to global health inequities, and of the human and economic costs of stripping vulnerable populations of access to health care due to migrating health professionals. For this reason, the RNAO supports the World Health Organization (WHO), the International Council of Nurses, and the Canadian Policy Research Network in calling for ethical international recruitment guidelines within the context of a responsible national and provincial health human resources strategy. At the same time, the RNAO acknowledges the right of individual nurses to migrate and the obligation to eliminate systemic barriers to internationally educated nurses with permanent status in Canada from practising their profession and serving the public.

Resolving Canada's nursing shortage requires a range of strategies, including: increasing the share of RNs working full-time; guaranteeing full-time employment for new graduates (most of whom experience great challenges securing full-time jobs despite a nursing shortage); programs to retain senior nurses; and equalizing remuneration and working conditions across the home care, long-term care, and acute care sectors. It also demands that nurses be able to work to their full scope of practice. This requires a dynamic legislative and regulatory environment, funding mechanisms, financial incentives, and practice environments that will enable current and future roles to strengthen medicare and improve timely access.

Protecting Medicare from Profit-seeking Ventures

Despite the solid evidence of the clinical, economic, and moral benefits of medicare, the forces of privatization continue to aggressively lobby the public and governments. We will always need to protect medicare from those who want to profit from the vulnerabilities of people. The data is unequivocal on the benefits of medicare, and we must continuously educate the public. For example, OECD countries with parallel private hospital systems have larger and longer public wait lists than countries with a single-payer system.

Parallel private systems do not increase the number of health care practitioners, rather, practitioners are split into two systems. This, in turn, creates an incentive for doctors to lengthen waiting lists in the public system. In 1999, administrative costs in the United States were $1,059 per capita as compared to $307 per capita in Canada. If US costs were streamlined to Canadian levels, far more than enough money would be saved to provide full insurance coverage for all of the 41.2 million Americans who were uninsured in 2001. Overhead costs for Canada's medicare system were 1.3 percent as compared to 13.2 percent for Canadian private insurers.

There is also considerable evidence on the differences of cost and outcomes between for-profit and not-for-profit delivery across sectors.[47] The most conclusive evidence comes from systematic reviews and meta-analyses of all available peer-reviewed literature on for-profit vs. not-for-profit health care, which found higher patient mortality rates in for-profit as compared to non-profit centres. Furthermore, research finds no cost benefits in for-profit delivery; in reality, a study found for-profit hospitals charge 19 percent *more* than not-for-profit hospitals. Canadian evidence, available from the long-term care sector, found that staffing levels were higher in not-for-profit facilities than in for-profit facilities and health outcomes were better in not-for-profit facilities. Moreover, a review of North American nursing home studies between 1990 and 2002 similarly concluded that for-profit homes appeared to deliver poorer quality care in a number of process and outcome areas.

Programs of alternative financing and procurement (AFPs) for hospitals and other public infrastructure are equally disturbing. These AFPs are forms of public–private partnerships (P3s) that roll together complex contracts to finance, design, build, and operate public facilities like hospitals. The Ontario government has implemented AFPs and claims that these are not P3s because they will remain publicly owned and controlled. However, they will be privately financed and partially operated by parallel private administrations.

Many of the problems associated with P3s arise from private financing and operation. A decision in December 2006 to exclude from AFPs "soft facility management services" such as laundry and housekeeping, reduces some of the immediate risk to staff and clients, but still carries the conflict of interest and inefficiency of running parallel private and public administrations. Studies show that costs of P3s tend to be higher, and often the quality of the service is reported to be poor. And, there are serious concerns about P3s' lack of transparency and public accountability, since sensitive financial and project information remains confidential. There is no way to verify the claims regarding the financial and risk gains from the AFP. Finally, AFPs introduce a privatizing force now working inside the framework of medicare and potentially forcing further erosion.

The message must be clear and concise: public funding and not-for-profit delivery work best. There is no other way to sustain medicare and provide universal access. To protect and expand medicare, we need to protect government's ability to regulate and make policies on the provision of health care services. The Trade, Investment and Labour Mobility Agreement (TILMA) between British Columbia and Alberta that comes into force this year will severely restrict governments' ability to make policies in the public interest. Since the health sector is not exempted from the agreement, it could severely restrict governments' abilities to regulate the health sector in the public interest and to regulate for-profit delivery. To build the next stage of medicare we must be watchful for, and advocate against, any mechanisms that would restrict our vision.

The Need to Build a National Pharmacare Program

Increasing and improving health care access, equity, and sustainability requires an expansion of medicare, rather than a retreat to
two-tier health care or for-profit delivery. A number of factors,
including shorter length of hospital stay, an aging population, and
cost structures call for an expansion of medicare to include a
national pharmacare program. Drugs are the second largest and
fastest growing category of health expenditures in Canada, after
hospital care.

Since 1997, calls for a pan-Canadian pharmacare program have
accelerated, including high-profile recommendations such as
those arising out of the Romanow Commission. Such a program
would provide equal access to prescription drugs across the country and keep the rising cost of drugs in check. Progress, tentative
as it may be, has been made on a national pharmacare plan by the
Federal/Provincial/Territorial Ministerial Task Force on the
National Pharmaceuticals Strategy, which was created out of the
2003 First Ministers' Accord on Health Care Renewal.

The Environment and Human Health

Nurses know that the environment is a major determinant of
health, and that people flourish best when they live in clean,
green, liveable environments. Canada can do much more to build
these environments, and the time to move on this front is now.
Evidence linking the environment to health outcomes is well
known. The WHO estimates that environmental factors account
for 24 percent of the world's burden of disease and 23 percent of
all deaths.

While the costs are higher in developing countries, environmental factors have a significant impact on the incidence of many
diseases across the globe. In developed regions, environmental factors accounted for 17 percent of deaths. In these regions,
environment plays a more significant role in chronic diseases such

as lung cancer (30 percent). These adverse health impacts are well recognized. For example, Environment Canada states that "asthma, lung cancer, cardiovascular disease, allergies, and many other human health problems have been linked to poor air quality." The international and Canadian evidence shows that these impacts are disproportionately borne by lower-income people. Environmental protection is not only a matter of health but also a matter of social justice.

Like all Canadians, nurses have become increasingly concerned about climate change and the impact of environmental toxins on the health of their families. As we build the next stage of medicare, we must include a focus on building healthier environments through addressing climate change, cleaner air, and reducing toxins in the environment and in our food.

Taxation, Fiscal Capacity, and the Future of Medicare
Spending on social programs, exclusive of health care, has dropped sharply in Ontario during the last decade, primarily as a result of the tax cuts implemented both at the federal and provincial levels. We know that these programs are the ones that have the largest impact on the health of Canadians — as they alleviate poverty, provide adequate housing, contribute to public health programs, and increase participation in our parks, schools, and community centres.

Preserving and enhancing Canada's social programs will require more public funding. Increasing Canada's fiscal capacity is not only achievable, but is also necessary if we are to enhance social programs and take care of our environment — and so improve the wellness and health of our nation. Thus, moving to the second stage of medicare will require that we face the tax cut agenda in Canada head on. We must continue to challenge this agenda as one that is tearing the social fabric of our country and endangering the health of Canadians.

Medicare and SDOH: Conflict or Complement?

We must be careful not to fall into the trap of following a health promotion and disease prevention agenda that focuses mainly on lifestyle choices and fails to address the systemic roots of illness embedded in SDOH. I say this because all too often we hear those who promote privatization and commercialization, also supporting health promotion. This is an individualistic approach that focuses only on one's responsibility to live a healthy life. Tommy Douglas's vision of building "a society in which we would have freedom from fear and freedom from want" speaks to our collective responsibility to tackle society's ailments — poverty, intolerance, social exclusion, a polluted environment — as essential to advance wellness. Tommy would also have added that, as we build a healthier society, we must continue to guard our illness-care services, so that when people do fall ill they are spared the financial burden.

A call for urgent action: we have a compelling agenda that speaks about building a healthier society and a stronger medicare. There are some who may be worried we are trying to cast too wide a net, that perhaps we should focus our limited energies on one new program at a time, or only on medicare so as not to diffuse our energies toward social programs, or vice versa. Nurses say this is not an ambitious agenda: that it is simply an agenda for social justice. Moving forward for us includes medicare, social programs, and environmental stewardship as inseparable elements in a nurturing, environmentally sustainable, and equitable vision of Canada.

Medicare requires both protection and expansion. Protecting medicare requires that we develop its next stage, focusing on prevention while also guarding, and where necessary strengthening, illness care. Thus, as we move forward and build a solid system of community health care, we will remain watchful that hospitals continue to deliver quality and safe care, and that they remain profit-free.

The time has come to break our silos and together engage the public. As Florence Nightingale said in 1892, "Let's create a public opinion which must drive the government, instead of the government having to drive us — an enlightened public opinion, wise in principles, wise in details."

NOTES

Part One: Tommy Douglas' Vision and the Future of Medicare

1   On the results, see http://www.cbc.ca/greatest.

2   Antonia Maioni, *Parting at the Crossroads: The Emergence of Health Insurance in the United States and Canada* (Princeton: Princeton University Press, 1998); Jacob Hacker, "The Historical Logic of National Health Insurance: Structure and Sequence in the Development of British, Canadian, and U.S. Medical Policy," *Studies in American Political Development* 12, no. 1 (1998): 57–130.

3   A.W. Johnson, *Dream No Little Dreams: A Biography of the Douglas Government of Saskatchewan, 1944–1961* (Toronto: University of Toronto Press, 2004).

4   Thomas H. McLeod and Ian McLeod, *Tommy Douglas: The Road to Jerusalem* (Edmonton: Hurtig, 1987):145.

5   R.F. Badgley and S. Wolfe, *Doctors' Strike: Medical Care and Conflict in Saskatchewan* (Toronto: Macmillan of Canada, 1967).

6   Tom Kent, *A Public Purpose* (Kingston and Montreal: McGill-Queen's University Press, 1988): 366.

7   Report on SOS Medicare Conference in *Canadian Labour* 24 (30 Nov. 1979): 6.

8   Tommy Douglas, from the 1982 film *Folks Call Me Tommy*, as quoted in Saskatchewan Health, *A Saskatchewan Vision for Health: A Framework for Change* (Regina: Saskatchewan Health, 1992).

9   The Health Insurance and Diagnostic Services Act (1957), and the Medical Care Act (1966).

10   The Established Program Financing Act (1977).

11   He also made other key recommendations, for example, that compulsory binding arbitration was essential to resolving fee disputes between doctors and their provincial government. Organized medicine opposed it ferociously. He also wanted health insurance premiums, where provinces had them, to be abolished.

12   Newfoundland, Prince Edward Island, and Nova Scotia were not penalized when the CHA came into effect in July 1984. Provincial penalties totalled some $245 million.

13   From 1975 to 1985, our ratio was 75 percent to 25 percent.

14   Joseph Heath, *The Efficient Society* (Toronto: Penguin Group (Canada), 2001).

15   Amartya Sen, "The Possibility of Social Choice," *American Economic Review* 89, no. 3 (1999): 349–78.

16   Ronald Labonte and Nazeem Muhajarine, "Healthy Populations Domain of the Canadian Index of Wellbeing" (2007 revision). In press.

17 Maggie Mahar, *Money-Driven Medicine* (New York; Harper Collins, 2006).
18 P.J. Devereaux and P.T.-L. Choi, "A Systematic Review and Meta-analysis of Studies Comparing Mortality Rates of Private for Profit and Private Not-for Profit Hospitals," *Canadian Medical Association Journal* 166 (2002): 1399–1406.
19 P.J. Devereaux and H.J. Schunemann, "Comparison of Mortality Between Private-for-Profit and Private Not-for-Profit Hemodialysis Centers: A Systematic Review and Meta-analysis," *Journal of the American Medical Association* 288 (2002): 2449–57.
20 Health Council of Canada: http://www.healthcouncilcanada.ca.
21 Lee Iacocca with Catherine Whitney, *Where Have All the Leaders Gone?* (New York: Scribner, 2007).

Part Two: The International Context

1 This is a more extensive version of a paper which originally appeared in the *Milken Institute Review* (Feb. 2007): 36-43.
2 See Milliman Medical Index 2006, http://www.milliman.com/pubs/Healthcare/content/mmi/Milliman-Medical-Index06-28-06.pdf (last viewed 2 February 2007).
3 US Bureau of the Census, FINC-01, "Selected Characteristics of Families by Total Money Income in 2005," http://pubdb3.census.gov/macro/032006/faminc/new01_001.htm (last viewed 3 February 2007).
4 Elizabeth A. McGlynn, et al., "The Quality of Health Care Delivered to Adults in the United States," *New England Journal of Medicine* 348, no. 26 (2003): 2635–45.
5 John E. Wennberg et al., Dartmouth Atlas of Health Care 1999 (AHA Press, 1999).
6 John H. Wennberg et al., "The Care of Patients with Severe Chronic Illness," in Dartmouth Atlas of Health Care 2006. http://www.dartmouthatlas.org/atlases/2006_Chronic_Care_Atlas.pdf (last viewed 8 February 2007).
7 See Elliott S. Fisher et al., "The Implications of Regional Variations in Medicare Spending, Parts 1 and 2," *Annals of Internal Medicine* 138, no. 4 (18 February 2003): 273–87 and 288–98.
8 Katherine Baicker and Amitabh Chandra "Medicare Spending, the Physician Workforce, And Beneficiaries' Quality of Care," *Health Affairs* Web Exclusive (7 April 2004): W4–184–97.
9 Cathy Schoen et al., "Taking the Pulse of Health Care Systems: Experiences of Patients with health Problems in Six Countries," *Health Affairs* Web Exclusive (3 November 2005): 509–25.
10 Institute of Medicine, *To Err is Human: Building a Safer Health System*

(Washington, DC: National Academy Press, 1999).

11   Cathy Schoen et al., "On the Front Lines of Care: Primary Care Doctors' Office Systems, Experiences and Views in Seven Countries," *Health Affairs Web Exclusive* (2 November 2006): W555–71.

12   See http://www1.va.gov/OPA/pressrel/pressrelease.cfm?id=532 (last viewed 12 February 2007).

13   Richard A. Rettig et al., *False Hope: Bone Marrow Transplantation for Breast Cancer* (Oxford: Oxford University Press, 2007).

14   McKinsey Global Institute, *Health Care Productivity* (Los Angeles: McKinsey & Co., 1996), Exhibit 5.

15   Steffie Woolhandler, Terry Campbell, and David U. Himmelstein, "Costs of Health Care Administration in the United States and in Canada," *New England Journal of Medicine* 349, no. 8 (21 August 2003): 768–75.

16   Henry J. Aaron, "The Cost of Health Care Administration in the United States and Canada – Questionable Answers to a Questionable Question," *New England Journal of Medicine* 349, no. 8 (21 August 2003): 801–3.

17   Lucette Lagnado, "Hospitals Try Extreme Measures to Collect their Overdue Debt," *Wall Street Journal* (30 October 2003): A1.

18   Federal Advisor on Wait Times, Final Report, Health Canada: June 2006 http://www.hc-sc.gc.ca/hcs-sss/alt_formats/hpb-dgps/pdf/pubs/2006-wait-attente/index_e.pdf (last viewed 10 February 2007).

19   Health Council of Canada, *Annual Report to Canadians 2005*, (Ottawa: Health Council of Canada February 2006).

20   C. David Naylor, "A Different View of Queues in Ontario," *Health Affairs* Fall (1991): 111–28.

21   Nadeem Esmail and Michael Walker, "Looking North for Inspiration," *Milken Review* (Dec. 2006): 32–9.

22   Michael L. Katz and Harvey S. Rosen, *Microeconomics*, (New York: McGraw-Hill, 1991):15

23   Institute of medicine, *Hidden Costs, Values Lost: Uninsurance in America* (Washington, DC: National Academy Press, 2003): 5.

24   http://www.kff.org/uninsured/upload/The-Uninsured-and-Their-Access-to-Health-Care-Oct-2004.pdf

25   Uwe E. Reinhardt, "Can Efficiency in Health Care be Left to the Market?" *Journal of Health Policy, Politics and Law* 26, no. 5 (October 2001): 967–92.

26   Ibid.

27   J. Hall and A. Maynard, "Healthcare Lessons from Australia: What can Michael Howard Learn from John Howard?" *British Medical Journal* 330 (2005): 357–9.

28   F. Colombo and N. Tapey, "Private Health Insurance," Health Working Paper 15 (Paris: Organisation for Economic Cooperation and Develop-

ment, 2004).

29 P. Kind, and A. Williams, "Measuring Success in Health Care: The Time
Has Come to Do it Properly," *Health Policy Matters* 9 (March 2004) University of York (accessible free of charge at
http://www.york.ac.uk/depts/healthsciences/pubs/hpmindex.htm).

30 Hall and Maynard, "Healthcare Lessons from Australia," 357–9.

31 Jon Johnson, "How Will International Trade Agreements Affect Canadian
Health Care?" in *Putting Health First: Canadian Health Care Reform in a
Globalizing World*, ed. Matthew Sanger and Scott Sinclair (Ottawa: Cana-
dian Centre for Policy Alternatives, 2004).

32 See Jim Grieshaber-Otto and Scott Sinclair, *Bad Medicine: Trade Treaties,
Privatization and Health Care Reform in Canada* (Ottawa: Canadian Centre
for Policy Alternatives, 2004).

33 The Annex I reservation applies against the NAFTA national treatment
(1102, 1202), most-favoured nation treatment (1103, 1203), local presence (1205), performance requirements (1106) and senior management
and board of directors (1107) articles.

34 See Barry Appleton, *Navigating NAFTA: A Concise Users' Guide to the
North American Free Trade Agreement* (Toronto: Carswell, 1994):161ff.

35 NAFTA Annex II-C-9 applies against the national treatment (1102,
1202), the services chapter's most-favoured nation treatment (1203), local
presence (1205), and senior management and board of directors (1107)
articles.

36 For a discussion of the differing views of Canadian and US governments
during the NAFTA sub-national reservations exercise, see Johnson,
Putting Health First, 13–15 endnote 1 and *Inside NAFTA*, 29 November,
1995.

37 See *Putting Health First*.

38 Damages were awarded against Canada in two cases, and a third (the
MMT case) was settled out of court with damages paid and legislation
withdrawn. See Scott Sinclair, "Table of NAFTA Investor-State Disputes," Canadian Centre for Policy Alternatives, March 2007, available at
http://www.policyalterntives.ca.

39 Roy J. Romanow, *Building on Values: The Future of Health Care in Canada*,
(Saskatoon: Commission on the Future of Health Care in Canada, 2002),
238.

40 It is, of course, very likely that US money is involved in the private clinics already established.

41 NAFTA's national treatment rules do not apply to subsidies (NAFTA
article 1108.7). In covered sectors such as health insurance, the GATS
does, however, guarantee foreign service providers access to the same
government subsidies and other advantages given to domestic service

providers.

Part Three: Privatization and the Principles of Medicare

1   Up–dated and expanded from "Political Wolves and Economic Sheep: The Sustainability of Public Health Insurance in Canada" in *The Public-Private Mix for Health*, ed. A. Maynard (London: The Nuffield Trust, 2005), 117–40

2   D.H. Meadows, D.I. Meadows, J. Randers, and W.W. Behrens III, *The Limits to Growth* (London: Earth Island, 1972).

3   The idea is not entirely new. H.G. Wells referred to civilization as a race between education and disaster, and Arnold Toynbee built a theory of history around the success or failure of different civilizations' responses to successive challenges.

4   T.F. Homer-Dixon, *The Ingenuity Gap* (Toronto: Alfred A. Knopf, 2000).

5   Advocates of market mechanisms tend to presume on a priori grounds that private markets always generate the right or "optimal" answer. This position is typically buttressed against empirical challenge by the implicit assumption that whatever outcome is generated by such markets is by definition optimal.

6   T.F. Homer-Dixon, J.H. Boutwell, and G.W. Rathjens, "Environmental Change and Violent Conflict," *Scientific American* 268, no. 2 (February 1993): 38–45.

7   The ingenuity requirement to manage an increasingly complex global environment — "tightly coupled" physically, financially, and even psychologically — does appear to be increasing rapidly, and it is far from clear that our political institutions in particular have the capacity or can even recognize the need to meet that growing demand.

8   R.G. Evans, "Healthy, Wealthy and Cunning? Profit and Loss from Health Care Reform," in *The Vancouver Institute: An Experiment in Public Education,* ed. P. N. Nemetz (Vancouver: JBA Press, 1998), 447–86.

9   Here and subsequently, calendar year data on GDP and health expenditure back to 1975 are from CIHI and data back to 1960 can be found in OECD; sources for pre-1960 data are given in M. L. Barer and R. G. Evans, "Riding North on a South-Bound Horse? Expenditures, Prices, Utilization and Incomes in the Canadian Health Care System," in *Medicine at Maturity: Achievements, Lessons and Challenges*, ed. R. G. Evans and G. L. Stoddart (Calgary: University of Calgary Press, 1986), 53–163.

10 R.G. Evans, "Health Care in Canada: Patterns of Funding and Regulation," in *The Public/Private Mix for Health: The Relevance and Effects of Change*, ed. G. McLachlan and A. Maynard (London: Nuffield Provincial Hospitals Trust, 1982), 371–424.

11 R.G. Evans, "Financing Health Care: Taxation and the Alternatives" in *Financing Health Care: Options for Europe*, ed. E. Mossialos, A. Dixon, J.

Figueras, and J. Kutzin (Buckingham: Open University Press, 2002), 39–58.

[12] J. White, *Competing Solutions: American Health Care Proposals and International Experience* (Washington, D.C.: Brookings, 1995).

[13] World Health Organization, *World Health Report* (Geneva: WHO, 2006). They exclude all countries with populations of less than a million, as well as those singled out in the Report as having unreliable data.

[14] The WHR data also show that while these average percentages have increased over the last five years, they have risen more than twice as fast in the countries with incomes over $15,000 in 2003.

[15] The pattern here is significantly dependent on the fact that countries are unweighted. China and India, each with populations well over a billion, also have unusually high rates of out-of-pocket payment. Weighting countries by population would increase the rate for low-income countries, but would not change the downtrend in high income countries.

[16] These are the official numbers. But private insurance in the United States (and in Canada) enjoys very favourable tax treatment, which, when accounted as indirect public expenditure, raises the public share of total health expenditures to nearly 69 percent and lowers private insurance to under 25 percent. S. Woolhandler and D.U. Himmelstein, "Paying for National Health Insurance – and Not Getting It," *Health Affairs* 21, no. 4 (2002): 88–99.

[17] R. G. Evans, "Tension, Compression, and Shear: Directions, Stresses, and Outcomes of Health Care Cost Control," *Journal of Health Politics, Policy and Law* 15, no. 1 (1990): 101–28.

[18] Even in the United States, the federal medicare program for those sixty-five and older has been more successful than private insurers in controlling hospital and medical costs over the long term. C. Boccuti and M. Moon, "Comparing Medicare and Private Insurers: Growth Rates in Spending over Three Decades," *Health Affairs* 22, no. 2 (2003): 230–237.

[19] The pharmaceutical industry and its advocates claim that this increase has made possible the reduction in hospital costs; the claim is spurious. It rests on little more than a correlation of trends, and cannot withstand any serious empirical scrutiny. But that again is another story.

[20] One should also note, however, that cross-national and interregional data show conclusively that higher levels of health spending are not necessarily associated with better health outcomes. Canadians are significantly healthier than Americans, and in the United States high utilization is associated with poorer quality of care and higher mortality. See references in R.G. Evans, "Economic Myths and Political Realities: The Inequality Agenda and the Sustainability of Medicare," CHSPR Working Paper, (University of British Columbia, July 2007).

[21] United States, *Projections of National Health Expenditures* (Washington,

      DC: Congressional Budget Office, October 1992).

22   J.A. Poisal, and the National Health Expenditure Accounts Projections
      Team, "Health Spending Projections through 2016: Modest Changes
      Obscure Part D's Impact," *Health Affairs* 26, no. 2 (2007): w242–w253.

23   J.F.R. Lu and W.C. Hsiao, "Does Universal Health Insurance Make
      Health care Unaffordable? Lessons from Taiwan," *Health Affairs* 22, no.3
      (2003): 77–88.

24   Canada's ratio of national debt to GDP was in 2005 the lowest among
      the major industrial countries of the G-7 — 26.3 percent. This ratio had
      fallen from its peak of 69.3 percent ten years earlier, and was on a steady
      downtrend.

25   Here and subsequently, fiscal year (FY) data on provincial and federal
      public accounts are from the federal Department of Finance, Fiscal Ref-
      erence Tables (Sept. 2006). FY health expenditures are from CIHI.

26   It is difficult to know how much of the rhetoric of "unsustainability" is
      simply part of the never-ending provincial campaign for larger federal
      transfers.

27   The provincial budget went from a $1.4 billion surplus in 2000/2001 to
      a $1.2 billion deficit in 2001/2002. A number of other fiscal changes
      were made, generally regressive in effect but not so directly linkable to
      income level.

28   The premium is discounted for those with incomes under $25,000,
      falling to zero at $15,000.

29   A *regressive* tax takes a larger share of the incomes of people lower down
      the income distribution, and rests more lightly on those with higher
      incomes. A *progressive* tax, by contrast, takes a larger share of the incomes
      of those with higher incomes.

30   This agenda was spelled out explicitly by Conrad Black (2001) in an edi-
      torial bitterly critical of Canadian governments for "taking money from
      people who have earned it and redistributing it to people who haven't." As
      owner at that time of most of the major newspapers in Canada he had
      taken the opportunity energetically to promote his personal political
      views. At the time of writing, Lord Black was convicted on three counts of
      fraud; his concept of "earning" may therefore be somewhat idiosyncratic.

31   M.C. Wolfson and B.B. Murphy, "New Views on Inequality Trends in
      Canada and the United States," *Monthly Labor Review* (United States,
      Bureau of Labor Statistics, April 1998), 3–21.

32   A. Sharpe, "Linkages between Economic Growth and Inequality: Intro-
      duction and Overview," *Canadian Public Policy* 29, Supplement, (January,
      2003): S1–S14; Statistics Canada, "Family Income 2001," *The Daily*, 25
      June 2003.

33   A. Wagstaff, E. van Doorslaer, H. van der Burg et al., "Equity in the

Finance of Health Care in Twelve OECD Countries," *Journal of Health Economics* 18, no. 3 (1999): 291–314; E. Van Doorslaer, A. Wagstaff, H. van der Burg et al. (1999) The Redistributive Effect of Health Care: Some Further International Comparisons," *Journal of Health Economics* 18, no. 3 (1999): 263–90.

34 C.A.M. Mustard, S. Shanahan, S. Derksen, "Use of Insured Health Care Services in Relation to Income in a Canadian Province," in *Health, Health Care and Health Economics: Perspectives on Distribution*, ed. M.L. Barer, T.E. Getzen, and G.L. Stoddart (Chichester: John Wiley, 1998): 157-178.

35 The share of market income paid in taxes is about 10 percent higher in the top decile than in the next highest, so the overall progressivity of the tax system accounts for part of the jump — but not much.

36 S. Woolhandler, T. Campbell and D.U. Himmelstein, "Costs of Health Care Administration in the United States and Canada," *New England Journal of Medicine* 349, no. 8 (2003): 768–75.

37 S. Woolhandler and D.U. Himmelstein, "Paying for National Health Insurance — and Not Getting It" *Health Affairs* 21, no. 4 (2002): 88–98.

38 The spread of "managed care" in the United States during the 1990s can be similarly interpreted as the application of ingenuity to deal with an increasingly unsatisfactory environment — somewhat less successfully.

39 Medical Savings Accounts provide a leading example. They would serve no useful purpose in the Canadian context, merely providing a cover for increases in both user charges and health expenditures. But de-bunking the claims of their advocates has taken up a significant amount of research effort (for example, J. Hurley, "Medical Savings Accounts: Approach with Caution," *Journal of Health Services Research and Policy* 5, no. 2 (2000): 30–32; and E. Forget, R. Deber, and L.L. Roos, "Medical Savings Accounts: Will They Reduce Cost?," *Canadian Medical Association Journal* 167, no. 2: 143–147), and diverted public attention from more constructive topics.

40 R.G. Evans, M.L. Barer, G.L. Stoddart, and V. Bhatia, *Who Are the Zombie Masters, and What Do They Want?* (Toronto: The Premier's Council on Health, Well-being and Social Justice, June 1994); M.L. Barer, R.G. Evans, C. Hertzman, and M. Johri, "Lies, Damned Lies, and Health Care Zombies: Discredited Ideas That Will Not Die" (HPI Discussion Paper #10, University of Texas-Houston Health Policy Institute, Houston, Texas, 1998), accessible at http://www.chspr.ubc.ca.

41 K. Bassett, "Anthropology, Clinical Pathology and the Electronic Fetal Monitor: Lessons from the Heart," *Social Science & Medicine* 42, no. 2 (1996): 281–92.

42 Accordingly, when technologies emerge that are both therapeutically

superior and less costly per patient treated, they are often associated with rapid proliferation — and increased total cost.

43   A similar pattern was observed in the United States when the Prospective Payment System was introduced in 1983. Patterns of care respond to economic incentives.

44   C.D. Furberg and the ALLHAT Investigators, "Major Outcomes in High-Risk Hypertensive Patients Randomized to Angiotensin-Converting Enzyme Inhibitor or Calcium Channel Blocker vs Diuretic," *Journal of the American Medical Association* 288, no. 23 (2002): 2981–97; J.E. Rossouw, and the Women's Health Initiative trial investigators, "Risks and Benefits of Estrogen Plus Progestin in Healthy Postmenopausal Women," *Journal of the American Medical Association* 288, no. 3 (2002): 321–333.

45   Families USA, *Off the Charts: Pay, Profits and Spending by Drug Companies* (Washington, DC: Families USA Foundation Publication no. 1–104, 2001).

46   B. Mintzes, M.L. Barer, R.L. Kravitz, K. Bassett, J.Lexchin, A. Kazanjian, R.G. Evans, R. Pan, and S.A. Marion, "How does Direct-To-Consumer Advertising (DTCA) Affect Prescribing? A Survey in Primary Care Environments with and without Legal DTCA," *Canadian Medical Association Journal* 169, no. 5, (2003): 405–412.

47   "The Pharmaceutical Research and Manufacturers of America, known as PhRMA, will spend at least $150 million in the coming year" on political lobbying activities including "spend[ing] $1 million for an '*intellectual echo chamber of economists — a standing network of economists and thought leaders to speak against federal price control regulations through articles and testimony, and to serve as a rapid response team.*'" and "allocates $1 million '*to change the Canadian health care system*'" (R. Pear, "Drug Companies Increase Spending to Lobby Congress and Governments," *New York Times* (1 June 2003): 33.

48   U.E. Reinhardt, "Commentary: On the Apocalypse of the Retiring Baby Boom," *Canadian Journal on Aging* 20, Supp. 1 (2001): 192–204.

49   Economists have been particularly helpful in this quest, being ingenious in providing rigorous demonstrations — from faulty assumptions — of the general benefit from smaller government and greater inequality. This ingenuity can be well rewarded.

50   Reinhardt, "Commentary: On the Apocalypse of the Retiring Baby Boom," 192–204.

51   This essay is a revised and updated version of the article which first appeared in the *Osgoode Hall Law Journal* 44, no.2 (2006): 273–310. I would like to thank Sasha Kontic and Lorian Hardcastle for their research and editorial assistance. I would also like to thank Tony Duggan, Sujit Choudhry, Greig Hinds, Marie-Claude Premont, Steven Lewis, Greg Marchildon, Duncan Sinclair, Lorne Sossin, Michael Trebilcock,

Roy Romanow, Robert McMurtry, and Kent Roach for their com-
ments. All errors and omissions remain mine.

52 See *Access to Care, Access to Justice: The Legal Debate Over Private Health
    Insurance in Canada* ed. Colleen M. Flood, Kent Roach, and Lorne Sossin
    (Toronto: University of Toronto Press, 2005).

53 Bernard M. Dickens, "The Chaoulli Judgment: Less Than Meets the Eye
    — or More" in *Access to Care*, Flood, Roach, and Sossin, ed.: 19.

54 Even the CBC played a documentary called "Medicare; Schmedicare" on
    Thursday, 8 December 2005. It is reported to have been filmed in private
    clinics in Montreal, Toronto, and Vancouver and compares the waiting
    times for those who use the private services to those who use the public
    system; online: CBC News — The Passionate Eye
    (http://www.cbc.ca/passionateeye/medicare.html).

55 *Charter of Human Rights and Freedoms*, R.S.Q. c. C-12 [Quebec Charter].

56 *Canadian Charter of Rights and Freedoms*, Part I of the Constitution Act,
    1982, being Schedule B to the Canada Act 1982 (U.K.), 1982, c. 11
    [Canadian Charter].

57 Canada, Senate, *The Health of Canadians — The Federal Role, vol. 3, Health
    Care Systems in Other Countries*, Interim Report of the Standing Senate
    Committee on Social Affairs, Science and Technology (Ottawa: The Sen-
    ate, 2001) (known as "the Kirby Report" after its chair, Senator Michael
    Kirby).

58 *Chaoulli v. Quebec (Attorney General)*, 2005 SCC 35 [*Chaoulli*], para. 140.

59 Colleen M. Flood, Mark Stabile, and Sasha Kontic, "Finding Health Poli-
    cy 'Arbitrary': The Evidence on Waiting, Dying, and Two-tier Systems,"
    in *Access to Care*, Flood, Roach, and Sossin, ed.: 307.

60 We discuss these in Flood, Stabile, and Kontic, "Finding Health Policy
    'Arbitrary'."

61 Organization for Economic Cooperation and Development (OECD),
    Health Data 2005 (Paris: OECD, 2005). Figures show that in both Cana-
    da and France private health insurance accounts for 12.7 percent of total
    health spending. Health care financed by private insurance is highest in
    the United States, at 36.7 percent, which reflects the fact that private
    insurance is the dominant form of coverage in this country. The Nether-
    lands, where private insurance is the primary payer for more than 30
    percent of the population, reports the second highest level of financing at
    17.2 percent. According to OECD statistics for 2003, private insurance
    accounts for less than 10 percent of total health expenditure in all
    remaining OECD countries supplying such information.

62 The comparison seems to originate from the following opinion piece: D.
    Gratzer, "Wanted: Credible Health Care Analysis," Fraser Institute Cana-

dian Student Review, 7, no. 2 (1998); online: The Fraser Institute (http://oldfraser.lexi.net/publications/csr/1998/september/health_care _analysis.html).

63 Colleen Flood and Tom Archibald, "The Illegality of Private Health Care in Canada," *Canadian Medical Association Journal* 164, no. 6 (2001): 825.

64 Chief Justice McLachlin and Justice Major further discount governmental arguments (and the evidence of expert witnesses) about the detrimental effect of a private tier on a public system and seem to accept that there is no downside to allowing a private tier.

65 *Chaoulli*, para. 140.

66 For example, a recent prima facie poor ranking for Canada by the World Health Organization has been roundly criticized and can be largely explained because a discount was factored in for educational attainment; in other words, because Canadians are more highly educated than, for example, the citizens of France, our otherwise excellent performance on health care outcomes like infant mortality and life expectancy was severely discounted — see Raisa Deber, "Why Did the World Health Organization Rate Canada's Health System as 30th? Some Thoughts on League Tables," *Longwoods Review* 2, no. 1 (2003): 2.

67 OECD, *Health Data 2005*. In 2003, Canada tied Greece for seventh place in the OECD in terms of total health care spending measured as a percentage of GDP.

68 See Alan Maynard, "How to Defend a Public Health Care System: Lessons From Abroad" in *Access to Care*, ed. Flood, Roach, and Sossin, 237.

69 Francesca Colombo and Nicole Tapay, "Private Health Insurance in OECD Countries: The Benefits and Costs for Individuals and Health Systems," 15 OECD Health Working Papers (2004), para. 20, online: http://www.oecd.org/dataoecd/34/56/33698043.pdf.

70 Canadian Institute for Health Information (CIHI), *Exploring the 70/30 Split: How Canada's Health Care System in Financed* (Ottawa: CIHI, 2005), online: http://secure.cihi.ca/cihiweb/dispPage.jsp?cw_page=AR_1282_E&cw_t opic=1282.

71 See Luigi Siciliani and Jeremy Hurst, "Explaining Waiting Times Variations for Elective Surgery Across OECD Countries," 7 OECD Health Working Papers (2003), online: http://www.oecd.org/dataoecd/31/10/ 17256025.pdf.

72 Carmen DeNavas-Walt, Bernadette D. Proctor, and Cheryl Hill Lee, US Census Bureau, Current Population Reports, P60–229, *Income, Poverty, and Health Insurance Coverage in the United States: 2004* (Washington DC: US Government Printing Office, 2005), online: US Census Bureau http://www.census.gov/prod/2005pubs/p60–229.pdf.

73 P. Dourgnon and C. Sermet, "Le tiers-payant est-il inflationniste?" CRE-

DES Working Paper (2000): 27, cited in Agnès Couffinhal, Valérie Paris, and CREDES, "Cost Sharing in France," CREDES Working Paper (2003): 4–5, online: IRDES http://www.irdes.fr/english/wp/CostSharing.pdf.

74 Carolyn Tuohy, Colleen Flood, and Mark Stabile have identified four basic models of structuring the relationship between public and private financing: parallel public and private systems; co-payment; group-based; and sectoral. See Carolyn Tuohy, Colleen Flood, and Mark Stabile, "How Does Private Finance Affect Public Health Care Systems? Marshalling the Evidence from OECD Nations," *Journal of Health Politics, Policy and Law* 29, no. 3 (2004): 359.

75 For a discussion see J. Wasem, S. Greß, and K.G.H. Okma, "The Role of Private Health Insurance in Social Health Insurance Countries" in *Social Health Insurance in Western Europe,* ed. R. Saltman, R. Busse, and J. Figueras, (London: Open University Press, 2004), 227.

76 This is similar to the mechanism employed in the provinces of Nova Scotia, Ontario and Manitoba to protect public medicare, namely preventing physicians charging more privately than they may publicly for the same essential services.

77 The Dutch Professional Guidelines for Doctors, found in the Individual Health Care Professions Act, states at article II.2 that doctors have to treat patients equally in equal cases (De arts zal patiënten in gelijke gevallen gelijk behandelen. Discriminatie wegens godsdienst, levensovertuiging, ras, geslacht of op welke grond dan ook, is niet toegestaan) — See J.E.M. Akveld, and H.E.G.M. Hermans, "Health Care in The Netherlands," in *International Encyclopaedia of Medical Law,* ed. H. Nys, (Leuven: Leuven University Press, 1995): 1.

78 Dourgnon and Sermet, "Le tiers-payant est-il inflationniste?": 4–5.

79 The only study that has explicitly measured equity in the finance of the French health care system was undertaken in the early 1990s. See E. van Doorslaer and A. Wagstaff, "Equity in the Finance of Health Care: Methods and Findings," in *Equity in the Finance and Delivery of Health Care. An International Perspective,* ed. E. van Doorslaer, A. Wagstaff, and F. Rutten, (Oxford: Oxford University Press, 1993): 20. The study has been referenced in Thomas C. Buchmueller and Agnes Couffinhal, "Private Health Insurance in France," OECD Health Working Papers No. 12 (2004), 7, online: http://www.oecd.org/dataoecd/35/11/30455292.pdf; and Couffinhal, Paris, and CREDES, "Cost Sharing in France,":12.

80 In France there is a plurality of health care delivery methods — either through public or private hospitals or by self-employed private physicians. The public and private sectors for the most part deliver different

types of care, and social insurance covers both public and private care. The private sector is not meant to be a second tier.

81 Since 1980, doctors in France have been able to extra-bill (or charge a "depassement") by choosing to be a Secteur 2 doctor. However, by 1990, only 68.2 percent of doctors were applying the negotiated tariff (57 percent of specialists), there was no proof of improved quality being offered by the Secteur 2 doctors, and the market provided little control over competitive pricing as the Secteur 2 fees were 45 percent higher than the conventional tariff — Jean-Pierre Poullier and Simone Sandier, "France," *Journal of Health Politics, Policy and Law* 899, 25:5 (2000): 902–3.

82 Buchmueller and Couffinhal, "Private Health Insurance in France," 10; and the World Health Organization, "Highlights on Health, France 2004," online: http://www.euro.who.int/eprise/main/who/progs/chhfra/system/20050131_1.

83 Couffinhal, Paris, and CREDES, "Cost Sharing in France," 14; and Buchmueller and Couffinhal, "Private Health Insurance in France,:10.

84 For a discussion see Tuohy, Flood, and Stabile, "How Does Private Finance Affect Public Health Care Systems?" 359.

85 See ibid.

86 Columbo and Tapay, "Private Health Insurance," 24.

87 Flood and Archibald, "The Illegality of Private Health Care in Canada," 825.

88 The dissent however was more sensitive to the complexity of health care financing in their treatment of evidence from other jurisdictions, They criticize the majority's treatment of this evidence in *Chaoulli*, para. 225–230.

89 United Kingdom, Select Committee on Health, "Memorandum by Professor David Light: Testimony on its Inquiry into Consultants' Contracts," Appendix 8 to *Health — Third Report* (London: House of Commons, 2000), online: http://www.publications.parliament.uk/pa/cm199900/cmselect/cmhealth/586/586ap17.htm.

90 See *Chaoulli*, para. 131, where McLachlin C.J.C. and Major J. say: "In order not to be arbitrary, the limit on life, liberty and security requires not only a theoretical connection between the limit and the legislative goal, but a real connection on the facts."

91 See *Chaoulli*, para. 63, Deschamps J.

92 See *Chaoulli*, para. 136, McLachlin C.J.C. and Major J.

93 The extent to which NZ wait times apparently seem to have fallen is due to a managerial sleight of hand rather than any substantive reform. The NZ booking system now requires that a patient not be put on a wait list unless the system has the resources to meet the need within six

months. If not, then the patient is referred back to his or her family doctor to "manage" the care until when (if ever) the system is able to meet the patient's need or the nature of the need changes so that it requires prioritization — in other words the patient gets much worse.

94 Medical Council of New Zealand, *The New Zealand Medical Workforce in 2000* (Wellington: Medical Council of New Zealand, 2000), 14, online: http://www.mcnz.org.nz/portals/1/publications/ workforce percent202000.pdf.

95 *The Commerce Commission v. The Ophthalmological Society of New Zealand* (2004), 10 T.C.L.R. 994 (H.C.).

96 Ibid., para. 67 on page 1013.

97 Alan Maynard and Karen Bloor, "Reforming the Consultant Contract Again?" *British Medical Journal* 329 (2004): 929.

98 United Kingdom, Select Committee on Health, *Health — Third Report: Minutes of Evidence — Volume II (HC 586–11)*, (London: House of Commons, 2000), online: http://www.publications.parliament.uk/pa/ cm199900/cmselect/cmhealth/586/586ap17.htm [*Third Report*].

99 Ibid., "Summary of Conclusions and Recommendations," Recommendation (o), para. 60.

100 Stephen J. Duckett, "Private Care and Public Waiting," *Australian Health Review* 29, no. 1 (2005): 87.

101 Carolyn DeCoster, Leonard MacWilliam, and Randy Walld, *Waiting Times for Surgery: 1997/98 and 1998/99 Update* (Winnipeg: Manitoba Centre for Health Policy and Evaluation, University of Manitoba, 1998), online: http://www.umanitoba.ca/centres/mchp/reports/pdfs/waits2.pdf.

102 See *Chaoulli*, para. 136, McLachlin C.J.C. and Major J.

103 Maynard and Bloor, "Reforming the Consultant Contract Again?" 929.

104 John Ibbitson, "Klein's Non-Partisan Health-Care Warnings," *Globe and Mail* (22 November 2005): A1.

105 See Bill Curray, "Not Opposed to Private Health Care, Layton Says," *Globe and Mail* (5 December 2005): A5.

106 See Steven Chase, "Layton defends his mid-'90s visit to private hernia clinic in Toronto," *Globe and Mail* (13 January 2006): A4.

107 See for example the Copeman Clinics online at: http://www.copeman-healthcare.com/.

108 Quoted in "How Quebec deals with its health plight," editorial, *Globe and Mail* (16 November 2005): A20.

109 Lysiane Gagnon, "A pill Quebec won't swallow," *Globe and Mail* (14 November 2005): A15.

110   Jeffrey Simpson, "Why Health-Care Posturing Won't Amount to a Hill of Beans," *Globe and Mail* (9 November 2005): A19.

111   See Noralou P. Roos et al., "Does Universal Comprehensive Insurance Encourage Unnecessary Use? Evidence From Manitoba Says 'No'," *Canadian Medical Association Journal* 170, no. 2 (2004): 210. A 1999 survey of residents in Winnipeg reveals in this paper that 70 percent of the population in the lowest use group consume just 10 percent of health care dollars, whereas just 10 percent of the population consume 74 percent of the dollars. Also note an earlier publication: Evelyn L. Forget, Raisa Deber, and Leslie L. Roos, "Medical Savings Accounts: Will They Reduce Costs?" *Canadian Medical Association Journal* 167, no. 2 (2002): 145. The study determines that over a three-year period between 1997 and 1999, the lowest-using 50 percent of the population only accounted for 4 percent of costs whereas the highest-using 1 percent of the population accounted for 26 percent of spending on hospital and physician care. The top 10 percent spending decile accounted for more that 70 percent of health care costs annually. Both studies show that only the public system can accommodate the catastrophic costs category because the costs associated with this kind of care far exceed the ability of any one individual to absorb them privately.

112   Editorial, "Private health care. Let's talk about it," *Globe and Mail* (7 December 2005): A26.

113   Those with vested interests in the private sector already have begun discussions on how to "better" the Canadian health care system in light of the *Chaoulli* decision. For example, the Canadian Independent Medical Clinics Association (an organization that represents private health care clinics) hosted a conference in Vancouver on November 11 and 12, 2005, called "Saving Medicare: Strategies & Solutions." The conference had a $1000 + registration fee and speakers included Reform Party founder Preston Manning, Senator Michael Kirby, Dr. Jacques Chaoulli, Ian McPherson (the CEO of New Zealand private health insurer Southern Cross), and Charles Auld (former CEO of UK based General Healthcare Group), as well as members of the legal community and doctors currently operating private clinics in British Columbia: http://www.uwindsor.ca/units/history/people.nsf/5f0f31d464ccc0df852 5698a0052c293/ff47d1a563fe48e585256aa40052808e?OpenDocument.

114   See Flood and Archibald, "The Illegality of Private Health Care in Canada," 825.

115   Ministry of Health and Long-Term Care, "Wait Time Strategy Overview," online: http://www.health.gov.on.ca/transformation/ wait_times/wt_strategy.html.

116   Patrick J. Monahan, "Wait Times Key to Saving Medicare," *Toronto Star*

(17 November 2005): A27.

117 Ibid.

118 For a discussion on appeal mechanisms in the province of Ontario see the paper by Caroline Pitfield and Colleen M. Flood, "Section 7 'Safety Valves': Appealing Wait Times Within a One-Tier System," in *Access to Care*, Flood, Roach, and Sossin, ed.: 477.

119 See: http://www.conservative.ca/EN/2023/37031: (accessed on 15 January 2006). See also http://www.hc-sc.gc.ca/hcs-sss/qual/acces/ wait-attente/index_e.html, which confirms the ten–year plan to strengthen health care.

120 See: Health Canada, News Release 20 November 2006, "Canada's new government launches historic first wait times guarantee in First Nations prenatal project," online: http://www.hc-sc.gc.ca/ahc-asc/media/ nr-cp/2006/2006_110_e.html (last time accessed on 29 June 2007).

121 Health Canada, News Release March 2007, "Patient Wait Times Guarantees," online: http://www.hc-sc.gc.ca/ahc-asc/media/nr-cp/2007/ 2007_wait-delai-bk1_e.html (accessed on 29 June 2007).

122 Office of the Prime Minister, News Release April 2007, "Canada's New Government announces Patient Wait Times Guarantees," online: http://www.pm.gc.ca/eng/media.asp?id=1611 (accessed on 29 June 2007).

123 Stanley H. Hartt, "Arbitrariness, Randomness and the Principles of Fundamental Justice," in *Access to Care*, ed. Flood, Roach, and Sossin: 505.

124 Within New Zealand there is indirect evidence of a loss of political support for public spending on services also covered by private insurance.

125 *Jacques Chaoulli et George Zeliotis c. Procureur général du Québec et Procureur général du Canada (Qc)* (4 August 2005), Supreme Court of Canada Rehearing — 29272, online: Supreme Court of Canada Bulletin of Proceedings http://www.lexum.umontreal.ca/csc-scc/en/bul/2005/html/ 05-08-12-bul.wpd.html. The judgment reads: "The motion for a partial rehearing is granted. The Court's judgment is stayed for a period of 12 months from the date such judgment was issued, namely June 9, 2005."

126 Aaron Derfel, "Montreal leads the country in offering private health care," *Montreal Gazette* (12 February 2005).

127 Canada, Office of the Auditor General of Canada, "Health Canada — Federal Support of Health Care Delivery," Status Report: Chapter 3 (Ottawa: Auditor General of Canada, 2002), online: 2002 Reports of the Auditor General of Canada http://www.oag-bvg.gc.ca/domino/ reports.nsf/html/20020903ce.html; Health Canada has recently addressed enforcement issues — see Health Canada, News Release, "Canadian Public Health Care Protection Initiative" (3 November 2005), online:

http://www.hc-sc.gc.ca/ahc-asc/media/notices-avis/
prop_e.html.

128   Henri Brun, Diane Demters, Patrice Garant, Andree Lajoie, Marie-Claude
      Premont, and Daniel Proulx, "Quebec Medicare Plan Is Not What the
      Supremes Ordered," *Montreal Gazette* (17 November 2005): A29.

129   Quebec, Ministry of Health and Social Services, *Guaranteeing Access:
      Meeting the challenges of equity, efficiency, and quality* (Quebec: 2006), online:
      http://publications.msss.gouv.qc.ca/acrobat/f/documentation/2005/05-
      721-01A.pdf.

130   Chantal Hebert, "Quebec Set to Pry Lid Off Medicare," *Toronto Star*, (8
      June 2007).

131   For a full discussion, see Tracey Epps and David Schneiderman, "Open-
      ing Medicare to Our Neighbours or Closing the Door on a Public
      System," in *Access to Care*, ed. Flood, Roach, and Sossin: 369.

132   Kelly Cryderman, "Waits for hip, knee surgery cut by 90 percent: Pilot
      project yields 'phenomenal results,'" *Edmonton Journal* (19 December
      2005): A1; Dawn Walton, "Alberta slashes wait times on some surgeries,"
      Globe and Mail (20 December 2005): A1.

133   Radio-Canada broke the news on 11 June 2007 that a regulation was
      about to be enacted where the list would grow to about thirty new
      medical acts, which could be carried out in Specialized Medical Centres.

134   "Public–private partnerships" is a term that has been used to describe a
      variety of contractual and commercial schemes that to one extent or
      another privatize the funding, establishment, ownership and/or operation
      of public infrastructure and services. As pointed out by the Ontario Hos-
      pital Association, although P3 structures may take many different legal
      forms, all P3 structures share the common basis of: "A relationship struc-
      tured between a government entity and a private entity whereby the
      private entity assumes a defined level of responsibility for the provision
      and/or operation of a facility or service which had previously been the
      sole responsibility of the government."

135   See for example, Diane Dawson, "The Private Finance Initiative: A Pub-
      lic Finance Illusion?", *UK Health Economics* 10, no. 6 (2001): 479–86;
      Allyson M Pollock, Jean Shaoul, Neil Vickers, "Private Finance and 'Value
      for Money'," in "NHS Hospitals: A Policy in Search of a Rationale?"
      British Medical Journal 324 (18 May 2002), bmj.com; P.J. Devereaux et al.,
      "A systematic review and metaanalysis of studies comparing mortality
      rates of private for-profit and private not-for-profit hospitals," *Canadian
      Medical Association Journal* 166, no. 11 (2002): 1399.

136   See R.G. Evans et. al, "Private Highway, One-Way Street: The DeKlein
      and Fall of Canadian Medicare?," Centre for Health Services and Policy

Research (CHSPR) Discussion Paper, University of British Columbia, March 2000, for an excellent analysis of how the objectives of private investors can collide with those medicare in the private hospital setting.

137 See "Summary of the William Osler Health Centre Project Agreement with the Healthcare Infrastructure Company of Canada," which can be found at http://www.williamoslerhc.on.ca/workfiles/Project_Agreement.pdf

138 In addition to the Project Agreement and schedules, there are several "Implementation Documents" (a defined term — see Schedule 1 to the PA), that are integral to the P3 scheme. These agreements and leases essentially define the relationship between the various private companies participating in the P3 scheme, rather than between the public hospital and the private consortium.

139 Other Canadian P3 hospital schemes are for longer terms, and in the case of the Royal Ottawa Hospital P3, may extend for sixty-six years.

140 Under article 17.7.2 of the Project Agreement only three types of business enterprises may not be established as part of the P3 hospital: 1) a casino or gaming operation; 2) an adult or sexually themed entertainment establishment; or 3) the sale of tobacco or alcoholic products.

141 Article 17.7.1.

142 Communication with Murray MacKenzie. Mr. MacKenzie served for many years as the CEO of the North York General Hospital, also served as the Chairman of the Cardiac Care Network of Ontario, past Chairman of the Ontario Hospital Association and an Assistant Professor in the Department of Health Policy, Management and Evaluation at the University of Toronto. He also served on the boards of several health-related organizations including: Cancer Care Ontario, Regional Geriatric Program of Metropolitan Toronto, and the Canadian Cancer Society.

143 In addition to this liability, and even where the private consortium defaults on its obligations under the scheme, the public hospital may still be obliged to compensate the consortium for the services contract if it is deemed to have a residual value.

144 Article 48.

145 See for example: Dawson, "The Private Finance Initiative"; A.M. Pollock, J. Shaoul, N. Vickers, "Private Finance and 'Value for Money' in NHS Hospitals: A Policy in Search of a Rationale?" *British Medical Journal* 324, no. 7347 (2002): 1205-1212; Devereaux et al., "A Systematic Review and Meta-analysis." 1389-1415.

146 The financial commitments of the government of Ontario are set out in a funding agreement negotiated with the WOHC, and authorized under the Public Hospital Acts. That agreement was disclosed in consequence of a challenge by several health care sector unions and the Ontario

Health Coalition to the lawfulness of the approvals and funding arrangements approved by the Ministry.

147 These figures are taken from a redacted version of the Financial Model to the Project Agreement for the WOHC P3, and may have since been revised somewhat.

148 S. Choudhry, N. K. Choudhry and A. D. Brown, "Unregulated Private Markets for Health Care in Canada? Rules of Professional Misconduct, Physician Kickbacks and Physician Self-referral," *Canadian Medical Association Journal* 170, no. 7(2004): 1115-1118.

149 Marie Claude Premont, "The Canada Health Act and the Future of Health Care Systems in Canada," Commission on the Future of Medicare, Discussion Paper #4, July 2002; and Joan Gilmour, "Regulation of Free-Standing Health Facilities: An Entrée for Privatization and For-Profit Delivery in Health Care," *Health Law Journal* 134, Special Edition (2003).

150 Choudhry, Choudhry, and Brown, "Unregulated Private Markets for Health Care."

151 See, for example, section 51 of the *By-Laws, Saskatchewan College of Physicians and Surgeons.*

152 Commission on the Future of Health Care in Canada, (R. Romanow, Comm'r.), *Building Values: The Future of Health Care in Canada* (Ottawa: The Commission, 2002) at p. 7. Available online at: http://finalreport.healthcarecommission.ca/

153 Canadian Institute for Health Information, "National Health Expenditure Trends, 1975–2005." (Ottawa: CIHI, 2005), 4–5, 99, as quoted by Health Canada, Government of Canada in "Canada's Health Care System, Health Expenditures" http://www.hc-sc.gc.ca/hcs-sss/pubs/system-regime/2005-hcs-sss/expen-depen_e.html#note1

154 For a comprehensive review of private health insurance, see Diana Gibson and Colleen Fuller, *The Bottom Line: The Truth about Private Health Insurance* (Edmonton: Parkland Institute and NuWest Press, 2007). Much of the information in this chapter is drawn from that book.

155 Dunn, Fred, Auditor General of Alberta, "Seniors and Care," (Edmonton: Government of Alberta, 9 May 2005), http://www.oag.ab.ca/files/oag/OAG_Seniors_2005.pdf (accessed 18 June 2007). This report found standards for Alberta's seniors facilities to be out of date and inadequate and that most facilities did not even meet those standards.

156 Flood, Stabile, and Kontic, "Finding Health Policy 'Arbitrary'": 304, as sourced in Gibson and Fuller, *The Bottom Line*: 27.

157 References for this data can be found in Gibson and Fuller, *The Bottom*

Line: 46.

Part Four: Health Care Reforms: Pharmacare, Home, Community, and Primary Care

1   C. Schoen, R. Osborn, P.T. Huynh, et al., "Taking the Pulse of Health Care Systems: Experiences with Health Problems in Six Countries," *Health Affairs* 10 (2005):w509–w525.

2   C.H. Houston, *Steps on the Road to Medicare* (Montreal: McGill-Queen's University Press, 2002).

3   M. Taylor, *Health Insurance and Canadian Public Policy: The Seven Decisions that created the Canadian Health Insurance System* (Montreal: McGill-Queen's University Press, 1978): 244; C.D. Naylor, *Private Practice, Public Payment: Canadian Medicine and the Politics of Health Insurance* (Montreal: McGill-Queen's University Press, 1986): 138–9.

4   For more details on the Swift Current Region see: http://scaa.usask.ca/gallery/medicare/en_swift-current.php. Accessed 10 April 2007; and also see: Houston, *Steps on the Road to Medicare*: 77–88.

5   Taylor, *Health Insurance and Canadian Public Policy:* 251–2; and Houston, *Steps on the Road to Medicare*: 85.

6   Houston, *Steps on the Road to Medicare*: 85.

7   A.D. Kelly, "The Swift Current Experiment," *Canadian Medical Association Journal* 58 (1948): 506–11.

8   Taylor, *Health Insurance and Canadian Public Policy*: 252; Naylor, *Private Practice, Public Payment:* 191.

9   Taylor, *Health Insurance and Canadian Public Policy*: 252; Naylor, *Private Practice, Public Payment:*178–9, 191.

10   This section draws from Taylor, *Health Insurance and Canadian Public Policy*: 239–330; Naylor, *Private Practice, Public Payment:* 176–213.

11   See: http://www.saskatooncommunityclinic.ca/.(accessed 15 June 2007).

12   See: http://www.ghc.on.ca/home.html (accessed 15 June 2007).

13   D. Murray, "The Group Health Centre Model – working to improve continuity, comprehensiveness and responsiveness in primary care," presentation to the Research Group on Equity of Access and Organization on Primary Health Care Services. Found at: http://www.greas.ca/publication/pdf/davidmurray.pdf. (accessed 2 November 2006).

14   For example, Group Health was given an award for innovation at the Ontario Ministry of Health and Long-term Care's Expo 2007. See: http://www.ghc.on.ca/news/news.html?ID=59 (accessed 20 June 2007).

15   J.E.F. Hastings, F.D. Mott, A. Barclay, D. Hewitt, "Prepaid group practice in Sault Ste. Marie, Ontario: Part I: Analysis of utilization records," *Medical Care* 11 (1973): 91–103.

16   F.D. Mott, J.E.F. Hastings, and A. Barclay, "Prepaid group practice in Sault
      Ste. Marie, Ontario. Part II: Evidence from the household survey," *Medical
      Care* 11 (1973): 173–88.

17   G.H. DeFriese, "On paying the fiddler to change the tune: Further evi-
      dence from Ontario regarding the impact of universal health insurance
      on the organization and patterns of medical practice," *Milbank Memorial
      Fund Quarterly* 53, no. 2 (1975): 117–48.

18   W.G. Manning, A. Leibowitz, G.A. Goldberg, W.H. Rogers, and J.P. New-
      house, "A controlled trial of the effect of a prepaid group practice on the
      use of services," *New England Journal of Medicine* 310 (1984): 1505–10.

19   J.E. Ware, W.H. Rogers, A.R. Davies AR, et al., "Comparison of health
      outcomes at a health maintenance organization with those of fee-for-
      service care," *Lancet* 328 (1986): 1017–22.

20   Organisation for Economic Cooperation and Development, "Frequently
      requested health statistics 2006," found at: http://www.oecd.org/
      dataoecd/20/51/37622205.xls (accessed 21 June 2007).

21   S. Woolhandler, T. Campbell, and D.U. Himmelstein, "Costs of health care
      administration in the United States and Canada," *New England Journal of
      Medicine* 349 (2003): 768–75.

22   US Institute of Medicine, "Health insurance is a family matter" (18 Sep-
      tember 2002), http://www.nap.edu/catalog/10503.html?onpi_newsdoc
      09182002 (accessed November 17, 2003).

23   A. Wordsworth, "Medical bills main culprit in bankruptcies: US study,"
      National Post (27 April 2000).

24   B. Purchase, "Health care and competitiveness," background paper for the
      National Health Policy Summit (Ottawa, 1996).

25   T.C. Douglas, "We must go forward," in *Medicare The Decisive Year*, ed. Lee
      Soderstrom (Ottawa: Canadian Centre for Policy Alternatives, 1984).

26   H. Gilmour and J. Park, "Dependency, chronic conditions, and pain in
      seniors," *Health Reports* supplement1 (2005): 21–31. Found at:
      http://www.statcan.ca/english/freepub/82-003-SIE/2005000/pdf/
      82-003-SIE20050007443.pdf (accessed 2 November 2006).

27   There is no recent comprehensive study of the cost of chronic disease in
      Canada but a recent study in Nova Scotia concluded that 60 percent of
      the province's health care costs were for chronic diseases. R. Colman, K.
      Hayward, A. Monette, et al., "The cost of chronic disease in Nova Scotia.
      GPI Atlantic." Found at: http://gov.ns.ca/health/downloads/chronic.pdf
      (accessed 2 October 2006). In 2004, the US Centers for Disease Control
      concluded that persons with chronic conditions consumed 75 percent of
      the costs of the system: http://www.cdc.gov/nccdphp/burdenbook2004/
      The higher figures could be due to some of the persons with chronic

conditions developing unrelated acute problems while the lower figure may be related to the exclusion of acute problems (such as falls in the elderly), which are often related to chronic problems.

28   C. Schoen, R. Osborn, P.T. Huynh, et al., "On the front lines of care: primary care doctors' office systems, experiences, and views in seven countries," *Health Affairs* 11 (2006): w555–w571. Found at: http://content.healthaffairs.org/cgi/content/full/hlthaff.25.w555/DC1. (accessed 2 November 2006).

29   M.J. Stampfer, F.B. Hu, J.E. Manson, et al., "Primary prevention of coronary heart disease in women through diet and lifestyle," *New England Journal of Medicine* 343 (2000): 16–22.

30   F.B. Hu, J.E. Manson, M.J. Stampfer, et al., "Diet, lifestyle, and the risk of type 2 diabetes mellitus in women," *New England Journal of Medicine* 345 (2001): 790–7.

31   R. Doll, R. Peto, K. Wheatley, et al., "Mortality in relation to smoking: 40 years' observations on male British doctors," *British Medical Journal* 309 (1994): 901–11.

32   From tabulations constructed from data from the Canadian Institute for Health Information. Found at: http://secure.cihi.ca/cihiweb/dispPage.jsp?cw_page=statistics_results_topic_hospital_e&cw_topic=Health percent20Services&cw_subtopic=Hospital percent20Discharges (accessed 10 November 2006). These conditions were responsible for 950,000 hospital days or roughly 2870 hospital beds (at 90 percent capacity).

33   The 2001 Saskatchewan Commission on Medicare chaired by long-time health administrator Ken Fyke noted: "Many attribute the quality problems to a lack of money. Evidence and analysis have convincingly refuted this claim. In health care, good quality often costs considerably less than poor quality." K.J. Fyke, "Caring for Medicare: sustaining a quality system," report of the Saskatchewan Commission on Medicare (Regina: The Commission, 2001).

34   R. T. Tsuyuki, M. Fradette, J.A. Johnson, et al., "A multicenter disease management program for hospitalized patients with heart failure," *Journal of Cardiac Failure* 10 (2004): 473–80.

35   Schoen, Osborn, Huynh et al., "Taking the pulse of health care systems."

36   Quote from speech by T.C. Douglas entitled "We Must Go Forward" in transcript of Canadian Centre for Policy Alternatives Conference proceedings entitled *Medicare: The Decisive Year* held on 12-13 November 1982 in Montreal. Copies of the 1982 conference proceedings may be obtained from the Canadian Centre of Policy Alternatives or the Canadian Health Coalition.

37   For one thing, it's pretty dangerous to be in hospital if you don't really

need to be there.

38   Found at: http://www.healthcouncilcanada.ca/en/index.php?option=
com_content&task=view&id=70&Itemid=72 (accessed 9 April 2007).

39   For examples, see the US Institute of Medicine, *Crossing the Quality
Chasm: A New Health System for the 21st Century* (Washington, DC:
National Academy Press, 2001).

40   G.R. Baker, P., G. Norton, V. Flinthoft, et al., "The Canadian Adverse
Events Study," *Canadian Medical Association Journal* 170 (2004): 1678–86.

41   C. H. Rojas-Fernandez, D. Carver, and R. Tonks, "Population trends in
the prevalence of benzodiazepine use in the older population of Nova
Scotia: A cause for concern?" *Canadian Journal of Clinical Pharmacology* 6,
no. 3 (1999): 149–56. See also, "Therapeutics Initiative. Use of Benzodi-
azepines ibn BC. Is it consistent with the recommendations?" Found at:
http://www.ti.ubc.ca/PDF/54.pdf (accessed 21 June 2007); and K. Tu,
M. Mamdani, J. Hux, and J. Tu, "Progressive Trends in the Prevalence of
Benzodiazepine Prescribing in Older People in Ontario, Canada," *Journal
of the American Geriatric Society* 49, no. 10 (October, 2001): 1341–5.

42   "Accessible, safe, client-centred, timely, efficient, and equitable," from the
Saskatchewan Health Quality Council Annual Report 2004/2005 (Regi-
na, 2005). Found at: http://www.hqc.sk.ca/download.jsp?DB3G1
GthpqzpLvJEazdYnX8xfpeDzqbvqhr5yD/Ts9e8cXBjtGTIzA==
(accessed 24 July 2006).

43   "Acceptability, accessibility, appropriateness, effectiveness, efficiency, and
safety," from the Alberta Quality Matrix for Health (Alberta Health
Quality Council). Found at: http://www.hqca.ca/index.php?id=87
(accessed 11 April 2007).

44   Ontario Health Quality Council 2006 Annual Report (Toronto, 2006).
Found at: http://www.ohqc.ca/pdfs/ohqc_report_2006en.pdf (accessed 6
June 2006).

45   US Institute of Medicine, *Crossing the Quality Chasm: A New Health System for the 21st Century* (Washington, DC: National Academy Press,
2001).

46   *Quebec Public Health Act* (updated 1 September 2003) http://publications
duquebec.gouv.qc.ca/dynamicSearch/telecharge.php?type=2&file=/
S_2_2/S2_2_A.html (accessed 26 September 2003); National Institute of
Public Health Act http://publi cationsduquebec.gouv.qc.ca/
dynamicSearch/telecharge.php?type=2&file=/I_13_1_1/I13_1_1_A.htm
l (accessed 26 September 2003).

47   See Pathways to Education: http://pathwaystoeducation.ca/
home-executive.html (accessed 12 April 2007).

48   Health Disparities Task Group of the Federal Provincial Territorial Advi-

sory Committee on Population Health and Health Security, "Health Disparities: Roles of the Health Sector" (2004). Found at: http://www.phac-aspc.gc.ca/ph-sp/disparities/pdf06/disparities_discussion_paper_e.pdf (accessed 23 September 2006).

49   Ibid.

50   Ibid.

51   "A population health strategy focuses on factors that enhance the health and well-being of the overall population. It views health as an asset that is a resource for everyday living, not simply the absence of disease. Population health concerns itself with the living and working conditions that enable and support people in making healthy choices, and the services that promote and maintain health," from Federal Provincial Territorial Advisory Committee on Population Health, "Strategies for Population Health: Investing in the Health of Canadians" (1994).

52   M. Lalonde, "A New Perspective on the Health of Canadians" (Ministry of Supply and Services,1974). Found at: http://www.phac-aspc.gc.ca/ph-sp/phdd/pdf/perspective.pdf (accessed 4 November 2005).

53   J. Epp, "Achieving Health for All: A Framework for Health Promotion," released at First International conference on Health Promotion (Ottawa, 1986). Found at: http://www.hc-sc.gc.ca/hcs-sss/pubs/care-soins/2001-frame-plan-promotion/index_e.html (accessed 7 September 2006).

54   B. Zimmerman and S. Globerman, "Complicated and Complex Systems: What Would Successful Reform of Medicare Look Like?" in *Health Care Services and the Process of Change*, ed. P.G. Forest, T. McIntosh, and G. Marchildon (Toronto: University of Toronto Press, 2004): 21–53.

55   Health Disparities Task Group of the Federal Provincial Territorial Advisory Committee on Population Health and Health Security, "Health Disparities: Roles of the Health Sector" (2004). Found at: http://www.phac-aspc.gc.ca/ph-sp/disparities/pdf06/disparities_discussion_paper_e.pdf (accessed 23 September 2006).

56   M. Lemura, C. Neudorf, and J. Opondo, "Health disparities by neighbourhood income," *Canadian Journal of Public Health* 97 (2006): 435–9.

57   See: http://www.saskatoonhealthregion.ca/news_you_need/media_centre/media/2006/news_091106.htm (accessed 11 April 2007).

58   Saskatchewan Hansard, 19 March 2007. Found at: http://www.legassembly.sk.ca/committees/HumanServices/Verbatim/070319HU.pdf (accessed 11 April 2007).

59   W. Langewitz, M. Denz, A. Keller, et al., "Spontaneous taking time at start of consultation in outclient clinic: cohort study," *British Medical Journal* 325 (2002): 682–3.

60   H. B. Beckman, and R. M. Frankel, "The effect of physician behavior on

the collection of data," *Annals of Internal Medicine* 101 (1984): 692–6.

61 M.K. Marvel, R.M. Epstein, K. Flowers, et al., "Soliciting the client's agenda: have we improved? " *Journal of the American Medical Association* 281 1999): 283–7.

62 C.H. Braddock, K.A. Edwards, N.M. Hasenberg, et al., "Informed decision making in outpatient practice: times to get back to basics," *Journal of the American Medical Association* 282 (1999): 2313–20.

63 J. Oxman-Martinez and J. Hanley, "Health and services for Canada's multicultural population: challenges to equity," Canada Citizenship and Immigration, in "Serving Canada's multicultural population for the future," discussion papers (2005). Found at: http://www.pch.gc.ca/multi/canada2017/PDFs/document_e.pdf (accessed 20 November 2006).

64 J. M. Anderson, "Ethnicity and illness experience: Ideological structures and the health care delivery system," *Social Science & Medicine* 22 (1986): 1277–83.

65 Oxman-Martinez and Hanley, "Health and services for Canada's multicultural population."

66 Schoen, Osborn, Huynh et al., "On the front lines of care."

67 See the website for the London Intercommunity Health Centre: http://www.lihc.on.ca/; or the Latin American Diabetes Program: http://www.pldiabetes.com/.

68 B. Harvey, "The diabetes epidemic from a CHC perspective," presentation to the annual meeting of the Association of Ontario Health Centres (Kingston, 5 June 2006).

69 R.S.A. Hayward, G.H. Guyatt, K.A. Moore, et al., "Canadian Physicians' attitudes about and preferences regarding clinical practice guidelines," *Canadian Medical Association Journal* 156 (1997): 1715–23.

70 B. Hutchison, C.A. Woodward, and G.R. Norman, et al., "Provision of preventive care to unannounced standardized clients," *Canadian Medical Association Journal* 158 (1998): 185–93.

71 Ontario Health Quality Council First Annual Report (Toronto, April 2006).

72 Schoen, Osborn, Huynh, et al., "Taking the pulse of health care systems."

73 Organization for Economic Cooperation and Development, "Health data set" (10 October 2006). Found at: http://www.oecd.org/dataoecd/20/51/37622205.xls (accessed 25 April 2007).

74 Ontario Health Quality Council 2007 Report (Toronto, 2007), 42. Also see: http://www.accessalliance.ca/.

75 M.M. Rachlis, "Public Solutions to Health Care Wait Lists" (Canadian Centre for Policy Alternatives: Ottawa, January 2006). Found at: http://policyalternatives.ca/documents/National_Office_Pubs/2005/Health_Care_Waitlists.pdf (accessed 12 January 2006).

76   For more details see the Health Quality Council's website: http://www.hqc.sk.ca.

77   N. Kates, A.M. Crustolo, S. Farrar, et al., "Mental health and nutrition: integrating specialists' services into primary care," *Canadian Family Physician* 48 (2002):1898–1903.

78   N. Kates, "Managing chronic mental health problems in primary care," presentation to Ministry of Health and Long-Term Care Expo" (Toronto, 19 April 2006).

79   Alberta hip and knee replacement project: Interim results (Alberta Bone and Joint Institute, December 2005). Found at: http://www.albertaboneandjoint.com/PDFs/Int_Rep_Dec_19_05.pdf (accessed 20 December 2005).

80   C.M. Hohl, J. Dankoff, A. Colacone, et al., "Polypharmacy, adverse drug-related events, and potential adverse drug interactions in elderly clients presenting to an emergency department," *Annals of Emergency Medicine* 38 (2001): 666–71.

81   R.M. Tamblyn, P.J. McLeod, M. Abrahamowicz, et al., "Questionable prescribing for elderly clients in Quebec," *Canadian Medical Association Journal* 150 (1994): 1801–9.

82   US Institute of Medicine, *To Err is Human: Building a Safer Health Care System*, eds. L.T. Kohn, J.M. Corrigan, and M.S. Donaldson (Washington, DC: National Academy Press, 2000).

83   Ibid.

84   See http://www.oscarmcmaster.ca for more details.

85   D. Chan, "Free/Libre Open Source Software (FLOSS) in Health Care: showcase of OSCAR, a Canadian product," presentation (12 November 2006).

86   See: http://www.caisi.ca/wiki/index.php/Main_Page (accessed 15 December 2006).

87   Rachlis, "Public Solutions to Health Care Wait Lists."

88   Statistics Canada, "2005 National Survey of the Work and Health of Nurses" (2006), Catalogue no-83-003-XIE.

89   S. Jenssen, and M. McCracken, *Trends in Illness and Injury Related Absenteeism and Overtime among Publicly Employed Registered Nurses* (Canadian Nurses Association: Ottawa, 2006).

90   Schoen, Osborn, Huynh, et al. "On the front lines of care."

91   Beth Jackson, Ann Pederson, and Madeline Boscoe, "Gender-Based Analysis and Wait Times: new Questions, New Knowledge," a discussion paper, available at http://www.cwhn.ca.

92   Manfred Huber, *The Need to Improve the Comparability of Long-Term Care Expenditure Data: Recent Estimates From a Selection of OECD Countries and Follow-Up Work* (Paris: OECD, 2005): 8.

93   Applied Management in association with Fraser Group Tristat Resources, "Canadians' access to insurance for prescription medicines: volume 2: the un-insured and under-insured" (Ottawa: Health Transition Fund, 2000).

94   Ministry of Health and Long-Term Care, *2005/05 Report Care for the Ontario Drug Benefit Program"* (Toronto, 2006).

95   W.J. Ungar, C. Daniels, T. McNeill, and M. Seyed, "Children in need of pharmacare: medication funding requests at the Toronto Hospital for Sick Children," *Canadian Journal of Public Health* 94 (2003): 121–6

96   J. Lexchin, "Income class and pharmaceutical expenditure in Canada: 1964–1990," *Canadian Journal of Public Health* 87 (1996): 46–50.

97   P. Grootendorst, D. Palfrey, D. Willison, and J. Hurley, "A review of the comprehensiveness of provincial drug coverage for Canadian seniors," *Canadian Journal on Aging* 22 (2003): 33–44.

98   S. Jacobzone, "Pharmaceutical policies in OECD countries: reconciling social and industrial goals," Labour market and social policy occasional papers No. 40 (Paris: OECD, 2000).

99   Standing Senate Committee on Social Affairs, Science and Technology, *The Health of Canadians: The Federal Role*, vol. 4: *Issues and Opinions* (Ottawa).

100 Commission on the Future of Health Care in Canada, *Building on Values: The Future of Health Care in Canada: Final Report* (Saskatoon: The Commission, 2002).

101 Federal/Provincial/Territorial Ministerial Task Force, *National Pharmaceuticals Strategy Progress Report* (Ottawa: Health Canada, 2006).

102 Federal/Provincial/Territorial Working Group on Drug Prices, *Cost Driver Analysis of Provincial Drug Plans. Ontario, 1992/93–1998/99* (Ottawa: Health Canada, 2000).

103 Robyn Tamblyn, Rejean Laprise, James A. Hanley, et al., "Adverse events associated with prescription drug cost-sharing among poor and elderly persons," *Journal of the American Medical Association* 285 (2001): 421–9.

104 C.L. Taylor, *The Corporate Response to Rising Health Care Costs* (Ottawa: Conference Board of Canada, 1996).

105 Palmer D'Angelo Consulting Inc, "National pharmacare cost impact study" (Ottawa, 1997).

106 Mark Stabile, "Impacts of private insurance on utilization," presented at Toward a National Strategy on Drug Insurance (Toronto, 2002).

107 Productivity Commission, "International pharmaceutical price differences: research report" (Canberra: AusInfo, 2001).

108 Pharmaceutical Management Agency, "Annual review 2005" (Wellington, 2006).

109 D.J. Graham, D. Campen, R. Hui, M. Spence, C. Cheetham, G. Levy, S.

Shoor, and W.A. Ray, "Risk of acute myocardial infarction and sudden cardiac death in patients treated with cyclo-oxygenase 2 selective and non-selective non-steroidal anti-inflammatory drugs: nested case-control study," *Lancet* 365 (2005): 475–81.

[110] This is a revised and updated version of an essay that first appeared in volume 18 of *Inroads* (2006): 94–108.

[111] Steve Morgan, "Drug Spending in Canada: Recent Trends and Causes," *Medical Care* 42 (2004): 640.

[112] *Building on Values: The Future of Health Care in Canada* (Saskatoon: Commission on the Future of Health Care in Canada, 2002), chapter 9.

[113] Gregory P. Marchildon, *Health System Profile: Canada* (Toronto: University of Toronto Press, 2006): table 4.4.

[114] Because of the Quebec drug plan's different funding and administrative structure, the Quebec plan data (under social security funds) have been added to the provincial/territorial drug plan data for the purposes of this analysis.

[115] A.H. Anix, D. Guh, and X. Wang, "A Dog's Breakfast: Prescription Drug Coverage Varies Widely across Canada," *Medical Care* 39 (2004): 315–324.

[116] Palmer D'Angelo Consulting Inc., *Cost Impact Study of a National Pharmacare Program for Canada: An Update to the 1997 Report* (Ottawa: Palmer D'Angelo Consulting Inc. for Health Canada, 2002).

[117] France St-Hilaire, "Fiscal Gaps and Imbalances: The New Fundamentals of Canadian Federalism," notes for a panel presentation, Institute of Intergovernmental Relations, Queen's University, updated 20 May 2005.

[118] Barbara Mintzes and Joel Lexchin, "Do Higher Drug Costs Lead to Better Health?" *Canadian Journal of Clinical Pharmacology* 12 (2005): 22–27.

[119] In this paper, I draw from a Manitoba Centre for Health Policy report on mental illness. P. Martens, R. Fransoo, N. McKeen, The Need to Know Team, E. Burland, L. Jebamani, C. Burchill, C. DeCoster, O. Ekuma, H. Prior, D. Chateau, R. Robinson, and C. Metge, "Patterns of Regional Mental Illness Disorder Diagnoses and Service Use in Manitoba: A Population-Based Study" (Winnipeg, MB: Manitoba Centre for Health Policy, September 2004). The full report is available at http://www.umanitoba.ca/centres/mchp/. It was truly a team effort, co-funded through the Canadian Institutes of Health Research and the MCHP/Manitoba Health contract. Our team is called The Need to Know Team – a group of top-level regional planners from the eleven Regional Health Authorities of Manitoba, planners from Manitoba Health, and University of Manitoba researchers at MCHP working together to produce research of relevance to decision makers. Descriptions of the team are available in various publications including: P.J. Martens and N.P. Roos, "When health services researchers and policy-

makers interact: Tales from the tectonic plates," *Healthcare Policy* 1, no. 1 (2005): 72–84; S. Bowenand P.J. Martens, and The Need to Know Team, "Demystifying 'Knowledge Translation': Learning from the Community," *Journal of Health Services Research & Policy* 10, no, 4 (2005): 203–211; and S. Bowen, P.J. Martens, "A model for collaborative evaluation of university-community partnerships," *Journal of Epidemiological and Community Health* 60, no.10 (2006): 902–907.

120 Martens, Fransoo, McKeen, et al., "Patterns of Regional Mental Illness Disorder Diagnoses and Service Use in Manitoba: A Population-Based Study"

121 P.J. Martens, R. Fransoo, The Need To Know Team, E. Burland, C. Burchill, H.J. Prior, and O. Ekuma, "Prevalence of mental illness and its impact on the use of home care and nursing homes: a population-based study of older adults in Manitoba, Canada," *Canadian Journal of Psychiatry* (in press, 2007).

122 The Standing Senate Committee on Social Affairs, Science and Technology, *Out of the Shadows at Last: Final Report of the Standing Senate Committee on Social Affairs, Science and Technology* [The Honourable Michael J.L. Kirby, Chair; the Honourable Wilbert Joseph Keon, Deputy Chair] (Government of Canada, May 2006).

123 The author would like to thank Freya Lilius for her contribution to this paper.

124 Tommy Douglas, "Keynote Address: SOS Medicare Conference" (Regina, Saskatchewan, 1979).

125 Monique Bégin, "Panel Presentation: SOS2 Medicare Conference" (Regina Saskatchewan, 2007).

126 Canadian Home Care Association (CHCA), *Home Care: A National Health Priority* (Position Statement, 2004).

127 Jane Aronson, "Elderly people's accounts of home care rationing: missing voices in long-term care policy debates," *Aging in Society* 22, no. 4 (2002): 399–418.

128 Marcus J. Hollander, "The National Evaluation of the Cost Effectiveness of Home Care. Substudy 1: Final Report of the Study on the Comparative Cost Analysis of Home Care and Residential Care Services" (2002) retrieved April 2007: http://www.homecarestudy.com/reports/full-text/substudy-01-final_report.pdf

129 Canada, *Report of the Royal Commission on Health Services* [Chair: Emmett Hall] (Ottawa: Queen's Printer, 1964).

130 Canadian Institute for Health Information (CIHI), *Exploring the 70/30 Split: How Canada's Health Care System is Financed,* (2005).

131 J. Eales, N. Keating, and J. Fast, "Analysis of the impact of federal, provincial and regional policies on the economic well-being of informal

caregivers of frail seniors," a report submitted to the Federal/Provin-
cial/Territorial Committee of Officials (Seniors) (2001).

[132] Susan Stobert and Kelly Cranswick, "Looking After Seniors: Who Does What For Whom?" *Canadian Social Trends,* vol. 74 (Statistics Canada, Autumn 2004).

[133] Canadian Home Care Human Resources Study, Final Report, 2003 (Co-chaired: Canadian Home Care Association, Human Resources Development, Canada)

[134] Neena L. Chappell, *Maintaining the Integrity of Home Care* 1, no. 4 (2000): 91–5.

[135] Health Canada, "National Profile of Family Caregivers in Canada, Final Report" (2002) http://www.hc-sc.gc.ca/

[136] Hollander, "The National Evaluation of the Cost–Effectiveness of Home Care."

Part Five: Inequality and Social Determinants of Health

[1] Robert G. Evans, "Introduction" in *Why Are Some People Healthy and Others Not?* ed. Robert G. Evans, Morris L. Barer, and Theodore R. Marmor (Hawthorne, NY: Aldine de Gruyter, 1994): 3–26.

[2] Robert Evans, *Interpreting and Addressing Inequalities in Health: From Black to Acheson to Blair to …?* (London: OHE and CIAR, 2002): 15.

[3] *The Solid* Facts, ed. Michael Marmot and Richard Wilkinson, 2 ed. (Copenhagen: WHO, 2003): 10.

[4] Louise Lemyre, et al., *Gradient in Psychological Stress by Executive Level in Canadian Civil Servants,* slide (Ottawa: GAP and University of Ottawa, 2002–2006).

[5] *Applying a Population Health Perspective to Health Planning and Decision-Making* (Ottawa: CPHI/CIHI, 2006), PowerPoint presentation 92 slides. This applies to the first five bullets.

[6] *Improving the Health of Canadians* (Ottawa: CPHI/CIHI, Sept. 2004): 80. This applies to the three last bullets.

[7] Official site of the Canadian Association of Food Banks/Association canadienne des banques alimentaires http://www.cafb-acba.ca.

[8] Senate Committee on Social Affairs, Science & Technology. RE: Study on the impact of the multiple factors and conditions that contribute to the health of Canada's population — known collectively as the social determinants of health, chaired by Senator Willie Keon.

[9] Armine Yalnizyan, *The Rich and the Rest of Us: The Changing Face of Canada's Growing Gap* (Toronto: Canadian Centre for Policy Alternatives, 2006): 29.

[10] Aboriginal and Northern Affairs; Culture, Heritage and Tourism; Education, Training and Youth; Family Services and Housing; Health; Justice;

and Status of Women. It is chaired by the minister of Health Living.

11   The project is led by Johan Fritzell, professor of Sociology, and Olle Lundberg, professor of Health Equity Studies.

12   David I Hay, *Economic Arguments for Action on the Social Determinants of Health* (Ottawa: Public Health Agency of Canada/Canadian Policy Research Network, 2006): 13.

13   This paper is excerpted from Dennis Raphael, *Poverty and Policy in Canada: Implications for Health and Quality of Life* (Toronto: Canadian Scholars' Press, 2007).

14   Innocenti Research Centre, *Child Poverty in Rich Nations, 2005. Report Card No. 6.* (Florence: Innocenti Research Centre, 2005).

15   Organization for Economic Cooperation and Development, *Society at a Glance: OECD Social Indicators 2005 Edition* (Paris, France: OECD, 2005).

16   D. Raphael, "Increasing poverty threatens the health of all Canadians," *Canadian Family Physician* 47 (2001): 1703–6.

17   K. Judge, and I. Paterson, *Treasury Working Paper: Poverty, Income Inequality and Health* (Wellington, NZ: Government of New Zealand, 2002).

18   T. Bryant, "Politics, public policy and population health," in *Staying Alive: Critical Perspectives on Health, Illness, and Health Care*, ed. D. Raphael, T. Bryant, and M. Rioux (Toronto: Canadian Scholars' Press, 2006): 193–216.

19   D. Brady, "The politics of poverty: Left political institutions, the welfare state, and poverty," *Social Forces* 82 (2003): 557–88.

20   Innocenti Research Centre, *Child Poverty in Rich Nations*.

21   R. Wilkins, J.M. Berthelot, and E. Ng, "Trends in mortality by neighbourhood income in urban Canada from 1971 to 1996," *Health Reports (Stats Can)* 13 Supplement (2002): 1–28.

22   Ibid.

23   Ibid.

24   G. Xi, I. McDowell, R. Nair, and R. Spasoff, "Income inequality and health in Ontario: A multilevel analysis," *Canadian Journal of Public Health* 96, no. 3 (2005): 206–11.

25   K. Humphries, and E. van Doorslaer, "Income related health inequality in Canada," *Social Science & Medicine* 50, no. 5 (2000): 663–71.

26   Canadian Institute on Children's Health, *The Health of Canada's Children: A CICH Profile 3rd Edition* (Ottawa: Canadian Institute on Children's Health, 2000).

27   R. Wilkins, C. Houle, J.-M. Berthelot, and D. P. Ross, "The changing health status of Canada's children," *ISUMA* 1, no. 2 (2000): 57–63.

28   Wilkins, Berthelot, and Ng, "Trends in mortality by neighbourhood income," 1–28.

29   D. Raphael, S. Anstice, and K. Raine, "The social determinants of the

incidence and management of Type 2 Diabetes Mellitus: Are we prepared to rethink our questions and redirect our research activities?" *Leadership in Health Services* 16 (2003): 10–20; and D. Raphael, and E. S. Farrell, "Beyond medicine and lifestyle: Addressing the societal determinants of cardiovascular disease in North America," *Leadership in Health Services* 15 (2002): 1–5.

30   Wilkins, Houle, Berthelot, and Ross, "The changing health status of Canada's children," 57–63.

31   D.P. Ross, and P. Roberts, *Income and Child Well-being: A New Perspective on the Poverty Debate* (Ottawa, Canada: Canadian Council on Social Development, 1999).

32   Canadian Institute on Children's Health, *The Health of Canada's Children.*

33   N. Auger, M. Raynault, R. Lessard, and R. Choinière, "Income and health in Canada," in *Social Determinants of Health: Canadian Perspectives*, ed. D. Raphael (Toronto: Canadian Scholars' Press, 2004).

34   G. Davey Smith, and D. Gordon, "Poverty across the life-course and health," in *Tackling Inequalities: Where Are We Now and What Can Be Done?* ed. C. Pantazis and D. Gordon (Bristol, UK: Policy Press, 2000).

35   G. Davey Smith, D. Grunnell, and Y. Ben-Shlomo, "Life-course approaches to socioeconomic differentials in cause-specific adult mortality," in *Poverty, Inequality and Health: An International Perspective*, ed. D. Leon and G. Walt (New York: Oxford Universtiy Press, 2001), 88–124.

36   M. Shields, and S. Tremblay, "The health of Canada's communities," *Health Reports* Supplement, 13 (July 2002): 9–13

37   S. Tremblay, N.A. Ross, and J.-M. Berthelot, (2002). "Regional Socio-economic Context and Health," *Health Reports* Supplement, 13 (2002): 1–12.

38   Government of British Columbia, *A Report on the Health of British Columbians* (Victoria, Canada: Government of British Columbia, 2000); Government of Ontario, *Wealth and Health, Health and Wealth* (Toronto, Canada: Government of Ontario, Queen's Printer for Ontario, 1994); N. Hamilton, and T. Bhatti, *Population Health Promotion: An Integrated Model of Population Health and Health Promotion* (Ottawa: Health Canada, 1996); Health Canada, "Taking Action on Population Health: A Position Paper for Health Promotion and Programs Branch Staff" (Ottawa: Health Canada, 1998).

39   Canadian Public Health Association, *Inequities in Health* (Ottawa, Canada: Canadian Public Health Association, 1993); Canadian Public Health Association, *The Health Impacts of Unemployment* (Ottawa, Canada: Canadian Public Health Association, 1996); Canadian Public Health Association, *Health Impacts of Social and Economic Conditions: Implications for Public Policy* (Ottawa, Canada: Canadian Public Health Association, 1997);

and Canadian Public Health Association, *Reducing poverty and its negative effects on health: resolution passed at the 2000 CPHA Annual Meeting* (2000), from http://www.cpha.ca/english/policy/resolu/2000s/2000/page2.htm.

40   P. M. Lantz, J. S. House, J. M. Lepkowski, D. R. Williams, R. P. Mero, and J.J. Chen, "Socioeconomic factors, health behaviors, and mortality," *Journal of the American Medical Association* 279, no. 21(1998): 1703–8.

41   R. Labonte, and S. Penfold, "Canadian perspectives in health promotion: A critique," *Health Education* 19(1981): 4–9.

42   M. Benzeval, K. Judge, and M. Whitehead, *Tackling Inequalities in Health: An Agenda for Action* (London: Kings Fund,1995).

43   M. J. Jarvis, and J. Wardle, "Social patterning of individual health behaviours: the case of cigarette smoking," in ed. M. G. Marmot and R. G. Wilkinson, *Social Determinants of Health* (Oxford, UK: Oxford University Press, 1999), 340–55.

44   D. Raphael, "Barriers to addressing the determinants of health: public health units and poverty in Ontario, Canada," *Health Promotion International* 18 (2003): 397–405.

45   R. Labonte, "Death of Program, Birth of Metaphor: The Development of Health Promotion in Canada," in *Health Promotion in Canada*, ed. A. Pederson, M. O'Neill and I. Rootman (Toronto: W.B. Saunders, 1994): 79.

46   S. Nettleton, "Surveillance, health promotion and the formation of a risk identity," in *Debates and Dilemmas in Promoting Health*, ed. M. Sidell, L. Jones, J. Katz, and A. Peberdy, (London, UK: Open University Press, 1997): 314–24.

47   D. Raphael, "Social determinants of health: Present status, unresolved questions, and future directions," *International Journal of Health Services* 36 (2006): 651–77.

48   Sudbury Health Unit, and Alder Group, *Determinants of health: Developing an action plan for public health* (Sudbury: The Sudbury and District Health Unit, 2006).

49   D. Raphael, J. Macdonald, R. Labonte, R. Colman, K. Hayward, and R. Torgerson, "Researching income and income distribution as a determinant of health in Canada: Gaps 236 Poverty and Policy in Canada between theoretical knowledge, research practice, and policy implementation," *Health Policy* 72 (2005): 217–32.

50   D. Coburn, "Income inequality, social cohesion and the health status of populations: The role of neo-liberalism," *Social Science & Medicine* 51, no. 1 (2000): 135–46; D. Coburn, "Beyond the income inequality hypothesis: Globalization, neo-liberalism, and health inequalities," *Social Science & Medicine* 58 no. 1 (2004): 41–56; G. Teeple, *Globalization and the Decline of Social Reform: Into the Twenty First Century* (Aurora, Ontario: Garamond Press, 2000).

51   R.J. Romanow, *Building on Values: The Future of Health Care in Canada* (Saskatoon: Commission on the Future of Health Care in Canada, 2002).

52   P. Freire, P., *Pedagogy of the Oppressed,* (New York:Seabury Press, 1970), p. 76.

53   D. Bohm, D., *Wholeness and the Implicate Order,* (New York,London: Routledge, 1980.)

54   W. Ermine, W., "Ethical Space: Transforming Relations," Commissioned Paper, (Heritage Canada, 2005); accessed at: http://www.traditions.gc.ca/docs/docs_disc_ermine_e.cfmavailable on Heritage Canada website;. R. Poole, R., *Towards Deep Subjectivity,* (London: Penguin Press, 1972).

55   G. Cajete, G., *Look to the Mountain: An Ecology of Indigenous Education,* 1st ed. (Durango, CO: Kivaki Press, 1994), p. 164.

56   D. Raphael, ed., *Social Determinants of Health: Canadian Perspectives* (Toronto: Canadian Scholars Press, 2004): 15; I. Kawachi, and B. Kennedy, *The Health of Nations: Why Inequality is Harmful to Your Health* (New York: New Press, 2002).

57   D. Bolm, *Unfolding Meaning: A Weekend of Dialogue with David Bohm* (London: Routledge, 1996).

Part Six: Getting There from Here

1   Roy J. Romanow, "A House Half Built," *The Walrus* (2006), available from: http://www.atkinsonfoundation.ca/files/ Walrus_RJR_pack_light.pdf.

2   Attorney General of Saskatchewan, cited in Supreme Court of Canada's *Reference re: Secession of Quebec,* [1998] 2 S.C.R. 217, available from: http://csc.lexum.umontreal.ca/en/1998/1998rcs2-217/ 1998rcs2-217.html

3   Government of Canada, *Canada Health Act* [R.S. c-6 1985].

4   Canadian Institute of Health Information, *Health Care in Canada 2006* (2006).

5   Canadian Institute of Health information, *Health Care in Canada: A First Annual Report* (2000).

6   Harriet Jackson and Alison McDermott, *Health Care Spending: Prospect and Retrospect, Analytical Note* (Economic and Fiscal Policy Branch, Department of Finance, 2004).

7   S. Landon, M.L. McMillan, V. Muralidharan, and M. Parsons, "Does Health Care Spending Crowd Out Other Provincial Government Expenditures?" *Canadian Public Policy* 32, no. 2 (2006): 121–42.

8   Canadian Institute for Health Information, 2006.

9   Cited in, Canadian Health Care Association, "A Strong Publicly-Funded

Health System: Keeping Canadians Healthy and Securing Our Place in a Competitive World," October 2006.

10   S. Woolhandler, T. Campbell, and D. Himmelstein, "Costs of Health Care Administration in the United States and Canada," *New England Journal of Medicine* 349, no. 8 (2003): 768–75.

11   Organisation for Economic Co-operation and Development, *A Comparative Analysis of 30 Countries* (Paris: OECD, 2006).

12   Some estimates project that US health care spending will increase to 20 percent of GDP in the next decade, see C. Borger, et al., "Health Spending Projections Through 2015: Changes on the Horizon," *Health Affairs Web Exclusive* W61: 22 February 2006. For Canada and US health spending figures see, Organisation for Economic Co-operation and Development, *OECD Health Data 2006:* (Paris: OECD, 2006).

13   US Census Bureau, *United States Census 2000* (2006).

14   D. Himmelstein, et al., "Illness and Injury as Contributors to Bankruptcy," *Health Affairs* 24, no. 1 (2005): 1.

15   Organisation for Economic Co-operation and Development, *A Comparitive Analysis fo 30 Countries.*

16   Canadian Health Care Association, "A Strong Publicly-Funded Health System."

17   Ibid.

18   Statistics Canada, *Access to Health Care Services in Canada: January to December 2005* (2005).

19   For an excellent analysis of contemporary debates about health care in Canada, see G. Marchildon, *Health Care in Canada and the United States: Consumer Good, Social Service or Right of Citizenship,* presented during the Roatch Global Lecture Series on Social Policy and Practice: Arizona State University (March 2006), available from: http://www.asu.edu/xed/roatch/index.html.

20   *Chaoulli v. Quebec* (Attorney General). [2005] SCC 35 (June 2005).

21   For a more in-depth discussion on the *Chaoulli* case, see *Access to Care, Access to Justice: The Legal Debate Over Private Health Insurance in Canada,* ed. (Colleen M. Flood, Lorne Sossin, and Kent Roach, Toronto: University of Toronto Press, 2005); and Theodore Marmor, "An American in Canada: Making Sense of the Supreme Court Decision on Health Care," in *Policy Options* (Montreal: Institute for Research in Public Policy, September 2005), 42.

22   Theodore Marmor, "Canada's Supreme Court and its National Health Insurance Program: Evaluating the Landmark Chaoulli Decision from an Imperative Prespective," *Osgoode Hall Law Journal* 44 (2006).

23   Roy J. Romanow, *Building on Values: The Future of Health Care in Canada* (Saskatoon: Commission on the Future of Health Care in Canada, 2002).

24 Ibid.

25 See, for example, Commission on the Future of Health Care in Canada, *Report on Citizens' Dialogue On the Future of Health Care in Canada* (June 2002).

26 See *e.g., Hunger v. Southam Inc.*, [1984] 2 S.C.R. 145.

27 See *e.g., RJR-MacDonald v. Canada (Attorney General)*, [1995] 3 S.C.R. 199.

28 See *e.g., R. v. Big M Drug Mart Ltd.*, [1985] 1 S.C.R. 295.

29 For example, the Supreme Court of Canada decided in *Re B.C. Motor Vehicle Act* to broaden its Charter powers by ignoring the clearly stated intention of the Charter's drafters and interpreting the "principles of fundamental justice" in section 7 as embracing substantive as well as procedural values: [1985] 2 S.C.R. 486.

30 [2005] 1 S.C.R. 791.

31 For a fuller discussion of the *Chaoulli* decision and the political nature of the Charter, see Andrew Petter, "Wealthcare: The Politics of the Charter Revisited" in *Access to Care, Access to Justice*, ed. Flood, Roach, and Sossin at 128–31.

32 Madame Justice B.M. McLachlin, Speech to the "25th Anniversary of the Charter Symposium," Toronto, 12 April 2007.

33 It might be hoped that such advocacy would also persuade politicians to invoke the notwithstanding clause in section 33 of the Charter should future court decisions go the wrong way. However, given the political constraints that have built up around its use, I doubt that that section 33 is a viable option. This is especially so given that, in order to be effective on this issue, section 33 would require all ten provincial legislatures to enact new legislation every five years.

34 Stuart N. Soroka, *A Report to the Health Council of Canada: Canadian Perceptions of the Health Care System* (Toronto: Health Council of Canada, 2007).

35 Ibid.:3.

36 Ibid.

37 Ibid.

38 Alicia Priest, Michael Rachlis, and Marcy Cohen, *Why Wait? Public Solutions to Cure Surgical Waitlists* (Vancouver, Canadian Center for Policy Alternatives, May 2007).

39 J. M. Murphy, *Residential Care Quality: A Review of the Literature on Nurse and Personal Care Staffing and Quality of Care*, (Victoria Nursing Directorate, British Columbia Ministry of Health, 2005); G. and B. Clarke, "How the Dutch do it: The role of the nursing home in the Netherlands," *Geriatrics Today: Journal of the Canadian Geriatrics Society* 7, no. 3 (2004). Online version accessed at: http://www.canadiangeriatrics.com/

pubs/GTSept2005/GTSept2004BethuneClarke.pdf

40 K. Tee, T.S. Ehmann, and G.W. MacEwan, "Early Psychosis Identification and Intervention Psychiatric Services," *Psychiatric Services* 54, no. 4 (2003): 573.

41 Marta Szebehely, "The Women Friendly Welfare State? Scandinavian Elder Care in Transition," paper presented at "Imagining Public Policy to Meet Women's Economic Needs" (Vancouver, Canadian Center for Policy Alternatives, October 2005).

42 Marcy Cohen, Democratizing Public Services, Lesson from Other Jurisdictions and Implications for Health Care Reform in BC," Vancouver, Canadian Centre for Policy Alternatives , 2005), accessed at: http://policyalternatives.ca/index.cfm?act=news&do=Article&call=1057&pA=a2286b2a&type=2,3,4,5,6,7

43 This paper draws on: RNAO, *Creating a Healthier Society: RNAO's Challenge to Ontario's Political Parties — Building Medicare's Next Stage* (Toronto: Registered Nurses' Association of Ontario, May 2007). This document, which includes complete references and data sources, can be downloaded from http://www.rnao.org.

44 Tommy Douglas, "Speech to the Canadian Labour Congress on the Public Healthcare System" (1970).

45 Tommy Douglas, "Speech on the State of the Medicare Program" (1982).

46 A detailed presentation can be found in: RNAO, *Creating a Healthier Society*.

47 All the references and data sources are provided in RNAO, *Creating a Healthier Society*.

Marcia Angell, MD, is senior lecturer in the Department of Social Medicine at Harvard Medical School. She stepped down as editor-in-chief of the *New England Journal of Medicine* in 2000 after more than twenty years with the *Journal*. She trained in both internal medicine and anatomic pathology and is a board-certified pathologist. Dr. Angell writes frequently in professional journals and the popular media on a wide range of health topics. Her most recent book is *The Truth About the Drug Companies: How They Deceive Us and What to Do About It* (Random House, 2004). Dr. Angell is a master of the American College of Physicians and a fellow of the American Association for the Advancement of Science. In 1997, *Time* magazine named Marcia Angell one of the twenty-five most influential Americans.

Pat Armstrong has served as chair of the Department of Sociology at York University, and the director of Canadian Studies at Carleton University. She is a partner in the National Network on Environment and Women's Health and chairs a working group on health reform that crosses the Centres of Excellence for Women's Health. She is also a site director for the Ontario Training Centre in Health Services and Policy Research and a board member of the Canadian Centre for Policy Alternatives. She is co-author or editor of many books including: *Women and Health Care Reform in Canada; Caring For/Caring About: Women, Home Care and Unpaid Caregiving; Heal Thyself: Managing Health Care Reform; Wasting Away: The Undermining of Canadian Health Care; Vital Signs: Nursing in Transition;* and *Take Care: Warning Signals for Canada's Health System.*

Elisabeth Ballermann was elected in 1995 as the president of the Health Sciences Association of Alberta (HSAA), which represents over 14,000 allied health professionals and support workers in over 150 occupations. She is a vice-president of the Alberta Federation of Labour and the National Union of Public and General Employees, and is a founding member of the Canadian Health Professionals Secretariat. She also represents HSAA as a member of the board of the Friends of Medicare (Alberta) and the Parkland Institute at the University of Alberta.

Maude Barlow is the national chairperson of The Council of Canadians. She is co-founder of the Blue Planet Project to stop the commodification of the world's water. She is a director of the San Francisco-based International Forum on Globalization and a fellow with the Washington-based Institute for Policy Studies. Maude Barlow is the author, or co-author, of fifteen books including: *Too Close for Comfort: Canada's Future Within Fortress North America* (McClelland & Stewart, 2005); and *Profit is Not the Cure: A Citizen's Guide to Saving Medicare* (McClelland and Stewart, 2002). She is the recipient of numerous awards and honourary doctorates. In 2005, she received the Right Livelihood Award given by the Swedish Parliament and widely referred to as "The Alternative Nobel."

Monique Bégin entered politics in 1972 as the first woman from Quebec elected to the House of Commons. She is best known as minister of national health and welfare in the Trudeau government (1977–84) and architect of the 1984 Canada Health Act. She was executive secretary of the Royal Commission on the Status of Women. She has been a university professor since leaving politics in 1984. She was the first holder of the Joint Chair in Women's Studies at Ottawa and Carleton Universities; dean of the Faculty of Health Sciences at the University of Ottawa; co-chair of the Royal Commission on Learning of Ontario; and a member of the International Independent Commission on Population and Quality of Life. She currently sits on the World Health Organization Commission on the Social Determinants of Health and is a visiting professor at the University of Ottawa School of Management and Health Administration.

Allan Blakeney was premier of Saskatchewan from 1971 to 1982. He served as a senior civil servant in Saskatchewan before entering politics and was a cabinet minister in the governments of Tommy Douglas and Woodrow S. Lloyd. As minister of public health, he played a crucial role in the development of medicare. On his retirement from political life in 1988, he was appointed Bora Laskin Professor of Constitutional Law, Osgoode Hall Law School (1988-90). In 1990, he was appointed the Inaugural Law Foundation of Saskatchewan Professor at the College of Law, and after completing his term Mr. Blakeney has remained at the college as a visiting scholar. In 1982 he was appointed to the Privy Council of Canada. In 1992, he was made an officer of the Order of Canada and in 2000 was awarded the Saskatchewan Order of Merit. In 2001, he was made a fellow of the Royal Society of Canada.

Bruce Campbell is executive director (since 1994) of the Canadian Centre for Policy Alternatives. Beyond his administrative responsibilities, he has spoken and written widely on public policy issues, and is a frequent media commentator. For many years he coordinated the Centre's *Alternative Federal Budget* project. He is co-author or editor of four books including: (with Maude Barlow) *Straight Through the Heart: How the Liberals Abandoned the Just Society* (HarperCollins, 1995); and *Living with Uncle: Canada-US Relations in an Age of Empire* (Lorimer, 2006). He was formerly a researcher with the North South Institute, a policy analyst with the federal NDP caucus, and a senior economist with the Canadian Labour Congress.

May Tsung-Mei Cheng is the executive editor and host of *International Forum,* a Princeton university television program on international affairs. She is the author, most recently, of a paper on Taiwan's National Health Insurance system. She is co-author (with Uwe Reinhardt) of "Section I: The Economics of Health Care Quality: Theory and Practice." She has an LLB from the National Taiwan University, and an MA in International Relations from Yale University.

Marcy Cohen is research and policy director at the BC Hospital Employees Union and research associate with the BC office of the Canadian Centre for Policy Alternatives (CCPA). She has in recent years led research projects on community health restructuring, the privatiza-

tion of support services, democratic governance of health care, public–private partnerships, and staffing issues in residential care. Her
current research focuses on positive strategies for reforming public
health: on wait lists and on community health services (home support,
home care, primary care, community mental health, and long-term
care). Marcy Cohen is the board chair of CCPA-BC and the Vancouver
Foundation Committee on Community Health Research.

Cathy Crowe calls herself a "street nurse" to remind politicians and
the public that the extent of homelessness and inadequate housing in this
country is obscene. For the past eighteen years she has been nursing and
organizing — on the streets and in shelters, drop-ins, and outdoor squats.
She believes that a national housing program is as vital to the health of
the nation as medicare. In 1998, she co-founded the Toronto Disaster
Relief Committee, which declared homelessness in Canada a national
disaster. She is a recipient of the Atkinson Charitable Foundation's Economic Justice Award. Cathy Crowe is co-author of *Dying for a Home:
Homeless Activists Speak Out* (Between the Lines Press, 2007).

Shirley Douglas was born to Irma and Tommy Douglas in 1934 in
Weyburn, Saskatchewan. It was there that Shirley witnessed the birth of
hospitalization and medicare and has since been determined that Canadians not lose what was so ferociously fought for. She is a celebrated
television, film, and stage actress, and renowned social activist. She has
traveled the continent speaking in church basements and local libraries,
at large public rallies, and international forums, on behalf of the Canadian Health Coalition. In Toronto, she founded a citizens' group
committed to protecting not-for-profit health services. In October
2003, she received the Order of Canada, and in 2004 she received a star
on Canada's Walk of Fame in Toronto.

Robert G. Evans is a Killam professor in the Department of Economics and a member of the Centre for Health Services and Policy
Research at the University of British Columbia. He is an institute fellow of the Canadian Institute for Advanced Research and founded its
program in population health. Dr. Evans has lectured and consulted

extensively with governments and other public agencies at home and abroad. He was a member of the British Columbia Royal Commission on Health Care and Costs (1990-91), and of the National Forum on Health, chaired by the prime minister of Canada (1994-97). He is an honorary life member of the Canadian College of Health Services Executives and of the Canadian Association for Health Services and Policy Research. He is an officer of the Order of Canada, a fellow of the Royal Society of Canada and of the Canadian Academy of Health Sciences, and a member of the National Academy of Social Insurance of the United States. In 2001, he was the first Canadian to win the Baxter International Foundation Prize for Health Services Research, awarded by the Association of University Programs in Health Administration.

Willie Ermine, a Cree from the Sturgeon Lake First Nation, is a writer and ethicist with the Indigenous Peoples' Health Research Centre and a professor at the First Nations University of Canada. He conducts research and writes in the areas of transforming knowledge and the ethics of research involving Indigenous Peoples and continues his "consuming pursuit to further understand Cree thought and practice."

Colleen Flood is an associate professor of law at the University of Toronto and is cross-appointed into the Department of Health Policy, Management, and Evaluation. She is a Canada Research Chair in Health Law and Policy and the scientific director of the Canadian Institute for Health Services and Policy Research. She has been consulted on comparative health policy and governance issues by the Senate Social Affairs Committee studying health care in Canada and the Romanow Commission on the Future of Health Care in Canada. She is the author of numerous articles, book chapters, and reports as well as the author or editor of four books, most recently, *Just Medicare: What's In, What's Out, How We Decide* (University of Toronto Press, 2006).

Diana Gibson is research director for the University of Alberta-based Parkland Institute. She has an extensive background in policy research on issues ranging from health care and education, to energy and international trade agreements. Diana Gibson has worked as a researcher and educator for various community organizations, colleges, trade unions, and the federal government. Her recent book, *The Bottom Line: The Truth About Private Health Insurance* (Newest Press, 2006) was a best seller in Alberta and helped defeat Ralph Klein's *Third Way for Health Care*.

Doris Grinspun has been executive director of the Registered Nurses' Association of Ontario (RNAO) since 1996. She is an assistant professor in the Faculty of Nursing at the University of Toronto; an adjunct professor at the School of Nursing, York University; an associate member of the Centre for Health Promotion at the University of Toronto; and an affiliate member of the Centre for Health Studies at York University. From 1996 to 1999, she was the chair of the Acquired Brain Injury Network of Metropolitan Toronto. From 1990 to 1996, Doris Grinspun served as director of nursing at Mount Sinai Hospital in Toronto. Doris Grinspun has received numerous professional and scholarly awards including the Order of Ontario.

France Gélinas is a licensed physiotherapist, a graduate of Laval University in Quebec. She has a master's degree in Business Administration from Laurentian University. For the last eleven years she has been executive director of the Francophone Community Health Centre in Sudbury, Ontario. She has served on the board of directors of the Association of Ontario Health Centres for the last six years and is currently president of that board as well as a board member of the Canadian Alliance of Community Health Centre Associations. She worked for over ten years in hospitals throughout Ontario. She has held positions in the Ministry of Health and Long Term Care of Ontario, mainly in the area of hospital restructuring.

Eber Hampton, Chickasaw, is principal investigator of the Indigenous Peoples' Health Research Centre, executive in residence at the Kenneth Levene Graduate School of Business and professor of business administration at the University of Regina. He is on the boards of the Saskatchewan Health Quality Council and the Aboriginal Health Research Network Secretariat. He holds an earned doctorate in Administration, Planning, and Social Policy from Harvard University and an honorary Doctor of Laws from Brock University. He was selected for a National Aboriginal Achievement Award in 2005.

Tom Kent was much involved both in establishing the Liberal Party's commitment to medicare, and in its implementation, along with other social policies by the Pearson government, which he served as co-ordinator of programming and policy secretary to the prime minister. His other activities have included war-time intelligence service, newspaper editor, deputy minister, crown corporation president, royal commission chairman, and university dean. He is the founding editor of *Policy Options*, the journal of the Institute for Research on Public Policy, and is a lifetime fellow of the Institute, as well as a fellow of the School of Policy Studies at Queen's University. He is a companion of the Order of Canada.

Stephen Lewis, former UN Special Envoy for HIV/AIDS in Africa (2001-06), is the inaugural scholar-in-residence at the Institute on Globalization and the Human Condition at McMaster University in Hamilton, Ontario. He is also a senior advisor to the Mailman School of Public Health at Columbia University in New York. Stephen Lewis is co-chair of the Leadership Programme Committee for the XVII International AIDS Conference, which will be held in Mexico City in August 2008. He also serves as a member of the board of directors of the International AIDS Vaccine Initiative, and is the chair of the board of the Stephen Lewis Foundation. His work with the United Nations spans more than two decades, including deputy executive director of UNICEF, coordinator for the Graça Machel study on the "Consequences of Armed Conflict on Children," and Canadian Ambassador to the United Nations. Stephen Lewis holds many distinguished awards and honorary degrees from Canadian universities and is a companion of the Order of Canada. In April 2005, *Time* magazine listed Stephen Lewis as one of the "100 most influential people in the world." His best-selling book, *Race Against Time* won the Canadian Booksellers Association's Libris Award for non-fiction book of the year in 2005.

Steven Lewis is a health policy and research consultant based in Saskatoon, and visiting scholar at Simon Fraser University in Vancouver (January to April 2007) as well as adjunct professor of health policy at the University of Calgary. Prior to resuming a full-time consulting practice he headed a health research granting agency and spent seven years as CEO of the Health Services Utilization and Research Commission in Saskatchewan. He has served on various boards and committees, including the Governing Council of the Canadian Institutes of Health Research, the Saskatchewan Health Quality Council, the Health Council of Canada, and the editorial boards of several journals. His published work covers topics such as strengthening medicare, improving health care quality, primary health care, regionalization, and the management of wait times.

Joel Lexchin, for the past nineteen years, has been an emergency physician at the University Health Network. He is currently a professor in the School of Health Policy and Management at York University and an associate professor in the Department of Family and Community Medicine at the University of Toronto. He has been a consultant on pharmaceutical issues for the province of Ontario, various agencies of the federal government, the World Health Organization, the government of New Zealand and the Australian National Prescribing Service. He is the author or co-author of over seventy peer-reviewed articles on topics such as physician prescribing behaviour, pharmaceutical patent issues, drug approval process, and prescription drug promotion.

Greg Marchildon is currently Canada Research Chair in Public Policy and Economic History at the Johnson-Shoyama Graduate School of Public Policy, University of Regina. He is a senior fellow at the School of Policy Studies, Queen's University, a mentor with the Trudeau Foundation, and the chair of the Saskatchewan Health Research Foundation. After receiving his PhD from the London School of Economics, he taught at the Johns Hopkins University School of Advanced International Studies in Washington. Dr. Marchildon served as cabinet secretary and deputy minister to the premier of Saskatchewan from

1996 to 2001. He was executive director of the Romanow Commission on the Future of Health Care. He is the author of *Health Systems in Transition: Canada* (University of Toronto Press, 2006) as well as other books and articles on Canadian health policy.

Patricia J. Martens is the director of the Manitoba Centre for Health Policy in the Department of Community Health Sciences of the Faculty of Medicine, University of Manitoba, and also an associate professor. Dr. Marten's research interests include projects on the health and health care use of Manitoba's rural and northern residents, children, and First Nations people, as well as projects on rural hospital indicators. She has also done extensive research on maternal/child health issues, including breastfeeding programs within Sagkeeng First Nation and in Manitoba's regional health authorities. Patricia Martens is a Canadian Institutes of Health Research New Investigator, and the 2004 recipient of the Winnipeg Rh Institute Award for high-impact health research. She directs a five-year CIHR grant called *The Need To Know* team, which is a collaboration of university academics as well as top-level planners from RHAs and Manitoba Health.

Danielle Martin is a comprehensive care family physician working in downtown Toronto and rural Northern Ontario. She is associate staff at Women's College Hospital and lecturer in the Department of Community and Family Medicine at the University of Toronto. A recipient of the Canadian Medical Association Award for Young Leaders, she sits on the Health Council of Canada and was founding co-chair of the New Health Professionals Network. In 2006, the Ontario College of Family Physicians recognized Danielle Martin as one of three New Family Doctors of the Year. In 2006, she was the founding chair of Canadian Doctors for Medicare, the voice of pro-medicare physicians who support a responsive, sustainable publicly funded health care system, and oppose privatization and two-tier medicine.

Alan Maynard is a professor of health economics at the University of York, England. He was founding director of the Centre for Health Economics at the University of York (1983-95) and currently teaches

economics in the Department of Health Sciences. He has written
and/or edited a dozen books, the most recent of which is a collection
of essays about national experiences of reform in countries including
Canada and the US, entitled *Public–Private Mix for Health: plus ca change;
plus ca meme chose* (Radcliffe, 2005). He is a specialist adviser to the Select
Committee on Health of the UK House of Commons (since 2006) and
has worked as a consultant in over two dozen countries for national and
international agencies such as the World Bank.

Robert McMurtry is professor of surgery at the University of Western Ontario and orthopedic consultant at St. Joseph's Health Care in
London, Ontario. His work involves an active clinical practice as well as
teaching and research. In October of 2003, he was appointed to the
Transition Advisory Board of the incoming provincial government of
Ontario. He is a member of the Health Council of Canada and chaired
the Wait Times and Accessibility Work Group (2004–2006). Dr.
McMurtry is the founding assistant deputy minister of the Population
and Public Health Branch of Health Canada. He was a special advisor
to the Romanow Commission. He was dean of medicine at the University of Western Ontario and subsequently dean of medicine and
dentistry from 1992 to 1999.

Andrew Petter is dean and professor of law at the University of Victoria. Prior to joining UVic Law in 1986, he taught at Osgoode Hall Law
School in Toronto and practised constitutional law with the government
of Saskatchewan. From 1991 to 2001, he served as a member of the Legislative Assembly of British Columbia and held numerous cabinet
portfolios including Attorney General, Advanced Education, Training
and Technology, Finance, and Health. His major fields of interest are constitutional law, civil liberties, and legislative and regulatory processes. He
has written and lectured extensively on these and related subjects.

Marie-Claude Prémont is professor of law, École nationale d'administration publique (ÉNAP), Québec, and former associate dean,
graduate studies, Faculty of Law, McGill University. She is a member of
the Quebec Bar and Quebec's Professional Order of Engineers (Ordre

des ingénieurs du Québec). Her research interests include health law, municipal governance, and legal history. She is a founding member of the Working Group on the Quebec health care system in the wake of the Supreme Court of Canada decision in the *Chaoulli* case. She is a frequent media commentator and has made presentations before public commissions of the Quebec legislature and the Parliament of Canada on health policy.

Dennis Raphael is associate professor and undergraduate program director at York University's School of Health Policy and Management. The most recent of his 100 scientific publications have been concerned with the health effects of income inequality, the quality of life of communities and individuals, and the impact of government decisions on Canadians' health and well-being. His policy research on current trends in social and health policy directly involves informed community members. His recent authored or edited books are *Poverty and Policy in Canada: Implications for Health and Quality of Life* (Canadian Scholars' Press, 2007); *Staying Alive: Critical Perspectives on Health, Illness, and Health Care* (Canadian Scholars' Press, 2006); and *Social Determinants of Health: Canadian Perspectives* (Canadian Scholars' Press, 2004).

Michael M. Rachlis practised family medicine at the South Riverdale Community Centre in Toronto from 1976 to 1984. He completed a residency in community medicine at McMaster University in 1988. Dr. Rachlis currently practises as a private consultant in health policy analysis. He has lectured widely on health care issues and has appeared before Canadian parliamentary and US congressional committees. He is a well known media commentator, and has authored three national best-selling books on Canada's health care system. His most recent book is *Prescription for Excellence: How Innovation is Saving Canada's Health Care System* (HarperCollins, 2005).

Uwe E. Reinhardt is James Madison Professor of Political Economy and professor of Economics and Public Affairs, Princeton University. He has served on a number of American government commissions and advisory boards including the National Advisory Council for the

Agency for Health Research and Quality, the US Department of Health
and Human Services, and the National Council on Health Care Technology. He is, or has been, a member of numerous editorial boards
including that of the *New England Journal of Medicine* and the *Journal of
the American Medical Association*.

Arnold S. Relman is currently professor emeritus of medicine and
social medicine at the Harvard Medical School and senior physician at
the Brigham and Women's Hospital in Boston. He was editor-in-chief
of the *New England Journal of Medicine* from 1977 to 1991 and before
that was chairman of the Department of Medicine at the University of
Pennsylvania's School of Medicine. Dr. Relman is a board certified
internist, a master of the American College of Physicians, and a fellow
of the Royal College of Physicians of London. He is a fellow of the
American Academy of Arts & Sciences and a senior member of the
Institute of Medicine of the National Academy of Sciences. His most
recent book, *Second Opinion: Rescuing American Health Care* (Public
Affairs, 2007), includes a chapter comparing the US and Canadian
health care systems.

Roy Romanow, former premier of Saskatchewan (1991–2001), was
appointed by Prime Minister Jean Chrétien, in 2001, to head the Royal
Commission on the Future of Health Care in Canada, whose mandate
was to recommend policies and measures to ensure the long-term sustainability of a universally accessible, high quality, publicly administered
health care system for all Canadians. The Commission's final report was
released November 28, 2002. In 2003, he received the Economic Justice
Award from the Atkinson foundation, and the Administration Award
from the Pan American Health Organization. He is a senior fellow in
Public Policy at the University of Saskatchewan and a visiting fellow at
the School of Policy Studies, Queen's University. Mr. Romanow is an
officer of the Order of Canada. Roy Romanow was first elected to the
Saskatchewan Legislature in 1967. Between 1971 and 1982, he served as
deputy premier of Saskatchewan, attorney general and minister of Intergovernmental Affairs.

Judith Shamian, PhD, is currently the president and CEO of the Victorian Order of Nurses. She formerly held the title of executive director of Nursing Policy with Health Canada and is a professor in the Faculty of Nursing at the University of Toronto. She was also the president of the Registered Nurses' Association of Ontario from 1998 to1999. Dr. Shamian is best known for shaping and influencing health policy both nationally and internationally. She is the 1995 recipient of the Ross Award for Nursing Leadership, was awarded the Golden Jubilee Medal in 2002 by the governor general of Canada, and is the recipient of two honorary doctorate degrees.

Steven Shrybman is a lawyer with the firm Sack, Goldblatt, Mitchell. His practice focuses on international trade and public interest legal issues, including those concerning the environment, health care, human and labour rights, the protection of public services, natural resources policy, and intellectual property rights. Steven Shrybman's legal opinions concerning the impact of trade law on diverse areas of Canadian policy and law have been widely disseminated. He has been involved in drafting, and working with international NGOs to promote, conventions on cultural diversity and access to water as a human right. He has published extensively both in Canada and internationally on the subject of international trade law.

Linda Silas is the elected president of the Canadian Federation of Nurses Unions, which represents more than 135,000 nurses in nine provinces. Ms Silas brings to the CFNU presidency years of experience as a nurse-leader, a public speaker, and a negotiator at the local, provincial, and national levels. Previously, she was president of the New Brunswick Nurses Union where she served for ten years. Linda Silas is a graduate of l'Université de Moncton where she earned a Bachelor of Science in Nursing. She has practised in New Brunswick at the l'Hôpital Dr. Georges L. Dumont: in ICU, Emergency, and Labour & Delivery.

Scott Sinclair is a senior researcher with the Canadian Centre for Policy Alternatives, where he coordinates the Centre's Trade and Investment Research Project. From 1994 to 1999 he was a senior trade policy

advisor to the government of British Columbia. He is an internationally respected authority on trade and investment agreements. He has
written extensively on the health policy implications of trade treaties
including: *Putting Health First: Canadian Health Care Reform, Trade Treaties
and Foreign Policy* (co-authored with Matthew Sanger) which was prepared for the Romanow Commission on the Future of Health Care in
Canada; and *Bad Medicine: Trade Treaties, Privatisation and Health Care
Reform in Canada* (co-authored with Jim Grieshaber-Otto).

Armine Yalnizyan is an economist and media commentator spe-
cializing in labour markets, social and budgetary policy. She has advised
governments at the federal, provincial, and local levels, taught economics at York University, and worked with international NGOs and
community-based organizations and coalitions. In 2002, she became the
first recipient of the Atkinson Foundation Award for Economic Justice
and received the Morley Gunderson Prize in 2003. She is currently
director of research with the Social Planning Council of Toronto. She is
also a research fellow with the Canadian Centre for Policy Alternatives.

INDEX